T0226822

Neuro-Oncology

Editors

EUDOCIA QUANT LEE
PATRICK Y. WEN

NEUROLOGIC CLINICS

www.neurologic.theclinics.com

Consulting Editor
RANDOLPH W. EVANS

August 2018 • Volume 36 • Number 3

ELSEVIER

1600 John F. Kennedy Boulevard • Suite 1800 • Philadelphia, Pennsylvania, 19103-2899

http://www.theclinics.com

NEUROLOGIC CLINICS Volume 36, Number 3
August 2018 ISSN 0733-8619, ISBN-13: 978-0-323-61402-3

Editor: Stacy Eastman
Developmental Editor: Donald Mumford

Neurologic Clinics (ISSN 0733-8619) is published quarterly by Elsevier Inc., 360 Park Avenue South, New York, NY 10010–1710. Months of issue are February, May, August, and November. Periodicals postage paid at New York, NY, and additional mailing offices. Subscription prices are $312.00 per year for US individuals, $631.00 per year for US institutions, $100.00 per year for US students, $390.00 per year for Canadian individuals, $765.00 per year for Canadian institutions, $423.00 per year for international individuals, $765.00 per year for international institutions, and $210.00 for Canadian and foreign students/residents. To receive student/resident rate, orders must be accompanied by name of affiliated institution, date of term, and the *signature* of program/residency coordinator on institution letterhead. Orders will be billed at individual rate until proof of status is received. Foreign air speed delivery is included in all *Clinics* subscription prices. All prices are subject to change without notice. **POSTMASTER:** Send address changes to *Neurologic Clinics*, Elsevier Health Sciences Division, Subscription Customer Service, 3251 Riverport Lane, Maryland Heights, MO 63043. **Customer Service: Telephone: 1-800-654-2452 (U.S. and Canada); 314-447-8871 (outside U.S. and Canada). Fax: 314-447-8029. E-mail: journalscustomerservice-usa@elsevier.com (for print support); journalsonlinesupport-usa@elsevier.com (for online support).**

Reprints. For copies of 100 or more of articles in this publication, please contact the Commercial Reprints Department, Elsevier Inc., 360 Park Avenue South, New York, New York, 10010-1710; Tel.: +1-212-633-3874; Fax: +1-212-633-3820, and E-mail: reprints@elsevier.com.

Neurologic Clinics is also published in Spanish by Nueva Editorial Interamericana S.A., Mexico City, Mexico.

Neurologic Clinics is covered in *Current Contents/Clinical Medicine, MEDLINE/PubMed (Index Medicus), EMBASE/Excerpta Medica, and PsycINFO, and ISI/BIOMED.*

Contributors

CONSULTING EDITOR

RANDOLPH W. EVANS, MD
Clinical Professor, Department of Neurology, Baylor College of Medicine, Houston, Texas, USA

EDITORS

EUDOCIA Q. LEE, MD, MPH
Center for Neuro-Oncology, Dana-Farber Cancer Institute, Division of Cancer Neurology, Department of Neurology, Brigham and Women's Hospital, Assistant Professor of Neurology, Harvard Medical School, Boston, Massachusetts, USA

PATRICK Y. WEN, MD
Center for Neuro-Oncology, Dana-Farber Cancer Institute, Division of Cancer Neurology, Department of Neurology, Brigham and Women's Hospital, Professor of Neurology, Harvard Medical School, Boston, Massachusetts, USA

AUTHORS

AYAL A. AIZER, MD, MHS
Department of Radiation Oncology, Brigham and Women's Hospital, Dana-Farber Cancer Institute, Harvard Medical School, Boston, Massachusetts, USA

KENNETH ALDAPE, MD
Professor, Pathology, MacFeeters-Hamilton Centre for Neuro-Oncology Research, Princess Margaret Cancer Centre, University of Toronto, Toronto, Ontario, Canada

BRIAN M. ALEXANDER, MD, MPH
Associate Professor, Brigham and Women's Hospital, Dana-Farber Cancer Institute, Harvard Medical School, Boston, Massachusetts, USA

ISABEL C. ARRILLAGA-ROMANY, MD, PhD
Stephen E. and Catherine Pappas Center for Neuro-Oncology, Massachusetts General Hospital, Harvard Medical School, Boston, Massachusetts, USA

JILL S. BARNHOLTZ-SLOAN, PhD
Sally S. Morley Designated Professor, Brain Tumor Research, Professor and Associate Director for Bioinformatics/Translational Informatics, Case Comprehensive Cancer Center, Institute for Computational Biology, Case Western Reserve University School of Medicine, Cleveland, Ohio, USA

FLORIS P. BARTHEL, MD
Department of Pathology, VU University Medical Center, Brain Tumor Center Amsterdam, Amsterdam, The Netherlands; The Jackson Laboratory for Genomic Medicine, Farmington, Connecticut, USA

TRACY BATCHELOR, MD, MPH
Departments of Neurology and Radiation Oncology, Division of Hematology and Oncology, Massachusetts General Hospital, Harvard Medical School, Boston, Massachusetts, USA

SUSAN M. CHANG, MD
Department of Neurosurgery, University of California, San Francisco, San Francisco, California, USA

DAVID COTE, BS
PhD Student, Department of Neurosurgery, Brigham and Women's Hospital, Harvard Medical School, Harvard T.H. Chan School of Public Health, Boston, Massachusetts, USA

JOSEP DALMAU, MD, PhD
ICREA Research Professor, Hospital Clínic/Institut d'Investigació Biomèdica August Pi i Sunyer (IDIBAPS), Barcelona, Spain; Adjunct Professor, Department of Neurology, University of Pennsylvania, USA

LISA M. DeANGELIS, MD
Chair, Department of Neurology, Memorial Sloan Kettering Cancer Center, Professor of Neurology, Weill Cornell Medical College, New York, New York, USA

PHEDIAS DIAMANDIS, MD, PhD
Assistant Professor, Pathology, MacFeeters-Hamilton Centre for Neuro-Oncology Research, Princess Margaret Cancer Centre, University of Toronto, Toronto, Ontario, Canada

CAMILO E. FADUL, MD
Division of Neuro-Oncology, University of Virginia Health System, Charlottesville, Virginia, USA

REBECCA A. HARRISON, MD
Assistant Professor, Department of Neuro-Oncology, The University of Texas MD Anderson Cancer Center, Houston, Texas, USA

KEVIN C. JOHNSON, PhD
The Jackson Laboratory for Genomic Medicine, Farmington, Connecticut, USA

JUSTIN T. JORDAN, MD, MPH
Department of Neurology and Cancer Center, Massachusetts General Hospital, Harvard Medical School, Boston, Massachusetts, USA

EUDOCIA Q. LEE, MD, MPH
Center for Neuro-Oncology, Dana-Farber Cancer Institute, Division of Cancer Neurology, Department of Neurology, Brigham and Women's Hospital, Assistant Professor of Neurology, Harvard Medical School, Boston, Massachusetts, USA

KIEN-NINH INA LY, MD
Stephen E. and Catherine Pappas Center for Neuro-Oncology, Massachusetts General Hospital, Harvard Medical School, Boston, Massachusetts, USA

JOE S. MENDEZ, MD
Fellow, Department of Neurology, Memorial Sloan Kettering Cancer Center, New York, New York, USA

QUINN T. OSTROM, PhD, MPH
Postdoctoral Associate, Department of Medicine, Section of Epidemiology and Population Sciences, Dan Duncan Comprehensive Cancer Center, Baylor College of Medicine, Houston, Texas, USA

ROGER J. PACKER, MD
Brain Tumor Institute, Center for Neuroscience and Behavioral Medicine, The Gilbert Family Neurofibromatosis Institute, Children's National Medical Center, Washington, DC, USA

KESTER A. PHILLIPS, MD
Department of Neuroscience, Inova Health System, Inova Fairfax Hospital, Falls Church, Virginia, USA

MICHAEL PLATTEN, MD
Professor of Neurology, Department of Neurology, Universitätsmedizin Mannheim, Medical Faculty Mannheim, Heidelberg University, Mannheim, Germany; Clinical Cooperation Unit Neuroimmunology and Brain Tumor Immunology, German Cancer Consortium (DKTK), German Cancer Research Center (DKFZ), Heidelberg, Germany

SCOTT R. PLOTKIN, MD, PhD
Department of Neurology and Cancer Center, Massachusetts General Hospital, Harvard Medical School, Boston, Massachusetts, USA

MYRNA R. ROSENFELD, MD, PhD
Neuroimmunology, Institut d'Investigació Biomèdica August Pi i Sunyer (IDIBAPS), Barcelona, Spain; Adjunct Professor, Department of Neurology, University of Pennsylvania, USA

DAVID SCHIFF, MD
Division of Neuro-Oncology, University of Virginia Health System, Charlottesville, Virginia, USA

KAYLYN SINICROPE, MD
Department of Neurology, Massachusetts General Hospital, Harvard Medical School, Boston, Massachusetts, USA

SHYAM K. TANGUTURI, MD
Instructor, Brigham and Women's Hospital, Dana-Farber Cancer Institute, Harvard Medical School, Boston, Massachusetts, USA

YOKO T. UDAKA, MD
Brain Tumor Institute, Division of Oncology, Center for Cancer and Blood Disorders, Center for Neuroscience and Behavioral Medicine, Children's National Medical Center, Washington, DC, USA

MARTIN J. VAN DEN BENT, MD
Brain Tumor Center, Erasmus MC Cancer Institute, Rotterdam, The Netherlands, USA

ROEL G.W. VERHAAK, PhD
The Jackson Laboratory for Genomic Medicine, Farmington, Connecticut, USA

JEFFREY S. WEFEL, PhD
Section of Neuropsychology, Associate Professor, Department of Neuro-Oncology, The University of Texas MD Anderson Cancer Center, Houston, Texas, USA

PIETER WESSELING, MD, PhD
Department of Pathology, VU University Medical Center, Brain Tumor Center Amsterdam, Amsterdam, The Netherlands; Department of Pathology, Princess Máxima Center for Pediatric Oncology and University Medical Center Utrecht, Utrecht, The Netherlands

WOLFGANG WICK, MD
Professor of Neurology/Neurooncology, Neurology Clinic, University of Heidelberg, Clinical Cooperation Unit (CCU) Neurooncology, German Cancer Consortium (DKTK), German Cancer Research Center (DKFZ), Heidelberg, Germany

Contents

Incidence, prevalence, and survival for brain tumors vary by histologic type, age at diagnosis, sex, and race/ethnicity. Significant progress has been made in identifying potential risk factors for brain tumors, although more research is warranted. The strongest risk factors that have been identified thus far include allergies/atopic disease, ionizing radiation, and heritable genetic factors. Further analysis of large, multi-center, epidemiologic studies, as well as well-annotated omic datasets (including genomic, epigenomic, transcriptomic, proteomic, or metabolomics data), can potentially lead to further understanding of the relationship between gene and environment in the process of brain tumor development.

Recent advances in molecular analysis and genome sequencing have prompted a paradigm shift in neuropathology. This article discusses the discovery and clinical relevance of molecular biomarkers in diffuse gliomas in adults and how these biomarkers led to revision of the World Health Organization classification of these tumors. The authors relate progress in clinical classification to an overview of studies using molecular profiling to study gene expression and DNA methylation to categorize diffuse gliomas in adults and issues dealing with intratumoral heterogeneity. These efforts will refine the taxonomy of diffuse gliomas, facilitate selection of appropriate treatment regimens, and ultimately improve patient's lives.

The recent update of the World Health Organization (WHO) classification of tumors of the central nervous system represents a paradigm shift. Previous iterations of the classification relied on morphologic features for classification. In the 2016 update, the definitions of specific neoplastic entities tumors now include precise molecularly defined entities. This article discusses this paradigm shift and focuses on the refinements in classification criteria, relations to previous editions, and their implication to neuropathology and neuro-oncology practice. The authors distinguish the criteria that were used to determine why molecular changes were included.

signaling pathway aberrations, and investigation of targeted systemic therapies.

Primary Central Nervous System Lymphoma

Kaylyn Sinicrope and Tracy Batchelor

Primary central nervous system lymphoma (PCNSL) is an aggressive form of non-Hodgkin lymphoma restricted to the central nervous system. Stereotactic biopsy is the gold standard for diagnosis of PCNSL. Extent of disease evaluation for patients with newly diagnosed PCNSL includes brain imaging, eye examination, cerebrospinal fluid assessment, body imaging, and bone marrow biopsy. Methotrexate-based chemotherapy is the standard induction for patients with PCNSL. Optimal consolidation therapy for PCNSL has not been defined, with several options feasible, including chemotherapy, high-dose chemotherapy, and autologous stem cell transplantation or whole-brain radiation therapy. Optimal treatment for relapsed and refractory PCNSL has not been defined.

Pediatric Brain Tumors

Yoko T. Udaka and Roger J. Packer

Pediatric central nervous system (CNS) tumors are the most common solid tumors in children and comprise 15% to 20% of all malignancies in children. Presentation, symptoms, and signs depend on tumor location and age of the patient at the time of diagnosis. This article summarizes the common childhood CNS tumors, presentations, classification, and recent updates in treatment approaches owing to the increased understanding of the molecular pathogenesis of pediatric brain tumors.

Brain Metastases

Ayal A. Aizer and Eudocia Q. Lee

Brain metastases from solid tumors are associated with increased morbidity and mortality. Standard treatment is local therapy with surgery and/or radiation therapy, although there is increasing interest in systemic therapies that can control both intracranial and extracranial disease. The authors review the most recent data for local therapy and systemic therapy options. Active areas of research within radiation oncology include hippocampal-sparing whole brain radiation therapy and stereotactic approaches for patients with more than 4 brain metastases. Newer targeted therapies with better central nervous system penetration and immunotherapies have demonstrated promising results in clinical trials of patients with brain metastases.

Metastatic Complications of Cancer Involving the Central and Peripheral Nervous Systems

Joe S. Mendez and Lisa M. DeAngelis

Neurologic complications of cancer may involve both the central nervous system and peripheral nervous system, manifesting as brain, leptomeningeal, intramedullary, intradural, epidural, plexus, and skull base metastases. Excluding brain involvement, neurologic complications affecting these other sites are relatively infrequent, but collectively they affect more than 25% of patients with metastatic cancer, causing significant

patient's demographics and risk factors for cancer. The presence of specific antineuronal antibodies can facilitate the diagnosis and suggest treatment strategies. Although some PNS are rarely responsive to therapies, other disorders are highly treatment responsive.

NEUROLOGIC CLINICS

Preface

The Interface Between Neurology and Oncology

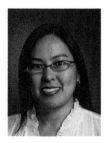 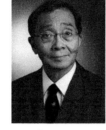

Eudocia Q. Lee, MD, MPH   Patrick Y. Wen, MD
Editors

This issue of *Neurologic Clinics* is devoted to nervous system tumors as well as neurologic complications of cancer and cancer therapy. Since the last issue devoted to neuro-oncology 10 years ago, increased understanding of the molecular underpinnings of primary brain tumors has led to the addition of molecular parameters for the first time to the WHO classification of central nervous system tumors. Therefore, the first half of this issue focuses on the molecular pathogenesis of gliomas, the reasoning behind the recent changes in WHO classification, and their implications for management of adult and pediatric brain tumors. We also review the epidemiology of brain tumors as well as the recent clinical and molecular advances in benign brain tumors and central nervous system lymphoma.

The second half of this issue reviews oncologic topics of interest to the general neurologist, including the neurologic and medical management of brain tumor patients, cancer metastases to the nervous system, neurologic complications of cancer therapy, neurocognitive dysfunction in patients with cancer, and paraneoplastic syndromes. These neurologic complications can significantly impact morbidity and mortality. Indeed, cancer treatment strategies increasingly aim at minimizing impact on neurocognition and quality of life. In addition, the central nervous system (particularly the brain) is a sanctuary site for cancer as many systemic therapies do not sufficiently penetrate the blood-brain barrier.

Neurol Clin 36 (2018) xiii–xiv
https://doi.org/10.1016/j.ncl.2018.05.001
0733-8619/18/© 2018 Published by Elsevier Inc.

neurologic.theclinics.com

We thank our authors for their outstanding contributions, the senior developmental editor, Donald Mumford, and the team at Elsevier for their help with this issue.

Eudocia Q. Lee, MD, MPH
Center for Neuro-Oncology
Dana-Farber Cancer Institute
450 Brookline Avenue, D2
Boston, MA 02215, USA

Division of Cancer Neurology
Department of Neurology
Brigham and Women's Hospital
Harvard Medical School
Boston, MA 02115, USA

Patrick Y. Wen, MD
Center for Neuro-Oncology
Dana-Farber Cancer Institute
450 Brookline Avenue, D2
Boston, MA 02215, USA

Division of Cancer Neurology
Department of Neurology
Brigham and Women's Hospital
Boston, MA 02115, USA

E-mail addresses:
eqlee@partners.org (E.Q. Lee)
pwen@partners.org (P.Y. Wen)

Epidemiology of Brain Tumors

Jill S. Barnholtz-Sloan, PhD[a],*, Quinn T. Ostrom, PhD, MPH[b], David Cote, BS[c]

KEYWORDS

- Brain tumors • Epidemiology • Incidence • Survival • Population based

KEY POINTS

- The most common type of nonmalignant brain and central nervous system (CNS) tumors are meningiomas, which represent approximately half of nonmalignant tumors diagnosed in the United States. The most common type of malignant tumors are gliomas, of which glioblastoma occurs with the greatest frequency.
- Overall age-adjusted incidence of brain and CNS tumors was 22.64 per 100,000 population in the United States between 2010 and 2014; however, incidence varies by histologic type of tumor, age at diagnosis, sex, and race/ethnicity. Overall, recent changes in incidence rates of brain and other CNS tumors have been small.
- The complete prevalence of primary malignant brain and CNS tumors in the United States in 2010 is estimated to be 47.6 per 100,000 (103,634 total cases).
- Overall 1-year relative survival after diagnosis with a malignant brain and CNS tumor was 56.6% between 2000 and 2010, with 5-year relative survival of 32.1%. Survival after diagnosis with a nonmalignant brain tumor is significantly higher, with 1-year relative survival of 94.5% and 5-year relative survival of 90.8%. Survival is poorest after diagnosis with glioblastoma, with 1-year survival of 37.4% and 5-year survival of 4.9%.
- Many environmental and genetic risk factors have been studied for brain tumors; consistent evidence has been found for ionizing radiation exposure and increased risk of brain tumors, for allergies and other atopic conditions and decreased risk of brain tumors, and for alleles at a specific set of 25 single nucleotide polymorphisms and increased risk of brain tumors.

Disclosure: There are no disclosures to report.
[a] Brain Tumor Research, Case Comprehensive Cancer Center, Institute for Computational Biology, Case Western Reserve University School of Medicine, 2-526 Wolstein Research Building, 103 Cornell Road, Cleveland, OH 44106-7295, USA; [b] Department of Medicine, Section of Epidemiology and Population Sciences, Dan Duncan Comprehensive Cancer Center, Baylor College of Medicine, One Baylor Plaza, Houston, TX 77030-3498, USA; [c] Department of Neurosurgery, Brigham and Women's Hospital, Harvard Medical School, Harvard T.H. Chan School of Public Health, 60 Fenwood Road, Boston, MA 02115, USA
* Corresponding author.
E-mail address: Jsb42@case.edu

INTRODUCTION

Brain and central nervous system (CNS) tumors represent approximately 1% of all newly diagnosed cancers in the United States, and about 2% of cancer deaths.[1,2] These are a heterogeneous group of diseases, and comprise more than 100 histologic types as defined by the *World Health Organization (WHO) Classification of Tumors of the Central Nervous System* based on cell of origin and other histopathologic features.[3,4] Brain and CNS tumors include tumors of the brain, cranial nerves, spinal nerves, spinal cord, and the meninges. Unlike most other cancer types, brain tumors are not staged. These tumors can be broadly classified as malignant and nonmalignant (or benign) tumors. The World Health Organization (WHO) classification specifies a grading system, ranging from grade I through grade IV. Grade I/II tumors are considered benign or low grade, whereas grade III/IV tumors are malignant or high grade. Most brain and CNS tumors that are diagnosed in the United States are nonmalignant (**Fig. 1**), and most of these are nonmalignant meningiomas. The most common type of malignant tumors are gliomas, of which glioblastoma occurs with the greatest frequency (see **Fig. 1**). With the newest revision in 2016 to the WHO classification system, histologic criteria for these tumors have become increasingly based on molecular markers, leading to more refined categorization of gliomas.

INCIDENCE OF PRIMARY BRAIN AND CENTRAL NERVOUS SYSTEM TUMORS

Overall age-adjusted incidence of brain and CNS tumors was 22.64 per 100,000 population in the United States between 2010 and 2014. This number is approximately the same as the incidence of thyroid cancer and melanoma. Approximately two-thirds of brain and CNS tumors are nonmalignant (**Table 1**).[1] Most malignant tumors are gliomas, which represent ~80% of all malignant brain tumors. More than half of gliomas diagnosed are glioblastomas (GBMs), or WHO grade IV astrocytomas. The most common type of nonmalignant brain and CNS tumors are meningioma, which represent approximately half of nonmalignant tumors diagnosed in the United States.

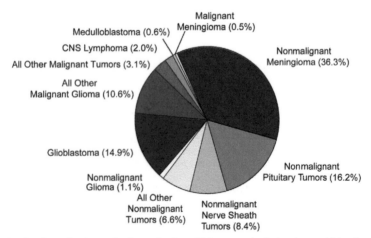

Fig. 1. Distribution of primary brain and other CNS tumors by behavior and histology. (*Data from* Ostrom QT, Gittleman H, Liao P, et al. CBTRUS statistical report: primary brain and other central nervous system tumors diagnosed in the United States in 2010–2014. Neuro Oncol 2017;19(suppl_5):v1–88.)

Table 1
Counts, annual age-adjusted incidence rates, and 95% confidence intervals for brain and CNS tumors overall and by behavior in the United States, 2010 to 2014

	All Brain and CNS Tumors			Malignant Brain and CNS Tumors			Nonmalignant Brain and CNS Tumors		
	Count	AAAIR	95% CI	Count	AAAIR	95% CI	Count	AAAIR	95% CI
Overall	379,848	22.64	22.56–22.71	119,674	7.15	7.10–7.19	260,174	15.49	15.43–15.55
Sex									
Male	160,077	20.34	20.24–20.44	66,300	8.39	8.32–8.45	93,777	11.95	11.87–12.03
Female	219,771	24.77	24.67–24.88	53,374	6.06	6.01–6.11	166,397	18.72	18.62–18.81
Age (y)									
0–14	16,941	5.54	5.46–5.63	11,589	3.79	3.72–3.86	5352	1.75	1.71–1.80
0–4	6011	6.02	5.87–6.18	4548	4.55	4.42–4.69	1463	1.47	1.39–1.55
5–9	5306	5.19	5.05–5.33	3747	3.66	3.55–3.78	1559	1.53	1.45–1.61
10–14	5624	5.44	5.30–5.58	3294	3.19	3.09–3.30	2330	2.24	2.15–2.34
15–39+	56,039	10.94	10.85–11.03	16,826	3.24	3.19–3.29	39,213	7.69	7.62–7.77
40+	306,868	40.82	40.67–40.96	91,259	12.04	11.96–12.12	215,609	28.77	28.65–28.90
Race									
White	313,998	22.75	22.67–22.83	104,978	7.64	7.59–7.68	209,020	15.11	15.04–15.18
Black	43,239	22.58	22.36–22.80	9073	4.54	4.44–4.64	34,166	18.05	17.85–18.24
AIAN	2463	14.18	13.58–14.80	670	3.67	3.37–3.98	1793	10.51	9.99–11.05
API	17,517	20.58	20.27–20.90	4091	4.83	4.68–4.98	13,426	15.76	15.48–16.03

Abbreviations: AAAIR, annual age-adjusted incidence rate; AIAN, American Indian/Alaska Native; API, Asian Pacific Islanders; CI, confidence interval.
From Ostrom QT, Gittleman H, Liao P, et al. CBTRUS statistical report: primary brain and other central nervous system tumors diagnosed in the United States in 2010–2014. Neuro Oncol 2017;19(suppl_5):v1–88; with permission.

Incidence by Sex

Overall incidence of brain and CNS tumors is higher among female patients compared with male patients (see **Table 1**).[1] Incidence of malignant brain and CNS tumors is higher in male patients (incidence ratio [IR] = 8.39 compared with IR = 6.06 for female]), whereas nonmalignant brains are more common in female patients (IR = 18.72 compared with IR = 11.95 for male). Glioma histologies (including GBM), medulloblastoma, and CNS lymphoma occur more commonly in male patients than in female. Malignant meningioma is slightly more common in female patients compared with male. Most nonmalignant histologies occur more often in female patients compared with male. Nonmalignant meningioma is more than twice as common in female patients. Pituitary tumors occur at slightly higher rates in female patients, whereas nonmalignant nerve sheath tumors occur at approximately equal rates in male and female.

Incidence by Age

Incidence of all brain and CNS tumors is highest in adults greater than 40 year old, and median age at diagnosis is 59 years.[1] Brain and CNS tumors are the most common solid tumors in children less than 15 years old, and most of these tumors are malignant.[5] Among children less than 15 years old, the highest incidence of brain and CNS tumors is in children aged 0 to 4 years (see **Table 1**).

Incidence of nonmalignant brain and CNS tumors increases with increasing age. Among adolescents and young adults (AYA; ages 15–39 years), nonmalignant tumors are more than twice as common as malignant tumors. Overall, brain and CNS tumors are the third most common types of cancer in AYA.[6] The most common types of malignant brain tumors in this age group are glioma, particularly lower grade gliomas (**Table 2**). Tumors of the pituitary are the most common type of nonmalignant tumor in AYA, as well as the most common tumor type overall (**Table 3**).

Among adults aged 40 years old or older, nonmalignant tumors are approximately 2.5 times as common as malignant brain and CNS tumors (see **Table 1**). The most common types of malignant brain tumor in older adults are gliomas, of which GBM is the most common (see **Table 2**). The most common type of nonmalignant tumor in older adults is nonmalignant meningioma, which represents more than half of all nonmalignant tumors. Tumors of the pituitary are the second most common nonmalignant tumors in older adults.

Incidence by Race

Brain and CNS tumors are most common among white people in the United States (see **Table 1**). Malignant brain and CNS tumors are nearly twice as common in white people compared with any other racial group. Nonmalignant tumors are most common among black people, in whom they are more than 4 times as common as malignant tumors. The most common types of malignant tumors among all groups are gliomas, which are nearly twice as common among white people as in any other group (see **Table 2**). Incidence of CNS lymphoma is highest among Asian Pacific Islanders (APIs) (see **Table 2**). The most common type of nonmalignant tumor in all groups is nonmalignant meningioma. These tumors are most common in black people (see **Table 3**). Tumors of the pituitary are the second most common type of nonmalignant tumor in all racial groups. These tumors are most common among black people, followed by API.

Global Incidence

Incidence of malignant brain tumors varies significantly by region of the globe. Incidence of these tumors is highest in northern Europe, followed by the

Table 2
Counts, annual age-adjusted incidence rates, and 95% confidence intervals for selected malignant histologies in the United States, 2010 to 2014

Group	All Glioma[a]			Glioblastoma			Malignant Meningioma			Medulloblastoma			CNS Lymphoma		
	Count	AAAIR	95% CI	Count	AAAIR	95% CI	Count	AAAIR	95% CI	Count	AAAIR	95% CI	Count	AAAIR	95% CI
Overall	96,559	5.74	5.71–5.78	56,421	3.20	3.17–3.23	1747	0.10	0.10–0.11	2208	0.15	0.15–0.16	7481	0.44	0.43–0.45
Sex															
Male	54,182	6.80	6.75–6.86	32,506	3.99	3.95–4.03	726	0.09	0.09–0.10	1389	0.19	0.18–0.20	3816	0.48	0.47–0.50
Female	42,377	4.83	4.78–4.87	23,915	2.52	2.49–2.56	1021	0.11	0.10–0.12	819	0.11	0.11–0.12	3665	0.40	0.38–0.41
Age (y)															
0–14	8200	2.68	2.62–2.74	481	0.16	0.14–0.17	18	0.01	0.00–0.01	1444	0.47	0.45–0.50	26	0.01	0.01–0.01
0–4	3029	3.03	2.92–3.14	119	0.12	0.10–0.14	b	b		528	0.53	0.48–0.58	b	b	b
5–9	2764	2.70	2.60–2.80	174	0.17	0.15–0.20	b	b		573	0.56	0.51–0.61	b	b	b
10–14	2407	2.33	2.24–2.43	188	0.18	0.16–0.21	b	b		343	0.33	0.30–0.37	b	b	b
15–39+	13,879	2.68	2.63–2.72	2564	0.51	0.49–0.53	129	0.03	0.02–0.03	608	0.11	0.10–0.12	506	0.10	0.09–0.11
40+	74,480	9.80	9.73–9.87	53,376	6.93	6.87–6.99	1600	0.21	0.20–0.22	156	0.02	0.02–0.03	6949	0.93	0.90–0.95
Race															
White	85,628	6.21	6.17–6.26	51,092	3.46	3.43–3.49	1386	0.10	0.09–0.10	1793	0.16	0.15–0.17	6356	0.44	0.43–0.45
Black	6812	3.38	3.30–3.47	3431	1.79	1.73–1.85	256	0.14	0.13–0.16	245	0.11	0.09–0.12	615	0.31	0.29–0.34
AIAN	502	2.75	2.49–3.02	221	1.47	1.26–1.69	b	b		22	0.09	0.06–0.14	45	0.27	0.19–0.36
API	2928	3.41	3.28–3.54	1332	1.61	1.52–1.70	86	0.11	0.09–0.14	119	0.14	0.11–0.16	400	0.49	0.44–0.54

[a] ICD-O-3 histology codes 9380 to 9384,9391 to 9460 and ICD-O-3 behavior code 3.
[b] Rate suppressed because there were fewer than 16 cases.
From Ostrom QT, Gittleman H, Liao P, et al. CBTRUS statistical report: primary brain and other central nervous system tumors diagnosed in the United States in 2010–2014. Neuro Oncol 2017;19(suppl_5):v1–88; with permission.

Table 3
Counts, annual age-adjusted incidence rates, and 95% confidence intervals for selected nonmalignant histologies in the United States, 2010 to 2014

	Nonmalignant Meningioma			Nerve Sheath Tumors			Tumors of the Pituitary		
	Count	AAAIR	95% CI	Count	AAAIR	95% CI	Count	AAAIR	95% CI
Overall	137,947	8.03	7.99–8.08	31,745	1.87	1.85–1.89	61,462	3.78	3.75–3.81
Sex									
Male	36,738	4.77	4.72–4.82	15,292	1.88	1.85–1.91	27,784	3.50	3.45–3.54
Female	101,209	10.90	10.83–10.97	16,453	1.87	1.84–1.90	33,678	4.14	4.10–4.19
Age (y)									
0–14	250	0.08	0.07–0.09	786	0.26	0.24–0.28	798	0.26	0.24–0.28
0–4	57	0.06	0.04–0.07	256	0.26	0.23–0.29	38	0.04	0.03–0.05
5–9	58	0.06	0.04–0.07	246	0.24	0.21–0.27	193	0.19	0.16–0.22
10–14	135	0.13	0.11–0.15	284	0.27	0.24–0.31	567	0.54	0.50–0.59
15–39+	8649	1.78	1.74–1.82	4815	0.96	0.93–0.98	17,916	3.46	3.41–3.51
40+	129,048	17.16	17.07–17.26	26,144	3.43	3.39–3.47	42,748	5.80	5.74–5.85
Race									
White	112,824	7.84	7.80–7.89	27,257	1.97	1.95–1.99	45,005	3.44	3.41–3.47
Black	17,205	9.47	9.32–9.61	1899	0.94	0.90–0.98	11,769	6.03	5.92–6.14
AIAN	784	5.15	4.77–5.55	206	1.09	0.93–1.25	557	2.97	2.71–3.25
API	6303	7.85	7.65–8.05	2074	2.28	2.18–2.38	3678	4.07	3.94–4.21

From Ostrom QT, Gittleman H, Liao P, et al. CBTRUS statistical report: primary brain and other central nervous system tumors diagnosed in the United States in 2010–2014. Neuro Oncol 2017;19(suppl_5):v1–88; with permission.

United States, Canada, and Australia (**Fig. 2**).[7,8] Incidence of malignant brain and CNS tumors also varies significantly by histologic type and age.[8] Incidence of gliomas, including astrocytic and oligodendroglial tumors, is highest in Australia, western Europe (annual age-adjusted incidence rate [AAIR] = 8.45; 95% confidence interval [CI], 8.3–8.59), and Canada (AAIR = 8.26; 95% CI, 8.04–8.48).

Incidence of these tumors is lowest southeast Asia, east Asia, and India. Malignant meningioma is most common in east Asia and southern Europe. Among children 0 to 14 years old, astrocytic tumors and medulloblastoma are the most common malignant brain and CNS tumors globally.

Incidence of pediatric medulloblastoma is highest in southern Europe and eastern Europe, whereas pediatric astrocytic tumors are most common in the United States and Canada.

Mortality caused by malignant brain and CNS tumors also varies across the globe (**Fig. 3**).[7] Mortality is highest in areas with highest brain and CNS tumor incidence, with the highest rates in northern Europe.

Incidence Time Trends

Time trends in cancer incidence rates are an important measure of the changing burden of cancer in a population over time. Incidence rates of cancer overall, and many specific cancer histologies, have decreased over time.[9] Overall, recent changes in incidence rates of brain and other CNS tumors have been small. In the United States and in other more developed countries, incidence of these tumors has been fairly steady in adults, whereas the incidence of brain tumors in children has been increasing.[1,10–12] Many things can affect incidence rates over time that are not related to true changes in incidence of these tumors, including demographic changes, changes in histologic classification, and changes in cancer registration procedures.

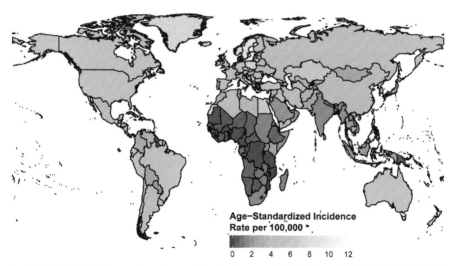

Fig. 2. Global incidence of malignant brain tumors. (*Data from* GLOBOCAN 2012 v1.0, Cancer incidence and mortality worldwide: IARC CancerBase no. 11. International Agency for Research on Cancer; 2013. Available at: http://globocan.iarc.fr. Accessed April 19, 2014.)

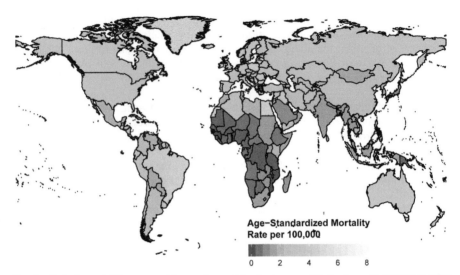

Fig. 3. Global mortalities caused by malignant brain tumors. (*Data from* GLOBOCAN 2012 v1.0, Cancer incidence and mortality worldwide: IARC CancerBase no. 11. International Agency for Research on Cancer; 2013. Available at: http://globocan.iarc.fr. Accessed April 19, 2014.)

PREVALENCE

Prevalence is the estimate of the total number of individuals with a disease alive within a population, compared with incidence that counts new diagnoses only. The International Agency for Research on Cancer's GLOBOCAN, project, which generates global cancer incidence and prevalence statistics using national cancer registry data, estimates the 5-year prevalence of malignant brain and CNS tumors to be 342,914 in 2012, with the largest number of prevalent cases occurring in Asia (186,866) and Europe (57,132).[7] The complete prevalence of primary malignant brain and CNS tumors in the United States in 2010 is estimated to be 47.6 per 100,000 (103,634 total cases).[13]

SURVIVAL

Overall 1-year relative survival after diagnosis with a malignant brain and CNS tumor was 56.6% between 2000 and 2010, with 5-year relative survival of 32.1% (**Table 4**). Survival after diagnosis with a nonmalignant brain tumor is significantly higher, with 1-year relative survival of 94.5% and 5-year relative survival of 90.8%. Survival is poorest after diagnosis with GBM, for which 1-year survival is 37.4% and 5-year survival is 4.9% (**Table 5**).

Survival by Sex

Survival after diagnosis with malignant brain tumor is similar between male and female patients, although female patients have slightly improved 5-year survival (33.7% compared with 30.8%) (see **Table 4**). Female patients also have slightly higher survival after diagnosis with a nonmalignant tumor. For both GBM and medulloblastoma, male patients have slightly higher 1-year survival compared with female, whereas female patients have longer 5-year survival (see **Table 5**). Both 1-year and 5-year survival are significantly higher among female patients compared with male (see **Table 5**).

Table 4
One-year and 5-year relative survival for brain and central nervous system tumors by behavior; sex; and age, Surveillance, Epidemiology, and End Results 2000 to 2014

Group	Malignant Brain and CNS Tumors			Nonmalignant Brain and CNS Tumors		
	Total Cases	1-y (95% CI)	5-y (95% CI)	Total Cases	1-y (95% CI)	5-y (95% CI)
Overall	86,703	56.6 (56.2–56.9)	32.1 (31.8–32.5)	142,989	94.5 (94.3–94.6)	90.8 (90.5–91.0)
Sex						
Male	48,380	56.7 (56.2–57.1)	30.8 (30.4–31.3)	51,463	93.8 (93.6–94.1)	90.1 (89.6–90.5)
Female	38,323	56.4 (55.9–56.9)	33.7 (33.2–34.3)	91,526	94.9 (94.7–95.0)	91.1 (90.8–91.5)
Age (y)						
0–14	9116	85.7 (85.0–86.5)	72.7 (71.7–73.7)	3099	98.5 (98.0–98.9)	96.7 (95.9–97.4)
0–4	3577	82.6 (81.3–83.8)	70.1 (68.5–71.7)	892	97.5 (96.1–98.4)	95.0 (93.0–96.5)
5–9	2979	85.0 (83.6–86.3)	71.1 (69.3–72.8)	880	98.1 (96.9–98.8)	96.3 (94.5–97.5)
10–14	2560	91.0 (89.8–92.1)	78.3 (76.5–80.0)	1327	99.4 (98.8–99.7)	98.0 (96.9–98.7)
15–39+	13,641	88.8 (88.2–89.3)	67.0 (66.1–67.9)	22,976	99.1 (99.0–99.3)	98.0 (97.7–98.2)
40+	63,946	45.5 (45.1–45.9)	18.5 (18.2–18.9)	116,914	93.5 (93.3–93.6)	89.2 (88.8–89.5)

From Surveillance Epidemiology and End Results (SEER) Program. SEER*Stat Database: Incidence - SEER 18 Regs Custom Data (with additional treatment fields), Nov 2016 Sub (2000–2014) <Katrina/Rita Population Adjustment > - Linked To County Attributes - Total U.S., 1969–2015 Counties, National Cancer Institute, DCCPS, Surveillance Research Program, released April 2017, based on the November 2016 submission. 2017; with permission.

Table 5
One-year and 5-year relative survival for malignant brain and central nervous system tumors by histology, sex and age, Surveillance, Epidemiology, and End Results 2000 to 2014

Group	Glioblastoma Total Cases	Glioblastoma 1-y (95% CI)	Glioblastoma 5-y (95% CI)	Medulloblastoma Total Cases	Medulloblastoma 1-y (95% CI)	Medulloblastoma 5-y (95% CI)	Malignant Meningioma Total Cases	Malignant Meningioma 1-y (95% CI)	Malignant Meningioma 5-y (95% CI)	Nonmalignant Meningioma Total Cases	Nonmalignant Meningioma 1-y (95% CI)	Nonmalignant Meningioma 5-y (95% CI)
Overall	39,529	37.4 (36.9–37.9)	4.9 (4.7–5.2)	1789	88.8 (87.2–90.2)	72.7 (70.3–74.9)	1432	81.5 (79.2–83.5)	64.4 (61.2–67.4)	74,334	92.6 (92.4–92.9)	86.8 (86.4–87.2)
Sex												
Male	22,934	38.6 (38.0–39.3)	4.9 (4.6–5.2)	1112	89.6 (87.6–91.3)	71.9 (68.9–74.7)	601	79.2 (75.4–82.4)	59.1 (54.1–63.8)	19,428	90.0 (89.5–90.5)	82.4 (81.5–83.2)
Female	16,595	35.8 (35.0–36.5)	5.0 (4.6–5.4)	677	87.4 (84.6–89.8)	74.0 (70.2–77.4)	831	83.1 (80.1–85.7)	68.1 (64.0–71.9)	54,906	93.6 (93.3–93.8)	88.4 (87.9–88.8)
Age (y)												
0–14	346	52.8 (47.2–58.0)	19.6 (15.1–24.5)	1123	88.2 (86.1–90.0)	72.5 (69.5–75.2)	a	a	a	139	97.8 (93.3–99.3)	96.9 (91.8–98.9)
0–4	87	59.1 (47.6–68.9)	39.6 (28.3–50.7)	441	80.0 (75.9–83.5)	63.6 (58.5–68.2)	a	a	a	a	a	a
5–9	126	42.6 (33.6–51.4)	11.7 (6.3–18.9)	454	92.4 (89.5–94.6)	75.8 (71.1–79.8)	a	a	a	a	a	a
10–14	133	58.4 (49.4–66.3)	15.3 (9.2–22.8)	228	95.9 (92.2–97.8)	83.3 (77.0–88.1)	a	a	a	a	a	a
15–39+	1981	72.4 (70.3–74.4)	22.1 (20.0–24.2)	542	91.0 (88.2–93.2)	74.3 (69.9–78.2)	128	97.7 (92.8–99.3)	90.6 (83.1–94.9)	4824	98.9 (98.6–99.2)	96.9 (96.2–97.5)
40+	37,202	35.4 (34.9–35.9)	3.8 (3.6–4.1)	124	84.3 (76.2–89.8)	67.6 (57.2–76.0)	1287	79.8 (77.3–82.1)	61.5 (58.1–64.7)	69,371	92.2 (91.9–92.4)	86.1 (85.6–86.5)

a Rate suppressed because there were fewer than 50 cases.
From Surveillance Epidemiology and End Results (SEER) Program. SEER*Stat Database: Incidence - SEER 18 Regs Custom Data (with additional treatment fields), Nov 2016 Sub (2000–2014) <Katrina/Rita Population Adjustment > – Linked To County Attributes - Total U.S., 1969–2015 Counties, National Cancer Institute, DCCPS, Surveillance Research Program, released April 2017, based on the November 2016 submission. 2017; with permission.

Survival by Age

Survival after diagnosis with both malignant and nonmalignant brain tumors is highest among AYA aged 15 to 39 years (see **Table 4**). Malignant brain tumor survival is poorest among persons 40 years of age and older, for whom 1-year survival is 45.5% and 5-year survival is 18.5%. GBM survival is highest among persons 15 to 39 years old, for whom 5-year survival is 22.1%. Among persons 40 years of age and older, 5-year survival after diagnosis with GBM is 3.8% (see **Table 5**).

ENVIRONMENTAL RISK FACTORS
Allergies

Well-designed epidemiologic studies have consistently suggested that allergic and atopic conditions such as asthma, hay fever, eczema, and food allergies reduce the risk of multiple CNS tumors, include glioma, meningioma, and vestibular schwannoma (a the summary of reported odds ratios for association between history of allergy or atopic disease and brain tumor is given in **Fig. 4**).[14–18] A large meta-analysis showed that allergies were associated with a 40% reduction in glioma risk. Proposed mechanisms for this association have varied. To control for the bias of self-report, investigators have recently evaluated more objective measures, such as immunoglobulin E (IgE) levels and genetic markers. Patients with glioma have repeatedly been shown to have lower levels of IgE, a biomarker of allergy. Specific single nucleotide polymorphisms (SNPs) associated with IgE have also been associated with glioma risk. In a 2013 meta-analysis, Sun and colleagues[19] showed that r20541 (within *IL13*) may be a genetic indicator of glioma risk. In a separate study, Schwartzbaum and colleagues[20] conducted a case-control study comparing 911 immune function genes and identified associations with the interleukin-2 receptor *CD25* gene.

Ionizing Radiation

One of the best-described risk factors for brain tumors is ionizing radiation (a summary of excess relative risk caused by ionizing radiation is given in **Fig. 5**).[21–24] Multiple studies have evaluated the association between even low doses of therapeutic radiation and brain tumors. In a 2005 study, Sadetzki and colleagues[21] showed that low doses averaging 1.5 Gy for tinea capitis of the scalp were associated with relative risks of 18, 10, and 3 for nerve sheath tumors, meningiomas, and gliomas, respectively. Among patients with glioblastoma or glioma, the incidence of prior therapeutic radiation has been reported to be as high as 17%, and other studies have identified

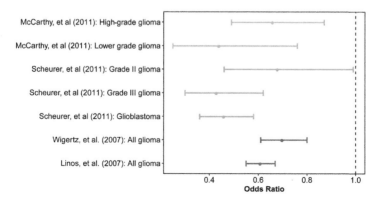

Fig. 4. Summary of recent studies of history of allergy and brain tumor risk.

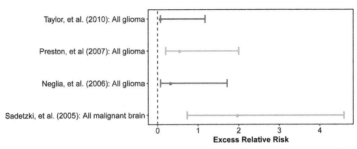

Fig. 5. Summary of recent studies of history of ionizing radiation exposure and brain tumor risk.

increased risk of brain tumors in patients who undergo radiation for acute lympho-blastic leukemia.[25]

As opposed to therapeutic doses of radiation, the effect of diagnostic radiation exposures on the development of brain tumors remains unclear. A recent 2011 study by Davis and colleagues[26] showed increased risk of glioma in patients undergoing 3 or more cumulative computed tomography (CT) scans to the head, only among patients with a family history of cancer. Two recent cohort studies of children undergoing CT scans suggested an increased risk of brain tumors.[27,28] This relationship was dose responsive, with one study reporting an increased incidence rate ratio of 0.16 per childhood CT scan. A 2012 consensus report by radiation experts concluded that there is good evidence that x-ray or gamma radiation doses of 10 to 50 mSv are associated with an increased risk of cancer.[29]

Cellular Phones

Cellular telephone technology was introduced in the 1980s, popularized and improved in the 1990s and early 2000s, and is now ubiquitous. The ubiquity of these devices has led to public concern over whether they could potentially be implicated in brain tumor risk. In response to these concerns, multiple large studies have evaluated the effect of cellular phone use on brain cancer risk, with mixed results (**Fig. 6** provides a summary of recent studies of the association between brain tumors and cellular phone use).[30–32] The International Agency for Research on Cancer (IARC) reviewed the available evidence in 2011, finding that radiofrequency fields produced by cellular phones can be considered possible carcinogens (IARC group 2B).[33] This conclusion was based mostly on findings that heavy users of cellular phones may be at higher risk of brain

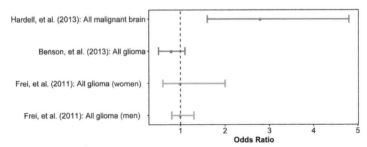

Fig. 6. Summary of recent studies of history of long-term cellular phone use and brain tumor risk.

tumors. In contrast, that same year, a separate review of the epidemiologic evidence published by Swerdlow and colleagues[34] concluded that the compiled studies did not support a relationship between cellular phone use and glioma risk.

In the intervening years, multiple additional studies have been published to attempt to clarify this issue further. Two cohort studies that have since been published used phone subscription records in Denmark and the United Kingdom and found no increase in glioma risk, even among those using cell phones daily or for longer than 10 years.[30,32] One case-control study published on this issue since the 2011 IARC report compared 593 malignant brain tumor cases with 1368 controls and found increased risk for use of cellular phone and increased odds for heavy users among patients with brain tumors. An additional case-control study performed in Korea identified no increased risk of glioma in mobile phone users but did show increased risk among ipsilateral cell phone users.[35]

Given that cellular phones are a recent innovation, any effect they may have on the incidence of brain tumors might be apparent in an analysis of incidence rates during the time period of their popularization. Three studies published since 2011 have evaluated this possibility by assessing incidence time trends in brain tumors, one in Nordic countries,[36] one in the United States,[37] and one in Israel.[38] All showed no significant increases in the incidence rates of glioma.

Although conflicted, the summation of evidence both before the 2011 IARC report and since shows little, if any, evidence of a significant association between mobile phone use and brain tumors. When interpreting the results of cellular phone studies and brain tumor risk, it is important to consider the source of cellular phone usage data.[39] Many of the case-control studies reporting a positive association have relied on self-reported cell phone usage data collected after brain tumor diagnosis, whereas cohort studies that have found null associations have relied on data collected prediagnosis. With the popularization of mobile phones earlier in life (eg, among children and adolescents), and the increased frequency of use throughout the life span, additional long-term follow-up studies relying on usage data rather than self-report will be useful in determining the true association between cellular phones and brain tumors.

Occupational Exposures

The effect of occupational exposures on the risk of brain tumors have been examined with largely inconsistent findings. As with all studies of brain tumors, studies of the effect of occupational exposures are made difficult by the small number of brain tumor cases and the methodological difficulties of examining the effects of individual exposures. In a study of 21 previously selected exposures of interest, Ruder and colleagues[40] showed in the 2012 Upper Midwest Health Study that only exposure to raw meat (eg, butchers) and possibly nonionizing radiation were associated with an increased risk of glioma. They found no association between risk of glioma and exposure to pesticides (eg, farmers), lead (eg, plumbers), polychlorinated biphenyls (eg, electrical workers), or N-nitroso compounds (eg, rubber workers).

The INTEROCC study was a multicenter case-control study that similarly evaluated the risk of brain tumors among participants with selected occupational exposures in 7 countries (Australia, Canada, France, Germany, Israel, New Zealand, and the United Kingdom). Selected exposures included solvents, combustion products, metals, dusts, formaldehyde, and sulfur dioxide, none of which showed a significant relationship with risk of glioma.[41] In a similar study of INTEROCC data, McLean and colleagues[42] reported that none of these exposures were associated with risk of meningioma.

Hormonal Risk Factors

Several studies support the role of reproductive factors and/or exogenous sex hormone exposure in meningioma, although there has been no consistently observed association in glioma.[43–46] Some association has been observed between meningioma growth and pregnancy, but increased parity has not been consistently associated with risk.[47,48] A recent meta-analysis of several previous case-control studies shows a significant increased risk of meningioma with increased used of estrogen-containing hormone replacement therapy (HRT).[44] There has been some suggestion that glioma risk increases with later menarche and menopause,[43] and that risk of glioma may decreased with exogenous estrogen exposure (eg, HRT and oral contraceptives). In contrast, meningioma risk may increase with HRT use. Another meta-analysis by the same investigators found a reduced risk of gliomas among women who previously used exogenous hormones.[49] In addition, a positive association between breast cancer and meningioma has been reported, but this has not been replicated in large cohort studies.[50]

Other Risk Factors

Many other potential risk factors have been explored for brain tumors, including diet, viruses, reproductive factors, head injury, and exposure to electromagnetic fields. Associations between these factors and risk of brain and CNS tumor have not been well replicated. Please see reviews by Baldi and colleagues[46] and Ostrom and colleagues[51] for further discussion of histology-specific risk factor research.

INHERITABLE GENETIC RISK FACTORS
Syndromic Brain Tumors

Approximately 5% of brain tumors are attributable to hereditary cancer syndromes (**Table 6** provides a brief summary of selected syndromes associated with development of brain tumors).[52,53] Neurofibromatosis type 1 (NF-1) and type 2 (NF-2) are perhaps the most well-known cancer syndromes associated with CNS tumors. NF-1, also known as von Recklinghausen disease, is an autosomal dominant single-gene disorder that occurs in approximately 1 of 3000 to 4000 live births. About half of patients with NF-1 have sporadic mutations in the locus 17q11.2. CNS lesions are commonly associated with NF-1, appearing in 4% to 45% of patients with the disorder, and include optic nerve gliomas, astrocytomas, ependymomas, acoustic neuromas, neurilemmomas, meningiomas, and neurofibromas. NF-2, also known as central neurofibromatosis, is rarer than NF-1, occurring in 1 in 25,000 to 40,000 live births. Loss of the NF-2 protein coded on the long arm of chromosome 22 results in impaired tumor suppression, resulting most commonly in vestibular schwannomas of cranial nerve VIII (nearly 100% of patients), spinal schwannomas, meningiomas, spinal ependymomas, and astrocytomas (approximately 53% of patients).

Several less common syndromes are also associated with the development of brain tumors, including:

- Tuberous sclerosis complex (TSC) is an autosomal dominant disorder occurring in approximately 1 in 6000 live births. TSC is associated with the development of subependymal giant cell astrocytomas (SEGA), and approximately 5% to 15% of those with TSC go on to develop SEGA.
- von Hippel-Lindau disease is a rare autosomal dominant multisystem disorder associated with a mutation in *VHL* on the short arm of chromosome 3. Occurring in 1 in 31,000 to 39,000 live births, VHL disease is associated with cerebellar hemangioblastoma of the CNS and visceral organs, retinal angiomatosis,

Table 6
Inherited syndromes associated with brain and other central nervous system tumors

Gene (Chromosome Location)	Disorder/Syndrome	Mode of Inheritance	Phenotypic Features	Associated Brain Tumors
NF1 (17q11.2)	Neurofibromatosis 1	Dominant	Neurofibromas, Schwannomas, café-au-lait macules	Astrocytoma, optic nerve glioma
NF2 (22q12.2)	Neurofibromatosis 2	Dominant	Acoustic neuromas, meningiomas, neurofibromas, eye lesions	Ependymoma
TSC1, TSC2 (9q34.14,16p13.3)	Tuberous sclerosis	Dominant	Development of multisystem nonmalignant tumors	Giant cell astrocytoma
MSH2, MLH1, MSH6, PMS2	Lynch syndrome	Dominant	Predisposition to gastrointestinal, endometrial and other cancers	Glioblastoma, other gliomas
TP53 (17p13.1)	Li-Fraumeni syndrome	Dominant	Predisposition to numerous cancers, especially breast, brain, and soft tissue sarcoma	Glioblastoma, other gliomas
CDKN2A (9p21.3)	Melanoma-neural system tumor syndrome	Dominant	Predisposition to malignant melanoma and malignant brain tumors	Glioma
IDH1/IDH2 (2q33.3/15q26.1)	Ollier disease	Acquired postzygotic mosaicism, dominant with reduced penetrance	Development of intraosseous benign cartilaginous tumors, cancer predisposition	Glioma

(continued on next page)

Table 6
(continued)

Gene (Chromosome Location)	Disorder/Syndrome	Mode of Inheritance	Phenotypic Features	Associated Brain Tumors
APC, MMR (5q21)	Turcot syndrome	Dominant	Development of multiple adenomatous colon polyps, predisposition to colorectal cancer and brain tumors	Medulloblastoma, glioma
PTCH1 (9q22.3)	Gorlin syndrome (nevoid basal cell carcinoma)	Dominant	Development of basal cell carcinomas, benign jaw tumors, fibromas of the heart or ovaries, and medulloblastoma	Medulloblastoma
RB1 (13q14)	Retinoblastoma	Dominant	Development of multiple tumors of the eye, increased risk of some brain tumors	Retinoblastoma, pineoblastoma, malignant glioma
VHL (3p25)	von Hippel-Lindau syndrome	Dominant	Predisposition to kidney cysts, renal cell carcinoma, pancreatic neuroendocrine tumors; pheochromocytomas, endolymphatic sac tumors and, brain tumors	Hemangioblastoma

Abbreviations: APC, adenomatous polyposis coli; *CDKN2A,* cyclin-dependent kinase inhibitor 2A; *IDH1,* isocitrate dehydrogenase 1; *IDH2,* isocitrate dehydrogenase 2; *MLH1,* MutL homolog 1; colon cancer, nonpolyposis type 2; *MSH2,* MutS protein homolog 2; *MSH6,* MutS protein homolog 6; *NF1,* Neurofibromin 1; *NF2,* Neurofibromin 2; *PMS2,* PMS1 homolog 2, mismatch repair system component; *PTCH1,* Patched 1; *RB1,* RB transcriptional corepressor 1; *TP53,* tumor protein p53; *TSC1,* TSC complex subunit 1; *TSC2,* TSC complex subunit 1; *VHL,* von Hippel-Lindau tumor suppressor.

Adapted from Farrell CJ, Plotkin SR. Genetic causes of brain tumors: neurofibromatosis, tuberous sclerosis, von Hippel-Lindau, and other syndromes. Neurol Clin 2007;25(4):925–46, viii; and Melean G, Sestini R, Ammannati F, et al. Genetic insights into familial tumors of the nervous system. Am J Med Genet C Semin Med Genet 2004;129C(1):74–84; with permission.

pancreatic cysts, and renal lesions. Approximately 20% to 38% of cerebellar hemangioblastomas are associated with VHL.

- Gorlin' syndrome, or nevoid basal cell carcinoma syndrome, is an autosomal dominant disorder occurring in approximately 1 in 57,000 to 164,000 live births associated with a germline mutation of Protein patched homolog 1 (*PTCH1*) on chromosome 9q. Among these patients, the lifetime risk of developing a medulloblastoma is ~5%, and approximately 2% of those with medulloblastoma are found to have Gorlin.
- Turcot syndrome is a syndromic association between brain tumors and colorectal polyposis. Among these patients, rates of brain tumors are extremely high: 60% develop medulloblastomas, 14% astrocytomas, and 10% ependymoma.
- Li-Fraumeni syndrome is a multisystem, autosomal dominant hereditary syndrome associated with germline p53 mutations. The result of these mutations is a familial syndrome associated with breast cancer, sarcomas, leukemia, and brain tumors.

Familial Aggregation of Brain Tumors

Almost all cases of glioma are sporadic but approximately 5% of gliomas are familial, meaning that a glioma has occurred multiple times within the same family.[54] Some epidemiologic studies have identified increased risk of developing a brain tumor for first-degree relatives (parents, children, and full siblings) in incident cases, but because of the rarity of glioma and further rarity of familial glioma the sample sizes for these studies are generally small.[54–58] Studies of first-degree relatives of persons with glioma have found that the incidence is 2 to 3 times higher than that in persons without a relative with glioma.[54,56] A study of the Swedish cancer registry estimated the risk of glioma among first-degree family members and spouses to estimate the genetic component of familial aggregation compared with shared environment, and found that having a first-degree relative with a brain tumor led to an increase in risk with no increased risk in spouses.[55] This finding suggests that there is a genetic component to familial aggregation, although this method does not account for shared environment in childhood. Some analyses have also shown increased risk of other nonbrain cancers in relatives of persons with brain tumors, including melanoma and sarcoma.[58,59]

Family studies have been conducted within affected glioma families (in which more than 1 person has been diagnosed with a glioma) but have had little success identifying genetic risk variants that are consistently associated with glioma.[60–63] Two early family-based linkage studies[62,63] of familial glioma found a single association at 15q23-q26.3[66] but were limited by small sample size. Analysis of families collected through the GLIOGENE consortium found a significant linkage peak at 17q12-21.32, which could not be replicated in a validation set, as well as other peaks that did not reach a logarithm of the odds (LOD) score of 3.[64] This region was further refined using a variable age-at-onset model to identify 2 separate peaks within the previous identified linkage region.[61] The initial GLIOGENE linkage analysis also found several loci nominally associated with glioma at 6p22.3, 12p13.33-12.1, 17q22-23.2, and 18q23.[60] When genotype frequencies of SNPs within these regions were compared between persons with a familial history of glioma and unaffected controls, there was a moderately significant association for 12 SNPs.[64] Additional analyses of these glioma families have found alterations in MutS protein homolog 2 (*MSH2*)[65] and protection of telomeres protein 1 (*POT1*)[66] that seem to be associated with glioma in a small number of families, but most mutations within glioma families seem to be specific to each family.

Table 7
Heritable variants associated with glioma risk from genome-wide association studies

Candidate Gene (Chromosome Location)	SNP Risk Allele	Odds Ratio[a]	RAF in Europeans[b]	Associated Glioma Subtype	Studies Detected
RAVER2 (1p31.3)	rs12752552-T	1.22	0.87	Glioblastoma	Melin et al,[67] 2017
MDM4 (1q32.1)	rs4252707-A	1.19	0.22	Lower grade glioma	Melin et al,[67] 2017
AKT3 (1q44)	rs12076373-G	1.23	0.84	Lower grade glioma	Melin et al,[67] 2017
C2orf80 (2q33.3)	rs7572263-A	1.20	0.76	Lower grade glioma	Melin et al,[67] 2017
LRIG1 (3p14.1)	rs11706832-C	1.15	0.46	Lower grade glioma	Melin et al,[67] 2017
TERT (5p15.33)	rs10069690-T	1.45	0.276	All glioma subtypes	Shete et al,[69] 2009 Wrensch et al,[76] 2009 Chen et al,[77] 2011 Sanson et al,[78] 2011 Rajamaran et al,[70] 2012 Melin et al,[67] 2017
EGFR (7p11.2)	rs75061358-G	1.42	0.099	All glioma subtypes	Jenkins et al,[79] 2011 Sanson et al,[78] 2011 Rajamaran et al,[70] 2012 Walsh et al,[80] 2013 Melin et al,[67] 2017
EGFR (7p11.2)	rs723527-A	1.25	0.573	Glioblastoma	Jenkins et al,[79] 2011 Sanson et al,[78] 2011 Rajamaran et al,[70] 2012 Walsh et al,[80] 2013 Melin et al,[67] 2017
CCDC26 (8q24.21)	rs55705857-G	3.39	0.05	Oligodendroglial tumors/IDH-mutant astrocytic tumors	Shete et al,[69] 2009 Jenkins et al,[79] 2011 Jenkins et al,[72] 2012 Rajamaran et al,[70] 2012 Enciso-Mora et al,[81] 2013 Melin et al,[67] 2017
CDKN2B (9p21.3)	rs634537-G	1.30	0.41	Astrocytic tumors, grades 2–4	Shete et al,[69] 2009 Wrensch et al,[76] 2009 Rajamaran et al,[70] 2012
STN1 (10q24.33)	rs11598018-C	1.14	0.462	Lower grade glioma	Melin et al,[67] 2017
VTI1A (10q25.2)	rs11599775-G	1.16	0.620	Lower grade glioma	Kinnersley et al,[68] 2015 Melin et al,[67] 2017
Intergenic (11q14.1)	rs11233250-C	1.24	0.868	Glioblastoma	Melin et al,[67] 2017

(continued on next page)

Table 7
(continued)

Candidate Gene (Chromosome Location)	SNP Risk Allele	Odds Ratio[a]	RAF in Europeans[b]	Associated Glioma Subtype	Studies Detected
MAML2 (11q21)	rs7107785-T	1.16	0.479	Lower grade glioma	Melin et al,[67] 2017
PHLDB1 (11q23.2)	rs648044-A	1.19	0.390	—	Shete et al,[69] 2009 Melin et al,[67] 2017
PHLDB1 (11q23.3)	rs498872-A	1.50	0.32	IDH-mutant gliomas	Shete et al,[69] 2009 Rajamaran et al,[70] 2012 Rice et al,[82] 2013
Intergenic (12q21.2)	rs1275600-T	1.16	0.595	Lower grade glioma	Kinnersley et al,[68] 2015 Melin et al,[67] 2017
AKAP6 (14q12)	rs10131032-G	1.33	0.916	Lower grade glioma	Melin et al,[67] 2017
ETFA (15q24.2)	rs1801591-A	1.35	0.086	Lower grade glioma	Kinnersley et al,[68] 2015 Melin et al,[67] 2017
RHBDF1 (16p13.3)	rs2562152-T	1.21	0.850	Glioblastoma	Melin et al,[67] 2017
RHBDF1 (16p13.3)	rs3751667-T	1.18	0.208	Lower grade glioma	Melin et al,[67] 2017
HEATR3 (16q12.1)	rs10852606-C	1.18	0.713	Glioblastoma	Melin et al,[67] 2017
TP53 (17p13.1)	rs78378222-C	2.70	0.01	All glioma subtypes	Rice et al,[83] 2011 Egan et al,[84] 2012 Enciso-Mora et al,[85] 2013 Melin et al,[67] 2017
RTEL1 (20q13.33)	rs2297440-C	1.36	0.796	All glioma subtypes	Shete et al,[69] 2009 Wrensch et al,[76] 2009 Chen et al,[77] 2011 Rajamaran et al,[70] 2012 Melin et al,[67] 2017
SLC16A8 (22q13.1)	rs2235573-G	1.15	0.51	Glioblastoma	Melin et al,[67] 2017

Abbreviations: AKAP6, A-kinase anchoring protein 6′; AKT3, AKT serine/threonine kinase 3; C2orf80, chromosome 2 open reading frame 80; CCDC26, coiled-coil domain containing 26; CDKN2B, cyclin-dependent kinase inhibitor 2B; EGFR, epidermal growth factor receptor; ETFA, electron transfer flavoprotein alpha subunit; HEATR3, HEAT repeat containing 3; MAML2, mastermind like transcriptional coactivator 2; MDM4, MDM4 p53 regulator; PHLDB1, pleckstrin homologylike domain family B, member 1; RAF, risk allele frequency; RAVER2, Ribonucleoprotein, PTB Binding 2; RHBDF1, rhomboid 5 homolog 1; RTEL1, regulator of telomere elongation helicase; SLC16A8, Solute carrier family 16 member 8; TERT, telomerase reverse transcriptase; TP53, tumor protein p53; VTI1A, vesicle transport through interaction with t-SNAREs 1A.

[a] Odds ratio estimates from Melin and colleagues,[67] 2017.
[b] Allele frequencies within European superpopulation within the 1000 Genomes Project.[86]

Genetic Risk Factors for Sporadic Glioma

Since the advances in technology that now allow rapid whole-genome genotyping, 6 genome-wide association studies of patients with glioma have been conducted.[54,67–70] Together these studies identified 25 genomic variants that increased glioma risk (**Table 7** provides a summary of these variants). An additional analysis using these 4 datasets estimated the proportion of incidence variance of glioma that is attributable to genetic factors to be 25%.[71] Many of these factors have stronger associations with specific grades and histologies of glioma, although some confer increased risk for all types. Although gliomas are known to be heterogeneous, most analyses have been conducted on all glioma types pooled or with classification based on histologically assigned type and grade. Because of their rarity, glioma case cohorts are often ascertained at multiple centers over multiple years, and availability of results from molecular tests may not be available on all cases. The variant near *CCDC26* is most strongly associated with oligodendroglial tumors with mutant isocitrate dehydrogenase 1/2 (*IDH1/2*) (OR = 5.1 and OR = 4.8, respectively), with no significant association for *IDH1/2* wild-type tumors.[72]

Genetic factors associated with risk for brain tumors other than glioma have not been as well studied. One risk locus within *MLLT10* has been associated with increased susceptibility to meningioma.[73,74] A recent meta-analysis pooled several case-control studies assessing associations between genetic variants and meningioma, and found that loci within MLLT10, MTRR, and MTHFR are associated with increased meningioma risk.[75]

SUMMARY

Incidence, prevalence, and survival for brain tumors varies by histologic type, age at diagnosis, sex, and race/ethnicity. Significant progress has been made in identifying potential risk factors for brain tumors, although more research is warranted. The strongest risk factors that have been identified thus far include allergies/atopic disease, ionizing radiation, and heritable genetic factors. Scientific evidence for an association between exposure to nonionizing radiation in the form of cellular phones and glioma risk is inconclusive. Modern genome-wide omic technologies (including genomic, epigenomic, transcriptomic, proteomic, or metabolomics data) provide the opportunity to examine risk factors while accounting for the heterogeneity of these tumors. Further analysis of large, multicenter epidemiologic studies, as well as well-annotated omic datasets, can potentially lead to further understanding of the relationship between gene and environment in the process of brain tumor development.

REFERENCES

1. Ostrom QT, Gittleman H, Liao P, et al. CBTRUS statistical report: primary brain and other central nervous system tumors diagnosed in the United States in 2010–2014. Neuro Oncol 2017;19(suppl_5):v1–88.
2. Siegel RL, Miller KD, Jemal A. Cancer statistics, 2017. CA Cancer J Clin 2017; 67(1):7–30.
3. Louis DN, Perry A, Reifenberger G, et al. The 2016 World Health Organization classification of tumors of the central nervous system: a summary. Acta Neuropathol 2016;131(6):803–20.
4. Louis DN, Ohgaki H, Wiestler OD, et al, editors. WHO classification of tumours of the central nervous system. Lyon (France): International Agency for Research on Cancer; 2007.

5. Ostrom QT, de Blank PM, Kruchko C, et al. Alex's Lemonade Stand Foundation infant and childhood primary brain and central nervous system tumors diagnosed in the United States in 2007-2011. Neuro-oncology 2015;16(Suppl 10):x1–36.
6. Ostrom QT, Gittleman H, de Blank PM, et al. American Brain Tumor Association adolescent and young adult primary brain and central nervous system tumors diagnosed in the United States in 2008-2012. Neuro-oncology 2016;18(Suppl 1):i1–50.
7. Ferlay J, Soerjomataram I, Ervik M, et al. GLOBOCAN 2012 v1.0, cancer incidence and mortality worldwide: IARC CancerBase no. 11. 2013. Available at: http://globocan.iarc.fr. Accessed August 18, 2017.
8. Leece R, Xu J, Ostrom QT, et al. Global incidence of malignant brain and other central nervous system tumors by histology, 2003-2007. Neuro Oncol 2017; 19(11):1553–64.
9. Siegel RL, Miller KD, Jemal A. Cancer statistics, 2016. CA Cancer J Clin 2016; 66(1):7–30.
10. GLOBOCAN 2012 v1.0, Cancer incidence and mortality worldwide: IARC CancerBase no. 11. International Agency for Research on Cancer; 2013. Available at: http://globocan.iarc.fr. Accessed February 19, 2014.
11. Gittleman HR, Ostrom QT, Rouse CD, et al. Trends in central nervous system tumor incidence relative to other common cancers in adults, adolescents, and children in the United States, 2000 to 2010. Cancer 2015;121(1):102–12.
12. Cancer incidence in five continents, Vol. X (electronic version). International Agency for Research on Cancer; 2013. Available at: http://ci5.iarc.fr. Accessed August 18, 2017.
13. Zhang AS, Ostrom QT, Kruchko C, et al. Complete prevalence of malignant primary brain tumors registry data in the United States compared with other common cancers, 2010. Neuro Oncol 2017;19(5):726–35.
14. Linos E, Raine T, Alonso A, et al. Atopy and risk of brain tumors: a meta-analysis. J Natl Cancer Inst 2007;99(20):1544–50.
15. Turner MC, Krewski D, Armstrong BK, et al. Allergy and brain tumors in the INTERPHONE study: pooled results from Australia, Canada, France, Israel, and New Zealand. Cancer Causes Control 2013;24(5):949–60.
16. McCarthy BJ, Rankin K, Il'yasova D, et al. Assessment of type of allergy and antihistamine use in the development of glioma. Cancer Epidemiol Biomarkers Prev 2011;20(2):370–8.
17. Scheurer ME, Amirian ES, Davlin SL, et al. Effects of antihistamine and anti-inflammatory medication use on risk of specific glioma histologies. Int J Cancer 2011;129(9):2290–6.
18. Wigertz A, Lönn S, Schwartzbaum J, et al. Allergic conditions and brain tumor risk. Am J Epidemiol 2007;166(8):941–50.
19. Sun G, Wang X, Shi L, et al. Association between polymorphisms in interleukin-4Ralpha and interleukin-13 and glioma risk: a meta-analysis. Cancer Epidemiol 2013;37(3):306–10.
20. Schwartzbaum JA, Huang K, Lawler S, et al. Allergy and inflammatory transcriptome is predominantly negatively correlated with CD133 expression in glioblastoma. Neuro-oncology 2010;12(4):320–7.
21. Sadetzki S, Chetrit A, Freedman L, et al. Long-term follow-up for brain tumor development after childhood exposure to ionizing radiation for tinea capitis. Radiat Res 2005;163(4):424–32.
22. Preston DL, Ron E, Tokuoka S, et al. Solid cancer incidence in atomic bomb survivors: 1958-1998. Radiat Res 2007;168(1):1–64.

23. Taylor AJ, Little MP, Winter DL, et al. Population-based risks of CNS tumors in survivors of childhood cancer: the British Childhood Cancer Survivor Study. J Clin Oncol 2010;28(36):5287–93.

24. Neglia JP, Robison LL, Stovall M, et al. New primary neoplasms of the central nervous system in survivors of childhood cancer: a report from the Childhood Cancer Survivor Study. J Natl Cancer Inst 2006;98(21):1528–37.

25. Perkins SM, Dewees T, Shinohara ET, et al. Risk of subsequent malignancies in survivors of childhood leukemia. J Cancer Surviv 2013;7(4):544–50.

26. Davis F, Il'yasova D, Rankin K, et al. Medical diagnostic radiation exposures and risk of gliomas. Radiat Res 2011;175(6):790–6.

27. Mathews JD, Forsythe AV, Brady Z, et al. Cancer risk in 680,000 people exposed to computed tomography scans in childhood or adolescence: data linkage study of 11 million Australians. BMJ 2013;346:f2360.

28. Pearce MS, Salotti JA, Little MP, et al. Radiation exposure from CT scans in childhood and subsequent risk of leukaemia and brain tumours: a retrospective cohort study. Lancet 2012;380(9840):499–505.

29. Linet MS, Slovis TL, Miller DL, et al. Cancer risks associated with external radiation from diagnostic imaging procedures. CA: a Cancer J clinicians 2012;62(2): 75–100.

30. Frei P, Poulsen AH, Johansen C, et al. Use of mobile phones and risk of brain tumours: update of Danish cohort study. BMJ 2011;343:d6387.

31. Hardell L, Carlberg M, Soderqvist F, et al. Case-control study of the association between malignant brain tumours diagnosed between 2007 and 2009 and mobile and cordless phone use. Int J Oncol 2013;43(6):1833–45.

32. Benson VS, Pirie K, Schuz J, et al. Mobile phone use and risk of brain neoplasms and other cancers: prospective study. Int J Epidemiol 2013;42(3):792–802.

33. Baan R, Grosse Y, Lauby-Secretan B, et al. Carcinogenicity of radiofrequency electromagnetic fields. Lancet Oncol 2011;12(7):624–6.

34. Swerdlow AJ, Feychting M, Green AC, et al, International Commission for Non-Ionizing Radiation Protection Standing Committee on Epidemiology. Mobile phones, brain tumors, and the interphone study: where are we now? Environ Health Perspect 2011;119(11):1534–8.

35. Yoon S, Choi JW, Lee E, et al. Mobile phone use and risk of glioma: a case-control study in Korea for 2002-2007. Environ Health Toxicol 2015;30:e2015015.

36. Deltour I, Auvinen A, Feychting M, et al. Mobile phone use and incidence of glioma in the Nordic countries 1979-2008: consistency check. Epidemiology 2012; 23(2):301–7.

37. Little MP, Rajaraman P, Curtis RE, et al. Mobile phone use and glioma risk: comparison of epidemiological study results with incidence trends in the United States. BMJ 2012;344:e1147.

38. Barchana M, Margaliot M, Liphshitz I. Changes in brain glioma incidence and laterality correlates with use of mobile phones–a nationwide population based study in Israel. Asian Pac J Cancer Prev 2012;13(11):5857–63.

39. Johansen C, Schuz J, Andreasen AS, et al. Study designs may influence results: the problems with questionnaire-based case-control studies on the epidemiology of glioma. Br J Cancer 2017;116(7):841–8.

40. Ruder AM, Waters MA, Carreon T, et al. The Upper Midwest Health Study: industry and occupation of glioma cases and controls. Am J Ind Med 2012; 55(9):747–55.

41. Lacourt A, Cardis E, Pintos J, et al. INTEROCC case-control study: lack of association between glioma tumors and occupational exposure to selected combustion products, dusts and other chemical agents. BMC Public Health 2013;13:340.

42. McLean D, Fleming S, Turner MC, et al. Occupational solvent exposure and risk of meningioma: results from the INTEROCC multicentre case-control study. Occup Environ Med 2014;71(4):253–8.

43. Hatch EE, Linet MS, Zhang J, et al. Reproductive and hormonal factors and risk of brain tumors in adult females. Int J Cancer 2005;114(5):797–805.

44. Qi ZY, Shao C, Huang YL, et al. Reproductive and exogenous hormone factors in relation to risk of meningioma in women: a meta-analysis. PLoS One 2013;8(12): e83261.

45. Lee E, Grutsch J, Persky V, et al. Association of meningioma with reproductive factors. Int J Cancer 2006;119(5):1152–7.

46. Baldi I, Engelhardt J, Bonnet C, et al. Epidemiology of meningiomas. Neurochirurgie 2018;64(1):5–14.

47. Anic GM, Madden MH, Nabors LB, et al. Reproductive factors and risk of primary brain tumors in women. J Neurooncol 2014;118(2):297–304.

48. Zong H, Xu H, Geng Z, et al. Reproductive factors in relation to risk of brain tumors in women: an updated meta-analysis of 27 independent studies. Tumour Biol 2014;35(11):11579–86.

49. Qi ZY, Shao C, Zhang X, et al. Exogenous and endogenous hormones in relation to glioma in women: a meta-analysis of 11 case-control studies. PLoS One 2013; 8(7):e68695.

50. Criscitiello C, Disalvatore D, Santangelo M, et al. No link between breast cancer and meningioma: results from a large monoinstitutional retrospective analysis. Cancer Epidemiol Biomarkers Prev 2014;23(1):215–7.

51. Ostrom QT, Bauchet L, Davis F, et al. The epidemiology of glioma in adults: a "state of the science" review. Neuro Oncol 2014;16(7):896–913.

52. Farrell CJ, Plotkin SR. Genetic causes of brain tumors: neurofibromatosis, tuberous sclerosis, von Hippel-Lindau, and other syndromes. Neurol Clin 2007;25(4): 925–46, viii.

53. Melean G, Sestini R, Ammannati F, et al. Genetic insights into familial tumors of the nervous system. Am J Med Genet C Semin Med Genet 2004;129C(1):74–84.

54. Wrensch M, Lee M, Miike R, et al. Familial and personal medical history of cancer and nervous system conditions among adults with glioma and controls. Am J Epidemiol 1997;145(7):581–93.

55. Malmer B, Henriksson R, Grönberg H. Familial brain tumours—genetics or environment? A nationwide cohort study of cancer risk in spouses and first-degree relatives of brain tumour patients. Int J Cancer 2003;106(2):260–3.

56. Malmer B, Grönberg H, Bergenheim AT, et al. Familial aggregation of astrocytoma in northern Sweden: an epidemiological cohort study. Int J Cancer 1999;81(3): 366–70.

57. Hill DA, Inskip PD, Shapiro WR, et al. Cancer in first-degree relatives and risk of glioma in adults. Cancer Epidemiol Biomarkers Prev 2003;12(12):1443–8.

58. Scheurer ME, Etzel CJ, Liu M, et al. Aggregation of cancer in first-degree relatives of patients with glioma. Cancer Epidemiol Biomarkers Prev 2007;16(11):2491–5.

59. Scheurer ME, Etzel CJ, Liu M, et al. Familial aggregation of glioma: a pooled analysis. Am J Epidemiol 2010;172(10):1099–107.

60. Shete S, Lau CC, Houlston RS, et al. Genome-wide high-density SNP linkage search for glioma susceptibility loci: results from the Gliogene Consortium. Cancer Res 2011;71(24):7568–75.

61. Sun X, Vengoechea J, Elston R, et al. A variable age of onset segregation model for linkage analysis, with correction for ascertainment, applied to glioma. Cancer Epidemiol Biomarkers Prev 2012;21(12):2242–51.

62. Paunu N, Lahermo P, Onkamo P, et al. A novel low-penetrance locus for familial glioma at 15q23-q26.3. Cancer Res 2002;62(13):3798–802.

63. Malmer B, Haraldsson S, Einarsdottir E, et al. Homozygosity mapping of familial glioma in northern Sweden. Acta Oncol 2005;44(2):114–9.

64. Liu Y, Melin BS, Rajaraman P, et al. Insight in glioma susceptibility through an analysis of 6p22.3, 12p13.33-12.1, 17q22-23.2 and 18q23 SNP genotypes in familial and non-familial glioma. Hum Genet 2012;131(9):1507–17.

65. Andersson U, Wibom C, Cederquist K, et al. Germline rearrangements in families with strong family history of glioma and malignant melanoma, colon, and breast cancer. Neuro Oncol 2014;16(10):1333–40.

66. Bainbridge MN, Armstrong GN, Gramatges MM, et al. Germline mutations in shelterin complex genes are associated with familial glioma. J Natl Cancer Inst 2014;107(1):384.

67. Melin BS, Barnholtz-Sloan JS, Wrensch MR, et al. Genome-wide association study of glioma subtypes identifies specific differences in genetic susceptibility to glioblastoma and non-glioblastoma tumors. Nat Genet 2017;49(5):789–94.

68. Kinnersley B, Labussiere M, Holroyd A, et al. Genome-wide association study identifies multiple susceptibility loci for glioma. Nat Commun 2015;6:8559.

69. Shete S, Hosking FJ, Robertson LB, et al. Genome-wide association study identifies five susceptibility loci for glioma. Nat Genet 2009;41(8):899–904.

70. Rajaraman P, Melin BS, Wang Z, et al. Genome-wide association study of glioma and meta-analysis. Hum Genet 2012;131(12):1877–88.

71. Kinnersley B, Mitchell JS, Gousias K, et al. Quantifying the heritability of glioma using genome-wide complex trait analysis. Sci Rep 2015;5:17267.

72. Jenkins RB, Xiao Y, Sicotte H, et al. A low-frequency variant at 8q24.21 is strongly associated with risk of oligodendroglial tumors and astrocytomas with IDH1 or IDH2 mutation. Nat Genet 2012;44(10):1122–5.

73. Dobbins SE, Broderick P, Melin B, et al. Common variation at 10p12.31 near MLLT10 influences meningioma risk. Nat Genet 2011;43(9):825–7.

74. Egan KM, Baskin R, Nabors LB, et al. Brain tumor risk according to germ-line variation in the MLLT10 locus. Eur J Hum Genet 2015;23(1):132–4.

75. Han XY, Wang W, Wang LL, et al. Genetic variants and increased risk of meningioma: an updated meta-analysis. OncoTargets Ther 2017;10:1875–88.

76. Wrensch M, Jenkins RB, Chang JS, et al. Variants in the CDKN2B and RTEL1 regions are associated with high-grade glioma susceptibility. Nat Genet 2009; 41(8):905–8.

77. Chen H, Chen Y, Zhao Y, et al. Association of sequence variants on chromosomes 20, 11, and 5 (20q13.33, 11q23.3, and 5p15.33) with glioma susceptibility in a Chinese population. Am J Epidemiol 2011;173(8):915–22.

78. Sanson M, Hosking FJ, Shete S, et al. Chromosome 7p11.2 (EGFR) variation influences glioma risk. Hum Mol Genet 2011;20(14):2897–904.

79. Jenkins RB, Wrensch MR, Johnson D, et al. Cancer genetics. Cancer Genet 2011;204(1):13–8.

80. Walsh KM, Anderson E, Hansen HM, et al. Analysis of 60 reported glioma risk SNPs replicates published GWAS findings but fails to replicate associations from published candidate-gene studies. Genet Epidemiol 2013;37(2):222–8.

81. Enciso-Mora V, Hosking FJ, Kinnersley B, et al. Deciphering the 8q24.21 association for glioma. Hum Mol Genet 2013;22(11):2293–302.

82. Rice T, Zheng S, Decker PA, et al. Inherited variant on chromosome 11q23 increases susceptibility to IDH-mutated but not IDH-normal gliomas regardless of grade or histology. Neuro Oncol 2013;15(5):535–41.
83. Stacey SN, Sulem P, Jonasdottir A, et al. A germline variant in the TP53 polyadenylation signal confers cancer susceptibility. Nat Genet 2011;43(11):1098–103.
84. Egan KM, Nabors LB, Olson JJ, et al. Rare TP53 genetic variant associated with glioma risk and outcome. J Med Genet 2012;49(7):420–1.
85. Enciso-Mora V, Hosking FJ, Di Stefano AL, et al. Low penetrance susceptibility to glioma is caused by the TP53 variant rs78378222. Br J Cancer 2013;108(10): 2178–85.
86. 1000 Genomes Project Consortium, Auton A, Brooks LD, Durbin RM, et al. A global reference for human genetic variation. Nature 2015;526(7571):68–74.

Evolving Insights into the Molecular Neuropathology of Diffuse Gliomas in Adults

Floris P. Barthel, MD[a,b], Kevin C. Johnson, PhD[b],
Pieter Wesseling, MD, PhD[a,c],*, Roel G.W. Verhaak, PhD[b],*

KEYWORDS

- Diffuse gliomas • Astrocytoma • Oligodendroglioma • IDH mutations
- 1p/19q codeletion

KEY POINTS

- Diffuse gliomas that are both IDH-mutant and 1p/19q-codeleted are classified as oligo-dendroglioma, whereas tumors lacking codeletion of these chromosome arms are classified as astrocytoma and are further separated based on IDH-status.
- Diffuse midline glioma, H3 K27M-mutant, was added in the WHO 2016 classification as a separate entity. These highly aggressive, diffuse infiltrative generally occur in children and are located in the midline of the CNS (brainstem, thalamus, cerebellum, and spinal cord).
- GBMs are classified into expression subtypes characteried by activation of distinct transcriptional pathways: "a mesenchymal" subtype enriched in angiogenesis and inflammatory genes, a "classical" subtype enriched in stem cell and cell cycle genes, and a "proneural" subtype enriched in neurodevelopmental genes. Recent data suggest that the previously defined "neural" subtype is not a glioma-intrinsic subtype and may reflect contamination from nontumor tissue.
- GBMs can also be classified by methylation subtypes: IDH (which carry *IDH1* mutations, display G-CIMP, and have a more favorable prognosis), RTK I (which frequently harbor *PDGFRA* amplification), mesenchymal (methylation profiles most similar to normal brain tissue despite substantial copy number changes and enriched for the mesenchymal gene expression cluster), and RTK II (characterized by high frequency of chromosome 7 gain and chromosome 10 loss).

This work was supported by grants from the National Institutes of Health R01 CA190121 and P30CA034196, the National Brain Tumor Society Oligo Research Fund, American Cancer Society PF-17-141-01-DMC and DefeatGBM Initiative, and grant 11026 from the Dutch Cancer Society KWF.
[a] Department of Pathology, VU University Medical Center, Brain Tumor Center Amsterdam, De Boelelaan 1117, Amsterdam 1081 HV, The Netherlands; [b] The Jackson Laboratory for Genomic Medicine, 10 Discovery Drive, Farmington, CT 06032, USA; [c] Department of Pathology, Princess Máxima Center for Pediatric Oncology and University Medical Center Utrecht, Lundlaan 6, 3584 EA Utrecht, The Netherlands
* Corresponding authors. The Jackson Laboratory for Genomic Medicine, 10 Discovery Drive, Farmington, CT 06032, USA.
E-mail addresses: p.wesseling@vumc.nl (P.W.); roel.verhaak@jax.org (R.G.W.V.)

Neurol Clin 36 (2018) 421–437
https://doi.org/10.1016/j.ncl.2018.04.002
neurologic.theclinics.com

EVOLUTION OF THE WORLD HEALTH ORGANIZATION CLASSIFICATION OF TUMORS OF THE CENTRAL NERVOUS SYSTEM

Gliomas are tumors of the central nervous system (CNS) whose neoplastic cells microscopically resemble nontumorous glial cells. Gliomas account for most tumors originating in the brain parenchyma.[1] The term "glioma" was introduced by the German pathologist Virchow[2] in the 1850s (**Fig. 1**), and in 1925 Bailey and Cushing[3] introduced the term glioblastoma multiforme (GBM) to describe a high-grade malignant glioma showing a wide range of histologic features (hence multiforme).

Later, (neuro) pathologists Ringertz, Scherer, Broders, and Kernohan provided important next building blocks for systematic histopathologic classification of gliomas.[4–8] Especially among adults, most of these tumors are diffuse gliomas, characterized by growth of tumor cells over long distances in the surrounding brain parenchyma (diffuse infiltrative growth). Traditionally, these diffuse gliomas were classified according to their microscopic similarities with (precursors of) glial cells and then designated as astrocytomas, oligodendrogliomas, or mixed diffuse glioma/oligoastrocytoma. Additionally, a malignancy grade (ranging from low-grade to high-grade) was assigned to these gliomas based on the presence or absence of particular histologic features.

Even after publication of the first edition of the World Health Organization (WHO) classification of tumors of the CNS in 1979, different schemes for typing and grading of diffuse gliomas were used in parallel.[9] However, the second edition of the WHO classification (published in 1993) was much more universally accepted as the standard for glioma classification.[10,11] For grading of astrocytomas, this latter classification incorporated elements of the St. Anne-Mayo grading approach in which absence or presence of mitotic activity, microvascular proliferation, and necrosis were used to assign a malignancy grade.[12]

The third and fourth editions of the WHO classification of CNS tumors (published 2000 and 2007) were built on essentially the same approach of histopathology-based diagnosis of diffuse gliomas, in some situations supported by the use of immunohistochemical markers.[13–17] However, despite being the time-honored diagnostic gold standard, it was increasingly clear that histopathologic classification of diffuse gliomas suffers from considerable interobserver and intraobserver variability, even among expert neuropathologists, and that the use of molecular markers had great potential to substantially improve the unequivocal discrimination of clinically relevant diffuse glioma subgroups.[18–23]

In the 1990s, the discovery that gliomas with a combined deletion of chromosome arms 1p and 19q (1p/19q codeletion) were associated with significantly improved survival and increased sensitivity to procarbazine-lomustine (CCNU)-vincristine (PCV) chemotherapy paved the way for molecular neuropathology of CNS tumors.[24–28] Typically, 1p/19q-codeleted tumors showed oligodendroglial histology, but the codeletion was reported to occur across different types and grades of diffuse gliomas with its favorable prognostic and predictive impact.[25] Of note, the apparent chemosensitivity of oligodendrogliomas was previously reported in 1988, years before a connection was made to 1p/19q codeletion in 1998.[29] The fact that 1p/19q-codeleted tumors responded well to PCV treatment led to introduction of 1p/19q-testing in clinical practice before this molecular marker became a part of the WHO diagnostic criteria for a subset of diffuse gliomas.[28]

Another finding with a major impact on the molecular neuropathology of diffuse gliomas is mutations of the isocitrate dehydrogenase 1 (*IDH1*) gene and the related *IDH2* gene.[30–32] IDH-mutant and IDH-wildtype astrocytomas are clinically different tumors despite overlapping histologic appearances. IDH mutations were first reported in

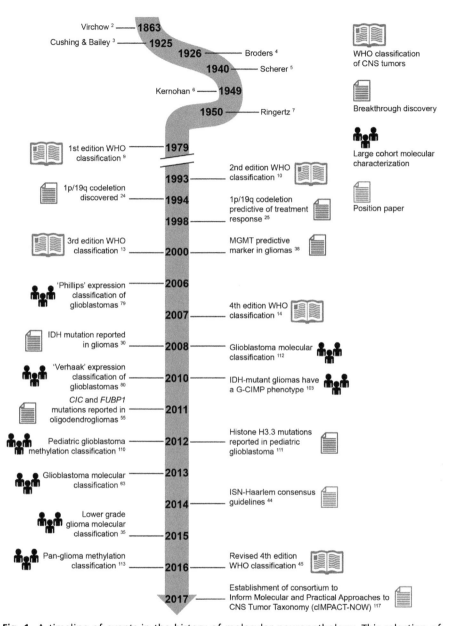

Fig. 1. A timeline of events in the history of molecular neuropathology. This selection of events is categorized into breakthrough discoveries, large cohort molecular characterizations, position papers, and different editions of the WHO classification of CNS tumors. ISN, International Society of Neuropathology; WHO, World Health Organization.

GBM and later discovered to be much more prevalent among lower grade (WHO grade II and III) gliomas.[31] IDH mutations contribute to gliomagenesis by activating alternative transcriptional programs via the genome-wide disruption of DNA methylation.[33] It has been proposed that this stochastic process is subject to careful selection to prioritize epigenetic changes that promote tumorigenesis.[34] Using modern genomic sequencing technologies, several groups independently reported that histologically similar gliomas could be subdivided into distinct tumor entities based on mutations in IDH and the 1p/19q codeletion, providing further fuel to the notion that a reclassification of these tumors is needed.[35–37]

Although the methylation status of the DNA repair enzyme O(6)-methylguanine-DNA methyltransferase (MGMT) does not distinguish between particular molecular subtypes of glioma, it is an important predictive biomarker. As was first reported in 2000, epigenetic silencing of the MGMT gene by methylation of the promoter seems to compromise conventional DNA repair mechanisms and thereby increases sensitivity to conventional chemotherapy using alkylating agents, such as temozolomide.[38–41] Especially in elderly patients with GBM lacking MGMT promoter methylation (ie, MGMT unmethylated), the benefit of temozolomide treatment often does not seem to outweigh the negative side effects.[42,43]

Because of increasing insights into the diagnostic potential of molecular markers in glial and other CNS tumors, a meeting was organized in Haarlem, Netherlands, in 2014 under the sponsorship of the International Society of Neuropathology to focus on how molecular information could be optimally incorporated into a next WHO classification. The paper that resulted from this meeting provided the basis for the design of an integrated histomolecular classification of especially glial and embryonal CNS tumors as represented in the 2016 revised fourth edition of the WHO classification.[44–46] Indeed, state-of-the-art diagnosis of diffuse gliomas now requires assessment of presence or absence of IDH mutation and 1p/19q codeletion. Meanwhile, a "Not Otherwise Specified" category was created for cases were information on these defining molecular features is lacking (eg, because molecular testing was not available, not informative, or not performed).

GLIOMA SUBCLASSIFICATION BASED ON MOLECULAR FEATURES

With the addition of molecular features to the 2016 WHO classification scheme, IDH mutation and 1p/19q codeletion status have become glioma subtype-defining features. Diffuse gliomas that are both IDH-mutant and 1p/19q-codeleted are classified as oligodendroglioma, whereas tumors lacking codeletion of these chromosome arms are classified as astrocytoma and are further separated based on IDH-status (**Fig. 2**). Because of this, the ambivalent oligoastrocytoma diagnosis is expected to largely disappear in favor of distinct molecularly defined subtypes, barring rare cases that contain a mixture of glioma cells carrying the codeletion with oligodendroglial appearance and astrocytic cells with retained 1p/19q.[47] In addition to subtype-defining molecular changes, gliomas are characterized by somatic mutations or copy number changes in several genes from various pathways, substantiating the hypothesis that the subtypes follow different gliomagenic trajectories and represent different biologies.

On average, IDH-mutant astrocytomas and GBMs are diagnosed at a median age of 38 years and demonstrate a median survival after diagnosis of 75 months overall, although this largely varies across WHO grades. IDH-mutant astrocytomas show frequent loss-of-function mutations or deletions in the Tumor Protein 53 (TP53) and Alpha Thalassemia/Mental Retardation Syndrome X-Linked (ATRX) genes. TP53 is well known as the "guardian of the genome" or "cellular gatekeeper" and functions to prevent cancer growth by activating a cascade leading to cell cycle arrest, senescence, and apoptosis.[48–50] Inactivation of the ATP-dependent helicase ATRX has been linked to recombination-driven alternative telomere maintenance mechanisms

Molecular category		IDH-wildtype	IDH-mutant & 1p/19q-non-codeleted	IDH-mutant & 1p/19q-codeleted
Histological type and WHO grade	Grade II	Diffuse astrocytoma	Diffuse astrocytoma	Oligodendroglioma
	Grade III	Anaplastic astrocytoma	Anaplastic astrocytoma	Anaplastic oligodendroglioma
	Grade IV	Glioblastoma	Glioblastoma	
Additional molecular features	Cell Cycle	*CDKN2A/B* 60% *TP53* 23% *CDK4* 15% *MDM4* 12% *RB1* 9% *MDM2* 8%	*TP53* 90% *CCND2* 9% *CDKN2A/B* 8%	
	RTK/PI3K	*EGFR* 54% *PTEN* 28% *PDGFRA* 13% *NF1* 13% *PIK3CA* 11% *PIK3R1* 7%		*PIK3CA* 12% *PIK3R1* 5%
	TMM	TPM 78%	*ATRX* 75%	TPM 98%
	Other			*CIC* 46% *FUBP1* 27% *NOTCH1* 14% *NIPBL* 7%

Oncogene
Tumor suppressor

Fig. 2. Groups of diffuse gliomas in adults classified according to IDH mutation and 1p/19q codeletion status demonstrate a distinct landscape of molecular features. Involved gene pathways (Cell Cycle, RTK/PI3K) are indicated in the second column. Genes in *orange* indicate genes preferentially targeted by gain-of-function (eg, hotspot) mutational events or amplification events. Genes marked in *blue* indicate genes commonly affected by loss-of-function mutation (eg, frameshift) or deletion events. Only features with frequencies greater than 5% are shown. Frequencies were derived from a recent publication.[113] PI3K, phosphoinositide-3 kinase; RTK, receptor tyrosine kinase; TMM, telomere maintenance mechanism; TPM, *TERT* promoter mutation.

and may provide glioma cells with unlimited proliferative capacity.[51–53] This molecular information may be helpful for diagnosing astrocytomas, even when molecular testing is not possible. For instance, a diffuse glioma that on immunohistochemical analysis lacks staining of tumor cell nuclei for ATRX and shows extensive and strong p53 staining of these nuclei (most likely representing the presence of respectively deactivating *ATRX* and *TP53* mutation) is highly indicative for an IDH-mutant, 1p/19q-noncodeleted astrocytoma. Obviously, acknowledging that about 90% of IDH-mutant diffuse gliomas carry the *IDH1* R132H mutation, immunohistochemistry for the IDH1 R132 mutant protein is a more direct way to test the IDH status of these tumors.[54]

With a median survival time of 116 months, IDH-mutant and 1p/19q-codeleted oligodendrogliomas demonstrate the highest survival rate among diffuse gliomas. With a median age at diagnosis of 46 years, patients with these tumors are generally older compared with those with IDH-mutant astrocytomas. IDH-mutant, 1p/19q-codeleted oligodendrogliomas commonly contain point mutations in 1p gene Capicua Transcriptional Repressor (*CIC*) and 19q gene Far Upstream Element Binding Protein 1 (*FUBP1*). Nearly 100% of gliomas in this category harbor mutations in the Telomerase Reverse Transcriptase (*TERT*) promoter. The mechanism for *CIC* and *FUBP1* mutations remains unknown, although *FUBP1* mutant tumors are associated with poorer outcomes.[37,55,56] *TERT* promoter mutations result in telomere maintenance and replicative immortality by constitutively activating the transcription of the enzymatic component of telomerase.[57–59]

In adults, IDH-wildtype diffuse gliomas are more frequently diagnosed in older patients (median age at diagnosis, 59 years) and show the least favorable prognosis with a median survival of 14.0 months. These IDH-wildtype tumors demonstrate higher mutational load than both IDH-mutant tumor types. Common events include *TERT* promoter mutations, loss-of-function mutations or deletions in phosphoinositide 3-kinase (PI3K) genes, phosphatase and tensin homolog (*PTEN*), and cell cycle regulator cyclin dependent kinase Inhibitor 2A (*CDKN2A*), and gain-of-function mutations and/or amplifications in receptor tyrosine kinases (RTKs) epidermal growth factor receptor (*EGFR*) and platelet-derived growth factor receptor alpha (*PDGFRA*). Deletions or loss-of-function mutations of the tumor suppressor *PTEN* are thought to promote tumorigenesis by antagonizing the suppression of RTKs including *EGFR* and *PDGFRA*.[60–62] Amplifications or gain-of-function mutations of the latter genes promote tumorigenesis by stimulating cellular proliferation through increased growth factor signaling.[63–66] Deletions of *CDKN2A* make tumor cells insensitive to growth-inhibitory signals and allow cells to bypass cellular senescence.[67–69]

TRANSCRIPTOME PROFILING AND INTRATUMORAL HETEROGENEITY

Tumor subtyping is a field that is of interest to clinicians and scientists alike because it has enabled the discovery of novel tumor entities that are biologically and clinically distinct. With the advent of array-based gene expression profiling in the late 1990s, many clinician-scientists were quick to use these methods across their in-house datasets. Expression subtyping was one of the earliest techniques that rapidly gained traction in the community. Microarray technologies, such as the AffyMetrix (Santa Clara, CA) U133 genechip, were at the forefront of the field and allowed one to simultaneously query the expression of thousands of genes in any given sample. The formation of large scientist-run and government-supported consortia, such as the Cancer Genome Atlas (TCGA), facilitated researchers from around the world to collaborate, share their data, and work with large and costly datasets otherwise outside the reach of single laboratories.

Using supervised statistical learning approaches in the early 2000s, several groups demonstrated that gene expression microarray analysis of glioma samples can reproduce histologic classification at high accuracy.[70–72] Moreover, they found that supervised statistical learning approaches were often better able to distinguish poor versus favorable outcome groups compared with conventional histopathology.[73,74] Studying the origin of genes associated with distinct clinical phenotypes, it was found that progression from low-grade to high-grade was associated with upregulation of cell cycle genes and that treatment resistance was associated with a self-renewal signature.[75,76]

Despite frequent difficulties in histologic classification, tumor samples from different broad histologic categories may demonstrate distinct transcriptional profiles.[77,78]

Building on this work researchers set out to use unsupervised learning approaches, where instead of trying to fit the molecular data to conform to a known histologic classification, they used techniques, such as principal component analysis and hierarchical clustering, to group samples independent of prior information and instead based on how similar they are to one another. Using these techniques, between 2006 and 2010, several groups were able to identify expression subtypes characterized by the activation of distinct transcriptional pathways, such as a "mesenchymal" subtype enriched in angiogenesis and inflammatory genes, a "classical" subtype enriched in stem cell and cell cycle genes, a "proneural" subtype enriched in neurodevelopmental genes, and a "neural" subtype enriched in adult neural markers.[79,80] Importantly, these groups driven by gene expression were found to be of independent prognostic importance beyond the existing histopathologic tumor groups, in part because of enrichment of the favorable outcome IDH-mutant GBM in the proneural group.

With the growing popularity of expression subtyping, tumor heterogeneity has become an increasingly important concern. Several multisector sequencing studies demonstrated that multiple samples from the same tumor can be classified according to different transcriptomic subtypes.[81–83] One study took multiple samples from a set of 10 tumors and found that in 60% of tumors multiple fragments from the same tumor were classified into at least two different expression subtypes.[81] A second study collected biopsies from the tumor core and tumor margin and reported that at the tumor margin samples generally classified as the neural subtype, whereas core samples were enriched in the three remaining subtypes.[82]

In a recent (2017) revision to the glioma subtypes, unsupervised learning was used to classify IDH-wildtype tumors after discarding a set of genes enriched in nontumor tissue and the previously described neural subtype was no longer detectable, suggesting this subtype was not a glioma-intrinsic subtype and reflected contamination from nontumor tissue.[84] Indeed, because of their diffuse infiltrative growth pattern, one can expect that diffuse gliomas contain a variable amount of contamination of nonneoplastic parenchymal cells.[85–87] In addition, data suggest that the mesenchymal subtype is a tumor-intrinsic phenotype and is further enriched by tumor-associated cells in the tumor microenvironment, such as immune cells and cellular components of the tumor microvasculature, some of which also contribute mesenchymal expression traits.[84] It has been shown that tumors can be highly immunogenic and recruit various immune effectors.[88–90] Similarly, it has been shown that tumor cells can activate angiogenic pathways and encourage vascular proliferation.[90–92] These studies underline the role of the microenvironment in gliomagenesis and its impact on determining transcriptional subtypes. Altogether, these studies highlight the importance of tumor heterogeneity in the transcriptional profiling in gliomas, and the need to take into account contributions from individual cell types (**Fig. 3**).

Transcriptomic studies from 2014 to 2017 have shown that individual cells from the same tumor may activate different transcriptional subtypes, highlighting heterogeneity at a single-cell level.[93–95] In a study using single-cell sequencing approaches to study oligodendrogliomas, researchers found cancer cells of oligodendroglial lineage, astrocytic lineage, and a limited population of neural stem cells to be present within the same tumor.[94] In a follow-up study, data suggested that more aggressive tumors can be characterized by a larger population of stem cells.[95] A recent study confirmed these findings using orthogonal approaches, identifying populations of slow-cycling stem-like cells, rapidly-cycling progenitor cells, and a large population of growth arrested cells in GBM xenograft models.[96] These studies reveal that in a

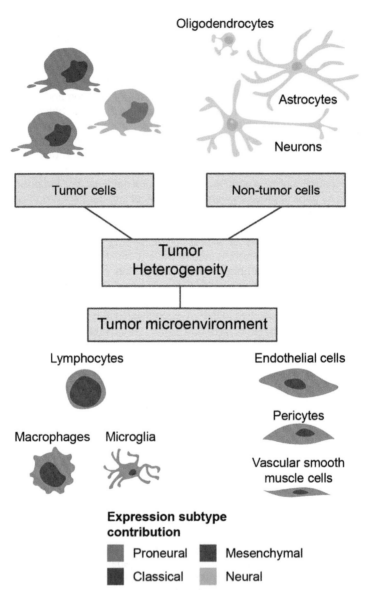

Fig. 3. Cell-type abundance is an important contributor to transcriptional subtypes. Tumor cells in diffuse gliomas can have a proneural, classical, or mesenchymal transcriptional profile. The now defunct neural subtype seemed to be the result of substantial admixture of nontumor cells in especially less cellular/more peripheral parts of diffuse gliomas. Cells from the tumor microenvironment including microvascular and immune cells contribute to the mesenchymal subtype.

bulk diffuse glioma sample, in addition to heterogeneity driven by the infiltration of immune and stromal cells and heterogeneity incurred from neighboring nonneoplastic brain tissue, there is considerable clonal heterogeneity within the population of cancer cells themselves with several distinct tumor clones at different stages of differentiation.

METHYLATION PROFILING AND THE IDENTIFICATION OF DNA METHYLATION-BASED SUBGROUPS

DNA methylation profiling has emerged as another method capable of distinguishing gliomas by tumor type and provides complementary molecular information to transcriptional profiles. DNA methylation refers to the covalent addition of a methyl group to the fifth position carbon of a cytosine nucleotide resulting in 5-methylcytosine. This epigenetic modification occurs primarily in the context of nucleotide-pairs in which cytosine is followed by guanine (ie, CpG dinucleotides) and is a critical regulator of gene expression.[97] Importantly, altered DNA methylation is a frequent event across cancers, including glioma.[98] Early studies of DNA methylation and glioma biology in the 1990s primarily focused on the methylation of single candidate genes, such as *MGMT*.[38–40] In the early 2000s, studies extended the search for candidate genes differentially methylated across histologically distinct glioma subtypes using real-time polymerase chain reaction methods, and reported that glioma tumor types demonstrated differential methylation patterns.[99,100] Cohort-level studies of glioma DNA methylation were transformed in the late 2000s by the introduction of methylation microarrays, such as the Illumina (San Diego, CA) GoldenGate cancer panel assaying 1505 CpG sites and the Illumina 27K array investigating roughly 27,000 CpGs sites.[101] These research tools enabled a more agnostic and expanded approach to studying disrupted genome-wide DNA methylation patterns. In an early analysis of methylation microarray data, a supervised clustering approach of 87 GBMs was the first study to reveal extensive glioma DNA methylation heterogeneity with some tumors exhibiting high levels of methylation, whereas others predominantly display low levels of methylation.[102] Genome-wide assessment of 272 GBMs in the TCGA dataset later identified that a subset of GBMs harbor a distinctive Glioma CpG Island Methylator Phenotype (G-CIMP), which reflected genome-wide patterns of hypermethylation.[103] The authors also discovered that the occurrence of G-CIMP was tightly associated with *IDH1* mutations and the proneural expression subtype, and that those patients with G-CIMP-positive tumors without *IDH1* mutations had a younger age at diagnosis.[103] In this same study, a small number of primary-recurrent IDH-mutant GBM pairs (n = 8) all retained their G-CIMP classification highlighting the stability of the phenotype.[103] The presence of a homogeneous G-CIMP DNA methylation profile across both IDH-mutant GBMs and lower grade gliomas was subsequently validated in a separate cohort.[104] These seminal contributions led to mechanistic follow-up studies, eventually establishing that *IDH1* mutations directly lead to genome-wide hypermethylation via the production of the oncometabolite 2-hydroxyglutarate and its inhibitory effect on the DNA demethylating enzyme ten-eleven translocation methylcytosine dioxygenase 1 (*TET1*).[105–108]

Glioma methylation subtypes display characteristic genetic features that are indicative of distinct biologic entities. In 2012, Sturm and colleagues[109] applied the more comprehensive Illumina 450K microarray to 151 GBMs and integrated these profiles with an expanded catalog of genetic alterations.[110] The authors then leveraged an unsupervised statistical learning method to cluster DNA methylomes based on the most variable methylation sites across the genome.[110] The resulting adult GBM classification revealed four methylation clusters: (1) IDH, (2) RTK I, (3) mesenchymal, and (4) RTK II. Diffuse gliomas in children and adolescents clustered in different categories that are enriched in mutations in the H3 Histone Family Member 3A (*H3F3A*) gene.[111] These methylation-based clusters were so named because of their association with the previously described GBM driver events.[112] For example, tumors in the IDH cluster carried *IDH1* mutations, displayed G-CIMP, and had a more favorable prognosis; RTK I tumors significantly more often harbored *PDGFRA* amplification; mesenchymal tumors had methylation profiles most similar to normal brain tissue despite substantial copy number changes and were enriched for the mesenchymal gene expression cluster; and RTK II tumors were characterized by high frequency of chromosome 7 gain and chromosome 10 loss.[110] Meanwhile, a few GBM catagories added on the basis of methyl. In 2016, the ultimate TCGA pan-glioma analysis analyzed 932 glioma samples (516 lower grade/WHO grade II and III gliomas and 129 GBMs with methylation data) to better define biologically distinct glioma subgroups.[113] Using the TCGA data (Illumina microarrays), our group selected 1300 tumor-specific methylated CpGs to define six clusters across gliomas, which we referred to as LGm1-6. LGm1-3 tumors were primarily *IDH1* or *IDH2* mutant tumors (99% of the tumors in these clusters combined) and were heavily enriched for low-grade gliomas (93% of tumors in these clusters). This largest glioma methylation study to date permitted the further subdivision of the IDH group identified in Sturm and colleagues into a 1p/19q codeleted cluster with elevated methylation (LGm3), a G-CIMP-high IDH-mutant noncodeleted cluster (LGm2), and a newly identified G-CIMP-low cluster with reduced methylation leading to gene expression changes and genetic aberrations in cell-cycle genes (LGm1). Patients with G-CIMP-low tumors demonstrated poorer overall survival when compared with the other IDH-mutant subgroups. The remaining DNA methylation clusters represented IDH-wildtype tumors. For example, LGm4 was described as "classic-like" similar to the Sturm RTK II classification, LGm5 was "mesenchymal-like" similar to the Sturm RTK I classification, and LGm6 was a subtype sharing epigenomic and genomic features with pilocytic astrocytoma despite a histologic diagnosis of diffuse glioma. The lower grade gliomas of LGm6 had near euploid copy number profiles and low frequency of typically observed GBM alterations (eg, *EGFR*, *CDKN2A*, and *PTEN*). Thus, the low-grade gliomas in LGm6 were referred to as pilocytic astrocytoma–like, whereas the GBM in this group were best described as LGm6-GBM. Finally, the study demonstrated that DNA methylation subtypes provided prognostic value independent of age and WHO grade that was assigned to these tumors.[113] Following this report, a retrospective central nervous system (CNS) tumor cohort (n = 2,801, Heidelberg cohort), including adult and pediatric gliomas, was profiled using microarray-based DNA methylation measurements (Capper et al. *Nature* 2018, PMID 29539639). The large dataset of 76 histopathological entities enabled the authors to classify diverse CNS tumor samples based on similar DNA methylation profiles. Their machine learning classification method revealed that a majority of CNS tumors have a DNA methylation profile that maps directly to established WHO entities, but strikingly that there also existed WHO entities that could be further subdivided based on DNA methylation as well as some potentially novel CNS tumor entities. The application of the Heidelberg classifier demonstrated a strong association with the previously defined TCGA classes LGm1-6 when applied to that same cohort.

DNA methylation profiles of longitudinally collected samples support epigenetic reprogramming as a driver of glioma recurrence.[113–116] In 2015, using 450K array data and multisector sampling, researchers demonstrated that IDH-mutant tumors tend to have homogeneous subtypes within a given tumor.[116] Yet, when examined over time the methylation profiles showed concerted changes as hypomethylation events led to an increase in the expression of cell cycle genes. In brain tumors where there was no observed loss of methylation at cell cycle genes these tumors displayed genetic alterations in these pathways suggesting the convergence of these disparate mechanisms on aberrant cell cycle activation.[116] It was recently estimated that between 10% and 40% of G-CIMP-high tumors recur with a G-CIMP-low phenotype, indicating that the G-CIMP-high to -low transition may be a marker of progression.[113,114] An improvement in sample number and genomic coverage of CpG sites was achieved in a 2017 study that measured 112 IDH-wildtype and 13 IDH-mutant primary-recurrent tumor pairs with reduced representation bisulfite sequencing (RRBS).[115] Use of a high coverage sequencing approach, such as RRBS, allowed for a between three- and five-fold increase in coverage for most samples under study. Similar to previous studies of primary-recurrent glioma samples, the authors discovered that relative hypomethylation was a striking feature at recurrence, and specifically that demethylation of Wnt signaling gene promoters was associated with worse prognosis.[115] Gliomas have been shown to display high levels of heterogeneity with subpopulations harboring distinct genetic and epigenetic alterations.[83,116] The authors applied the single-allele methylation resolution of the RRBS technology to quantify the epigenetic heterogeneity of each tumor sample and found extensive epigenetic heterogeneity across individual tumors.

SUMMARY

The integration of molecular features with neuropathologic assessment has yielded invaluable insights into the underpinnings of diffuse gliomas. Past studies have helped to identify glioma-initiating events, revealed potentially targetable oncogenic proteins, defined co-occurrences of molecular alterations in specific tumor subgroups, demonstrated that epigenetic inactivation of genes is predictive of therapeutic response, and that there exists a dynamic molecular landscape in glioma progression. The resulting molecular evidence has enabled the further refinement of tumor subgroups that would have previously been indiscernible using histopathologic assessment alone.

The ability to separate tumors based on molecular alterations possesses clear clinical relevance. The unsupervised learning approaches applied to sequencing data do not suffer from the interobserver variability that can hinder adequate recognition of histologically defined diagnostic entities. Indeed, diagnostic entities that were once histologically ambiguous can now often be accurately classified into molecular subgroups that display different clinical behavior. Tumor classification improvements can be made even to well-understood diagnostic entities, such as IDH-mutant tumors. For example, combining multiple molecular data, such as mutations and DNA methylation, further parsed IDH-mutant tumors into subgroups with unique clinical and molecular characteristics. As sequencing costs drop and more tumors are comprehensively profiled, the sensitivity to detect new molecular subtypes increases. In response to the rapid changes to tumor classifications the Consortium to Inform Molecular and Practical Approaches to CNS Tumor Taxonomy (cIMPACT-NOW) has been launched to evaluate the value of molecular markers for CNS tumor classification with greater frequency than allowed by the current WHO timeline.[117] In parallel, efforts using DNA methylation profiling to characterize tumors, such as the online platform for next-generation neuropathology (MolecularNeuropathology.org), are at the forefront of innovation in molecular neuropathology.

Future advancement in glioma classification will require additional research to more fully understand the contribution of diverse molecular alterations that may exist within different regions of a tumor mass. In this regard, recent results from multisector, longitudinal, and single-cell experiments are challenging the notion that a tumor is represented by single molecular subtype. These studies have made it clear that a given tumor often encompasses multiple molecular subtypes over space and time. Thus, it is likely that future clinically relevant biomarkers will need to provide information on not only the classification of the tumor as a whole, but also on the proportions of molecularly different single tumor cell types within a glioma. Thus, additional high-resolution modeling of (including extrachromosomal) genetic, transcriptomic, and epigenetic intratumoral heterogeneity is needed to facilitate the development of yet more precise biomarkers.[118] The further characterization of diffuse gliomas in space and time will serve to improve therapeutic results in individual patients through a more comprehensive understanding of their unique disease.

ACKNOWLEDGMENTS

The authors thank members of the Verhaak laboratory for insightful discussion and valuable input. The authors thank Zoë Reifsnyder of the Jackson Laboratory creative team for artwork.

REFERENCES

1. Ostrom QT, Gittleman H, Fulop J, et al. CBTRUS statistical report: primary brain and central nervous system tumors diagnosed in the United States in 2008-2012. Neuro Oncol 2015;17(Suppl 4):iv1–62.
2. Virchow R. Die krankhaften Geschwülste. Dreissig Vorlesungen, gehalten während des Wintersemesters 1862-1863 an Der Universität Zu Berlin. Berlin: A. Hirschwald; 1863.
3. Bailey P, Cushing H. Microchemical color reactions as an aid to the identification and classification of brain tumors. Proc Natl Acad Sci U S A 1925;11(1):82–4.
4. Broders AC. Carcinoma: grading the malignancy of carcinoma, grading and practical application. Arch Pathol Lab Med 1926;2:376.
5. Scherer HJ. A critical review: the pathology of cerebral gliomas. J Neurol Psychiatry 1940;3(2):147–77.
6. Kernohan JW, Mabon RF, et al. A simplified classification of the gliomas. Proc Staff Meet Mayo Clin 1949;24(3):71–5.
7. Ringertz N. Grading of gliomas. Acta Pathol Microbiol Scand 1950;27(1):51–64.
8. Louis DN, von Deimling A. Grading of diffuse astrocytic gliomas: Broders, Kernohan, Zülch, the WHO… and Shakespeare. Acta Neuropathol 2017; 134(4):517–20.
9. Zülch K. Histologic typing of tumours of the central nervous system. Geneva (Switzerland): World Health Organization; 1979.
10. Kleihues P, Burger P, Scheithauer B. Histological typing of tumours of the central nervous system. World Health Organization international histological classification of tumours. 2nd edition. Berlin: Springer Verlag; 1993.
11. Kleihues P, Burger PC, Scheithauer BW. The new WHO classification of brain tumours. Brain Pathol 1993;3(3):255–68.
12. Daumas-Duport C, Scheithauer B, O'Fallon J, et al. Grading of astrocytomas. A simple and reproducible method. Cancer 1988;62(10):2152–65.
13. Kleihues P, Cavenee W. World Health Organisation classification of tumours: pathology and genetics of tumours of the nervous system. Lyon (France): IARC Press; 2000.
14. Louis DN, Ohgaki H, Wiestler OD, et al. WHO classification of tumours of the central nervous system. Lyon (France): IARC Press; 2007.
15. Kleihues P, Sobin LH. World Health Organization classification of tumors. Cancer 2000;88(12):2887.
16. Louis DN, Ohgaki H, Wiestler OD, et al. The 2007 WHO classification of tumours of the central nervous system. Acta Neuropathol 2007;114(2):97–109.
17. Scheithauer BW. Development of the WHO classification of tumors of the central nervous system: a historical perspective. Brain Pathol 2009;19(4):551–64.
18. van den Bent MJ. Interobserver variation of the histopathological diagnosis in clinical trials on glioma: a clinician's perspective. Acta Neuropathol 2010; 120(3):297–304.

19. Coons SW, Johnson PC, Scheithauer BW, et al. Improving diagnostic accuracy and interobserver concordance in the classification and grading of primary gliomas. Cancer 1997;79(7):1381–93.

20. Aldape K, Simmons ML, Davis RL, et al. Discrepancies in diagnoses of neuroepithelial neoplasms: the San Francisco Bay Area Adult Glioma Study. Cancer 2000;88(10):2342–9.

21. Kros JM, Troost D, van Eden CG, et al. Oligodendroglioma. A comparison of two grading systems. Cancer 1988;61(11):2251–9.

22. Kros JM, Gorlia T, Kouwenhoven MC, et al. Panel review of anaplastic oligodendroglioma from European Organization for Research and Treatment of Cancer Trial 26951: assessment of consensus in diagnosis, influence of 1p/19q loss, and correlations with outcome. J Neuropathol Exp Neurol 2007;66(6):545–51.

23. Kros JM. Grading of gliomas: the road from eminence to evidence. J Neuropathol Exp Neurol 2011;70(2):101–9.

24. Reifenberger J, Reifenberger G, Liu L, et al. Molecular genetic analysis of oligodendroglial tumors shows preferential allelic deletions on 19q and 1p. Am J Pathol 1994;145(5):1175–90.

25. Cairncross JG, Ueki K, Zlatescu MC, et al. Specific genetic predictors of chemotherapeutic response and survival in patients with anaplastic oligodendrogliomas. J Natl Cancer Inst 1998;90(19):1473–9.

26. Kraus JA, Koopmann J, Kaskel P, et al. Shared allelic losses on chromosomes 1p and 19q suggest a common origin of oligodendroglioma and oligoastrocytoma. J Neuropathol Exp Neurol 1995;54(1):91–5.

27. von Deimling A, Louis DN, von Ammon K, et al. Evidence for a tumor suppressor gene on chromosome 19q associated with human astrocytomas, oligodendrogliomas, and mixed gliomas. Cancer Res 1992;52(15):4277–9.

28. Cairncross G, Wang M, Shaw E, et al. Phase III trial of chemoradiotherapy for anaplastic oligodendroglioma: long-term results of RTOG 9402. J Clin Oncol 2013;31(3):337–43.

29. Cairncross JG, Macdonald DR. Successful chemotherapy for recurrent malignant oligodendroglioma. Ann Neurol 1988;23(4):360–4.

30. Parsons DW, Jones S, Zhang X, et al. An integrated genomic analysis of human glioblastoma multiforme. Science 2008;321(5897):1807–12.

31. Watanabe T, Nobusawa S, Kleihues P, et al. IDH1 mutations are early events in the development of astrocytomas and oligodendrogliomas. Am J Pathol 2009; 174(4):1149–53.

32. Yan H, Parsons DW, Jin G, et al. IDH1 and IDH2 mutations in gliomas. N Engl J Med 2009;360(8):765–73.

33. Flavahan WA, Drier Y, Liau BB, et al. Insulator dysfunction and oncogene activation in IDH mutant gliomas. Nature 2016;529(7584):110–4.

34. Flavahan WA, Gaskell E, Bernstein BE. Epigenetic plasticity and the hallmarks of cancer. Science 2017;357(6348):eaal2380.

35. Cancer Genome Atlas Research Network, Brat DJ, Verhaak RGW, et al. Comprehensive, integrative genomic analysis of diffuse lower-grade gliomas. N Engl J Med 2015;372(26):2481–98.

36. Eckel-Passow JE, Lachance DH, Molinaro AM, et al. Glioma groups based on 1p/19q, IDH, and TERT promoter mutations in tumors. N Engl J Med 2015; 372(26):2499–508.

37. Jiao Y, Killela PJ, Reitman ZJ, et al. Frequent ATRX, CIC, FUBP1 and IDH1 mutations refine the classification of malignant gliomas. Oncotarget 2012;3(7):709–22.

38. Esteller M, Garcia-Foncillas J, Andion E, et al. Inactivation of the DNA-repair gene MGMT and the clinical response of gliomas to alkylating agents. N Engl J Med 2000;343(19):1350–4.

39. Esteller M, Hamilton SR, Burger PC, et al. Inactivation of the DNA repair gene O6-methylguanine-DNA methyltransferase by promoter hypermethylation is a common event in primary human neoplasia. Cancer Res 1999;59(4):793–7.

40. Costello JF, Futscher BW, Tano K, et al. Graded methylation in the promoter and body of the O6-methylguanine DNA methyltransferase (MGMT) gene correlates with MGMT expression in human glioma cells. J Biol Chem 1994;269(25):17228–37.

41. Hegi ME, Diserens A-C, Gorlia T, et al. MGMT gene silencing and benefit from temozolomide in glioblastoma. N Engl J Med 2005;352(10):997–1003.

42. Wick W, Platten M, Meisner C, et al. Temozolomide chemotherapy alone versus radiotherapy alone for malignant astrocytoma in the elderly: the NOA-08 randomised, phase 3 trial. Lancet Oncol 2012;13(7):707–15.

43. Wick W, Weller M, van den Bent M, et al. MGMT testing-the challenges for biomarker-based glioma treatment. Nat Rev Neurol 2014;10(7):372–85.

44. Louis DN, Perry A, Burger P, et al. International Society of Neuropathology–Haarlem consensus guidelines for nervous system tumor classification and grading. Brain Pathol 2014;24(5):429–35.

45. Louis DN, Ohgaki H, Wiestler OD, et al. WHO classification of tumours of the central nervous system. Lyon (France): IARC Press; 2016.

46. Louis DN, Perry A, Reifenberger G, et al. The 2016 World Health Organization classification of tumors of the central nervous system: a summary. Acta Neuropathol 2016;131(6):803–20.

47. Barresi V, Lionti S, Valori L, et al. Dual-genotype diffuse low-grade glioma: is it really time to abandon oligoastrocytoma as a distinct entity? J Neuropathol Exp Neurol 2017;76(5):342–6.

48. Harris SL, Levine AJ. The p53 pathway: positive and negative feedback loops. Oncogene 2005;24(17):2899–908.

49. Lane DP. Cancer. p53, guardian of the genome. Nature 1992;358(6381):15–6.

50. Levine AJ. p53, the cellular gatekeeper for growth and division. Cell 1997;88(3):323–31.

51. Barthel FP, Wei W, Tang M, et al. Systematic analysis of telomere length and somatic alterations in 31 cancer types. Nat Genet 2017;49(3):349–57.

52. Clynes D, Jelinska C, Xella B, et al. Suppression of the alternative lengthening of telomere pathway by the chromatin remodelling factor ATRX. Nat Commun 2015;6:7538.

53. Heaphy CM, de Wilde RF, Jiao Y, et al. Altered telomeres in tumors with ATRX and DAXX mutations. Science 2011;333(6041):425.

54. Reuss DE, Sahm F, Schrimpf D, et al. ATRX and IDH1-R132H immunohistochemistry with subsequent copy number analysis and IDH sequencing as a basis for an "integrated" diagnostic approach for adult astrocytoma, oligodendroglioma and glioblastoma. Acta Neuropathol 2015;129(1):133–46.

55. Bettegowda C, Agrawal N, Jiao Y, et al. Mutations in CIC and FUBP1 contribute to human oligodendroglioma. Science 2011;333(6048):1453–5.

56. Hu X, Martinez-Ledesma E, Zheng S, et al. Multigene signature for predicting prognosis of patients with 1p19q co-deletion diffuse glioma. Neuro Oncol 2017;19(6):786–95.

57. Chiba K, Lorbeer FK, Shain AH, et al. Mutations in the promoter of the telomerase gene TERT contribute to tumorigenesis by a two-step mechanism. Science 2017;357(6358):1416–20.

58. Bell RJA, Rube HT, Kreig A, et al. The transcription factor GABP selectively binds and activates the mutant TERT promoter in cancer. Science 2015; 348(6238):1036–9.
59. Killela PJ, Reitman ZJ, Jiao Y, et al. TERT promoter mutations occur frequently in gliomas and a subset of tumors derived from cells with low rates of self-renewal. Proc Natl Acad Sci U S A 2013;110(15):6021–6.
60. Li J, Yen C, Liaw D, et al. PTEN, a putative protein tyrosine phosphatase gene mutated in human brain, breast, and prostate cancer. Science 1997; 275(5308):1943–7.
61. Steck PA, Pershouse MA, Jasser SA, et al. Identification of a candidate tumour suppressor gene, MMAC1, at chromosome 10q23.3 that is mutated in multiple advanced cancers. Nat Genet 1997;15(4):356–62.
62. Pennisi E. New tumor suppressor found–twice. Science 1997;275(5308):1876–8.
63. Brennan CW, Verhaak RG, McKenna A, et al. The somatic genomic landscape of glioblastoma. Cell 2013;155(2):462–77.
64. Nishikawa R, Ji XD, Harmon RC, et al. A mutant epidermal growth factor receptor common in human glioma confers enhanced tumorigenicity. Proc Natl Acad Sci U S A 1994;91(16):7727–31.
65. Cohen S. The stimulation of epidermal proliferation by a specific protein (EGF). Dev Biol 1965;12(3):394–407.
66. Andrae J, Gallini R, Betsholtz C. Role of platelet-derived growth factors in physiology and medicine. Genes Dev 2008;22(10):1276–312.
67. Uhrbom L, Dai C, Celestino JC, et al. Ink4a-Arf loss cooperates with KRas activation in astrocytes and neural progenitors to generate glioblastomas of various morphologies depending on activated Akt. Cancer Res 2002;62(19):5551–8.
68. Uhrbom L, Nister M, Westermark B. Induction of senescence in human malignant glioma cells by p16INK4A. Oncogene 1997;15(5):505–14.
69. Campisi J, d'Adda di Fagagna F. Cellular senescence: when bad things happen to good cells. Nat Rev Mol Cell Biol 2007;8(9):729–40.
70. Rickman DS, Bobek MP, Misek DE, et al. Distinctive molecular profiles of high-grade and low-grade gliomas based on oligonucleotide microarray analysis. Cancer Res 2001;61(18):6885–91.
71. Godard S, Getz G, Delorenzi M, et al. Classification of human astrocytic gliomas on the basis of gene expression: a correlated group of genes with angiogenic activity emerges as a strong predictor of subtypes. Cancer Res 2003;63(20):6613–25.
72. van den Boom J, Wolter M, Kuick R, et al. Characterization of gene expression profiles associated with glioma progression using oligonucleotide-based microarray analysis and real-time reverse transcription-polymerase chain reaction. Am J Pathol 2003;163(3):1033–43.
73. Nutt CL, Mani DR, Betensky RA, et al. Gene expression-based classification of malignant gliomas correlates better with survival than histological classification. Cancer Res 2003;63(7):1602–7.
74. Freije WA, Castro-Vargas FE, Fang Z, et al. Gene expression profiling of gliomas strongly predicts survival. Cancer Res 2004;64(18):6503–10.
75. Tso CL, Freije WA, Day A, et al. Distinct transcription profiles of primary and secondary glioblastoma subgroups. Cancer Res 2006;66(1):159–67.
76. Murat A, Migliavacca E, Gorlia T, et al. Stem cell-related "self-renewal" signature and high epidermal growth factor receptor expression associated with resistance to concomitant chemoradiotherapy in glioblastoma. J Clin Oncol 2008; 26(18):3015–24.

77. Shai R, Shi T, Kremen TJ, et al. Gene expression profiling identifies molecular subtypes of gliomas. Oncogene 2003;22(31):4918–23.

78. Liang Y, Diehn M, Watson N, et al. Gene expression profiling reveals molecularly and clinically distinct subtypes of glioblastoma multiforme. Proc Natl Acad Sci U S A 2005;102(16):5814–9.

79. Phillips HS, Kharbanda S, Chen R, et al. Molecular subclasses of high-grade glioma predict prognosis, delineate a pattern of disease progression, and resemble stages in neurogenesis. Cancer Cell 2006;9(3):157–73.

80. Verhaak RG, Hoadley KA, Purdom E, et al. Integrated genomic analysis identifies clinically relevant subtypes of glioblastoma characterized by abnormalities in PDGFRA, IDH1, EGFR, and NF1. Cancer Cell 2010;17(1):98–110.

81. Sottoriva A, Spiteri I, Piccirillo SG, et al. Intratumor heterogeneity in human glioblastoma reflects cancer evolutionary dynamics. Proc Natl Acad Sci U S A 2013; 110(10):4009–14.

82. Gill BJ, Pisapia DJ, Malone HR, et al. MRI-localized biopsies reveal subtype-specific differences in molecular and cellular composition at the margins of glioblastoma. Proc Natl Acad Sci U S A 2014;111(34):12550–5.

83. Kim H, Zheng S, Amini SS, et al. Whole-genome and multisector exome sequencing of primary and post-treatment glioblastoma reveals patterns of tumor evolution. Genome Res 2015;25(3):316–27.

84. Wang Q, Hu B, Hu X, et al. Tumor evolution of glioma-intrinsic gene expression subtypes associates with immunological changes in the microenvironment. Cancer Cell 2017;32(1):42–56.e6.

85. Van Loo P, Campbell PJ. Absolute cancer genomics. Nat Biotechnol 2012;30(7): 620–1.

86. Carter SL, Cibulskis K, Helman E, et al. Absolute quantification of somatic DNA alterations in human cancer. Nat Biotechnol 2012;30(5):413–21.

87. Aran D, Sirota M, Butte AJ. Systematic pan-cancer analysis of tumour purity. Nat Commun 2015;6:8971.

88. Fridman WH, Pages F, Sautes-Fridman C, et al. The immune contexture in human tumours: impact on clinical outcome. Nat Rev Cancer 2012;12(4):298–306.

89. Yoshihara K, Shahmoradgoli M, Martinez E, et al. Inferring tumour purity and stromal and immune cell admixture from expression data. Nat Commun 2013;4:2612.

90. Charles NA, Holland EC, Gilbertson R, et al. The brain tumor microenvironment. Glia 2011;59(8):1169–80.

91. Shweiki D, Itin A, Soffer D, et al. Vascular endothelial growth factor induced by hypoxia may mediate hypoxia-initiated angiogenesis. Nature 1992;359(6398):843–5.

92. Jain RK, di Tomaso E, Duda DG, et al. Angiogenesis in brain tumours. Nat Rev Neurosci 2007;8(8):610–22.

93. Patel AP, Tirosh I, Trombetta JJ, et al. Single-cell RNA-seq highlights intratumoral heterogeneity in primary glioblastoma. Science 2014;344(6190):1396–401.

94. Tirosh I, Venteicher AS, Hebert C, et al. Single-cell RNA-seq supports a developmental hierarchy in human oligodendroglioma. Nature 2016;539(7628):309–13.

95. Venteicher AS, Tirosh I, Hebert C, et al. Decoupling genetics, lineages, and microenvironment in IDH-mutant gliomas by single-cell RNA-seq. Science 2017;355(6332) [pii:eaai8478].

96. Lan X, Jorg DJ, Cavalli FMG, et al. Fate mapping of human glioblastoma reveals an invariant stem cell hierarchy. Nature 2017;549(7671):227–32.

97. Deaton AM, Bird A. CpG islands and the regulation of transcription. Genes Dev 2011;25(10):1010–22.

98. Jones PA, Baylin SB. The epigenomics of cancer. Cell 2007;128(4):683–92.

99. Stone AR, Bobo W, Brat DJ, et al. Aberrant methylation and down-regulation of TMS1/ASC in human glioblastoma. Am J Pathol 2004;165(4):1151–61.
100. Uhlmann K, Rohde K, Zeller C, et al. Distinct methylation profiles of glioma subtypes. Int J Cancer 2003;106(1):52–9.
101. Bibikova M, Le J, Barnes B, et al. Genome-wide DNA methylation profiling using Infinium(R) assay. Epigenomics 2009;1(1):177–200.
102. Martinez R, Martin-Subero JI, Rohde V, et al. A microarray-based DNA methylation study of glioblastoma multiforme. Epigenetics 2009;4(4):255–64.
103. Noushmehr H, Weisenberger DJ, Diefes K, et al. Identification of a CpG island methylator phenotype that defines a distinct subgroup of glioma. Cancer Cell 2010;17(5):510–22.
104. Christensen BC, Smith AA, Zheng S, et al. DNA methylation, isocitrate dehydrogenase mutation, and survival in glioma. J Natl Cancer Inst 2011;103(2):143–53.
105. Xu W, Yang H, Liu Y, et al. Oncometabolite 2-hydroxyglutarate is a competitive inhibitor of alpha-ketoglutarate-dependent dioxygenases. Cancer Cell 2011; 19(1):17–30.
106. Lu C, Ward PS, Kapoor GS, et al. IDH mutation impairs histone demethylation and results in a block to cell differentiation. Nature 2012;483(7390):474–8.
107. McCarthy N. Metabolism: unmasking an oncometabolite. Nat Rev Cancer 2012; 12(4):229.
108. Turcan S, Rohle D, Goenka A, et al. IDH1 mutation is sufficient to establish the glioma hypermethylator phenotype. Nature 2012;483(7390):479–83.
109. Sturm D, Witt H, Hovestadt V, et al. Hotspot mutations in H3F3A and IDH1 define distinct epigenetic and biological subgroups of glioblastoma. Cancer Cell 2012; 22(4):425–37.
110. Sandoval J, Heyn H, Moran S, et al. Validation of a DNA methylation microarray for 450,000 CpG sites in the human genome. Epigenetics 2011;6(6):692–702.
111. Schwartzentruber J, Korshunov A, Liu XY, et al. Driver mutations in histone H3.3 and chromatin remodelling genes in paediatric glioblastoma. Nature 2012; 482(7384):226–31.
112. The Cancer Genome Atlas Research Network. Comprehensive genomic characterization defines human glioblastoma genes and core pathways. Nature 2008; 455(7216):1061–8.
113. Ceccarelli M, Barthel FP, Malta TM, et al. Molecular profiling reveals biologically discrete subsets and pathways of progression in diffuse glioma. Cell 2016; 164(3):550–63.
114. de Souza CF, Sabedot TS, Malta TM, et al. Distinct epigenetic shift in a subset of Glioma CpG island methylator phenotype (G-CIMP) during tumor recurrence. bioRxiv 2017.
115. Klughammer J, Kiesel B, Roetzer T, et al. The DNA methylation landscape of glioblastoma disease progression shows extensive heterogeneity in time and space. bioRxiv 2017.
116. Mazor T, Pankov A, Johnson BE, et al. DNA methylation and somatic mutations converge on the cell cycle and define similar evolutionary histories in brain tumors. Cancer Cell 2015;28(3):307–17.
117. Louis DN, Aldape K, Brat DJ, et al. Announcing cIMPACT-NOW: the consortium to inform molecular and practical approaches to CNS tumor taxonomy. Acta Neuropathol 2017;133(1):1–3.
118. Smallwood SA, Lee HJ, Angermueller C, et al. Single-cell genome-wide bisulfite sequencing for assessing epigenetic heterogeneity. Nat Methods 2014;11(8): 817–20.

World Health Organization 2016 Classification of Central Nervous System Tumors

Phedias Diamandis, MD, PhD, Kenneth Aldape, MD*

KEYWORDS

- World Health Organization • Brain tumors • Neuropathology • Classification
- Molecular pathology

KEY POINTS

- The recent update of the World Health Organization (WHO) classification of tumors of the central nervous system represents a paradigm shift.
- Previous iterations of the classification relied solely on morphologic features for classification.
- In the 2016 update, for the first time, the definitions of specific neoplastic entities tumors are not exclusively subgrouped based on morphologic features but now include precise molecularly defined entities.
- This article discusses this paradigm shift, and focuses on the refinements in classification criteria, relations to previous editions, and their implication to neuropathology and neuro-oncology practice.
- The authors distinguish the criteria that were used to determine why molecular changes were included while other recent and important molecular discoveries were seemingly omitted from the classification system.
- The authors further discuss emerging and complementary efforts that aim to better harmonize the rapidly evolving genomic landscape of cancer with routine clinical practice.

INTRODUCTION

The classification of central nervous system (CNS) tumors represents a critical component of the epidemiologic, clinical, and basic-level understanding of a diverse array of neoplasms. The World Health Organization (WHO) has historically played a central role in providing guidance and a standardized set of pathologic criteria for consistent classification of these lesions at different international centers. Given their mission and widespread use, updates to these WHO guidelines require a

MacFeeters Hamilton Centre for Neuro-Oncology Research, Princess Margaret Cancer Centre, 101 College Street, 14–601, Toronto, Ontario M5G 1L7, Canada
* Corresponding author.
E-mail address: kaldape@gmail.com

Neurol Clin 36 (2018) 439–447
https://doi.org/10.1016/j.ncl.2018.04.003
0733-8619/18/© 2018 Elsevier Inc. All rights reserved.
neurologic.theclinics.com

prudent balance of integrating novel insights into brain tumor classification with criteria that are applicable to the international community at large. Historically, brain tumor classification was exclusively carried out based on histomorphologic features of tumors,[1] an approach compatible within the capabilities of most clinical centers throughout the world. Although emerging molecular tests could help provide support for particular diagnoses, it was thought that morphology alone was sufficient to accurately subgroup lesions into entities with common biological drivers and clinical outcomes. The maturing and evolving journey into the molecular era has, however, now dramatically improved the understanding of brain tumors since the previous morphology-centric 2007 WHO Classification of Tumors of the Central Nervous System (2007 CNS WHO). Advances in molecular understanding of brain tumors that have occurred since 2007 have driven the concept that incorporation of clinically relevant molecular markers can provide a biologic basis for classification, that, when integrated with morphologic features, may result in a classification that promotes increase accuracy and precision. As a result, the recent 2016 update of the WHO Classification of Tumors of the Central Nervous System (2016 CNS WHO) represents a revolutionary shift from previous iterations by having, for the first time, tumor classes defined not only by their histomorphologic features, but also by key diagnostic molecular parameters[2,3] (**Fig. 1**). The development of this update presented the unique challenge of embracing a growing number of molecular alterations while acknowledging the current limited accessibility and practicality of a purely molecularly driven classification system. Some of these key changes to the 2016 CNS WHO are summarized in **Table 1**[3] and allow for, where clinically applicable, incorporation of biologically based parameters into superior the classification CNS tumors.[4–7] An example of this can be seen in the emphasis, in the 2007 edition and earlier, in the primary distinction of astrocytic versus oligodendroglial tumors, on the basis of morphology. The current understanding now indicates a close biologic relationship of a subset of diffuse oligodendroglial and astrocytic tumors on the basis on IDH mutations, while other astrocytic tumors are biologically quite distinct.

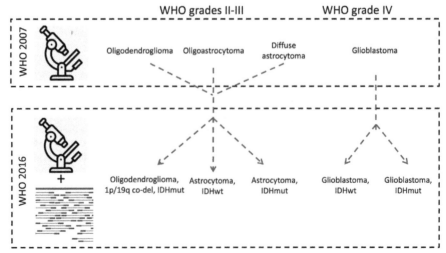

Fig. 1. The 2016 update of the WHO classification of tumors of the central nervous system represents a shift from previous iterations by adding key diagnostic molecular parameters to define tumor classes.

Table 1
Selected changes to the 2016 CNS WHO Classification Update

2007 CNS WHO	2016 CNS WHO
Diffuse Astrocytic and Oligodendroglial Tumors	Diffuse Astrocytic and Oligodendroglial Tumors
Diffuse astrocytoma	Diffuse astrocytoma, NOS Diffuse Astrocytoma, IDH-wildtype Diffuse Astrocytoma, IDH-mutant
Anaplastic astrocytoma	Anaplastic astrocytoma, NOS Anaplastic Astrocytoma, IDH-wildtype Anaplastic astrocytoma, IDH-mutant
Glioblastoma	Glioblastoma, NOS Glioblastoma, IDH-wildtype Glioblastoma, IDH-mutant Diffuse midline glioma, H3 K27M-mutant
Oligodendroglioma	Oligodendroglioma, NOS Oligodendroglioma, IDH-mutant 1p19q-codeleted
Anaplastic Oligodendroglioma	Anaplastic Oligodendroglioma, NOS Anaplastic Oligodendroglioma, IDH-mutant, 1p19q-codeleted
Oligoastrocytoma	Oligoastrocytoma, NOS
Anaplastic Oligoastrocytoma	Anaplastic Oligoastrocytoma, NOS
Ependymal Tumors	Ependymal Tumors
Subependymoma	Subependymoma
Myxopapillary Ependymoma	Myxopapillary Ependymoma
Ependymoma	Ependymoma Ependymoma, RELA fusion-positive
Anaplastic ependymoma	Anaplastic ependymoma
Embryonal tumors	Embryonal tumors
Medulloblastoma NOS	Medulloblastoma NOS
	Medulloblastoma, Genetically Defined Medulloblastoma, WNT-activated Medulloblastoma, SHH-activated and TP53-mutant Medulloblastoma, SHH-activated and TP53-wildtype Medulloblastoma, non-WNT/non-SHH
Medulloblastoma	Medulloblastoma, histologically defined
Medulloblastoma, classic	Medulloblastoma, classic
Medulloblastoma, desmoplastic/nodular	Medulloblastoma, desmoplastic/nodular
Medulloblastoma with extensive nodularity	Medulloblastoma with extensive nodularity
Medulloblastoma large cell anaplastic	Medulloblastoma large cell anaplastic
CNS primitive neuroectodermal tumor	Embryonal tumor with multilayered rosettes, NOS
Ependymoblastoma	Embryonal tumor with multilayered rosettes, C19MC-altered
Medulloepithelioma	Medulloepithelioma

A recent survey of the neuro-oncology community showed overall strong support for the update, although the reception of the changes has been somewhat mixed among different subspecialties.[8] Here are highlighted some of the major changes to the 2016 CNS WHO, and discussion of them in the context of diagnostic neuropathology, clinical management, and a refined brain tumor classification system. It is hoped that this discussion reinforces some of the decisions to which molecular changes were ultimately included in the updated 2016 CNS WHO. Also discussed are some of the practical difficulties needed to implement these and additional changes into their clinical practice (eg, workload, test availability, and timing). The authors further highlight emerging and complementary initiatives that try to harmonize the need for a widely adoptable brain tumor classification with the desire for more prompt and generous incorporation of the new and rapidly evolving molecular literature.

WORLD HEALTH ORGANIZATION CLASSIFICATION SYSTEM: PURPOSE AND RECENT CHANGES

To understand the motivation behind the changes to the 2016 CNS WHO, it is important to re-emphasize that the purpose of this initiative. The WHO classification system is not meant to summarize the complete body of information of each tumor type, but rather define biologically distinguishable groups that have substantially different clinical outcomes.

For example, among infiltrating adult gliomas, distinct neoplasms can now be distinguished by evaluating combinations of IDH mutations and 1p19q codeletions. In pediatric and adolescent forms, segregation of gliomas harboring H3 K27M mutations also reveal a subset with a substantially worse prognosis.[9,10] As such, these biologically, clinically, and molecularly distinct subgroups were incorporated into the updated classification scheme.

In addition to these groups, the 2016 CNS WHO expanded and codified a "not otherwise specified, NOS" category for cases in which the recommended molecular testing could not be completed (ie, because of test availability or sample quality). This group provides an important undefined or uncharacterized class where tumors lacking molecular information could be triaged. Not only is this group needed to foster participation of a larger number of centers without access to routine molecular testing, it also provides a practical solution to many challenging cases. For example, there are some pediatric tumors that, although they resemble oligodendrogliomas, do not harbor 1p19q-codeletions. Similarly, there are cases where available material is insufficient to initiate molecular testing. The NOS category provides a place for these cases that cannot be fully profiled with the recommended molecular analysis.

Similar reasoning motivated the persistence of the controversial oligoastrocytoma entity. Oligoastrocytoma is a morphologic class that has proven difficult to classify as it suffers from interobserver consistency and clinical heterogeneity.[11,12] These difficulties have now been molecularly resolved, as this group has been shown to be comprised of molecular alterations that correlate with either astrocytomas or oligodendrogliomas. No specific molecular alteration was found to correlate with histologically defined oligoastrocytoma, and such cases, for the most part, can now be resolved using on IDH and 1p19q molecular testing,[5,13,14] with only extremely rare cases showing a heterogenous tumor composition.[15,16] Although discouraged, this diagnosis of oligoastrocytomas can still be made in the absence of molecular information. To highlight this principle, this entity only exists as a NOS class, signifying the incomplete molecular information associated with this tumor group.

As an important feature of IDH mutation testing, note is made of the fact that although the most common mutation (R132H mutation in IDH1) is easily detected by immunohistochemistry, a negative immunohistochemistry stain with the R132H IDH1 antibody cannot rule out a noncanonical mutation. The corollary of this point is that for practical purposes, the diagnosis of astrocytoma, IDH-wildtype requires that the possibility of an IDH mutation (both canonical and noncanonical) be ruled out.

A consistent and similar approach was also used with the introduction of the molecular subclassification of medulloblastoma (eg, WNT-, SHH-activated, Group 3 and Group 4[17]), and ependymal (RELA fusion-positive[18,19]) tumors. Similar to gliomas, each subdivided class is meant to highlight a unique and clinically distinct group of tumors among a previously larger morphologic class. The inclusion of a NOS class allows centers without access to molecular testing to still use the histologic classification system while cautioning the molecular uncertainty of the lesion. This balance helps maintain consistency with previous editions while incorporating robust molecular changes with reproducible differences in biology.

The same rationale was also used to collapse and converge tumor entities that may show morphologic distinction, but common molecular underpinnings. For example, historically defined morphologic groups that have since proven to provide little clinical and biologic relevance (eg, protoplasmic vs fibrillary astrocytoma) have now been removed. Similarly, molecular information has allowed merging of certain tumor types that share specific molecular events and an apparent similar clinical course. For example, the morphologically distinct embryonal tumors with abundant neuropil and multilayer rosettes, ependymoblastomas, and medulloepitheliomas, all share a grim prognosis and show common C19MC amplifications. As such, they have now been grouped into a unified class referred to as embryonal tumors with multilayered rosettes, C19MC-altered. This update was emblematic of additional changes that were incorporated in pediatric brain tumors, including a shift in the conceptualization of embryonal tumors, such as primitive neuroectodermal tumor (PNET). The PNET concept lumped a variety of entities based on a similar morphologic appearance (primitive-appearing histology, often with a "small round blue cell" appearance). Molecular characterization has not shown a unifying signature that corresponds to this apparent histologic similarity, and it is increasingly recognized that many such small round blue cell tumors, upon molecular characterization, can fit into variants and patterns of other known entities.

IMPORTANT MOLECULAR CHANGES THAT DID NOT APPEAR IN THE 2016 CENTRAL NERVOUS SYSTEM WORLD HEALTH ORGANIZATION

There were many recent and seminal molecular insights of brain tumor biology that did not appear in the updated 2016 CNS WHO, for a variety of reasons. Issues related to molecular platform, extensive experience/validation of findings, and test availability were relevant to some of these decisions. BRAF and beta-catenin mutations found exclusively in the papillary and adamantinomatous forms of craniopharyngiomas, respectively, were not incorporated into the names of these entity like other molecular changes discussed previously (eg, IDH, H3K27M, 1p19q), perhaps because this finding was recent and has not been verified on a large number of cases. The important distinction here is that these mutations are uniformly present within their morphologic class and thus offer little for further subclassification of these brain tumor classes. Without this distinction, each and every molecular change would need to be appended with the morphologic name descriptor of each tumor. Such a requirement would serve a major hindrance to diagnostic neuropathology practice with little if any benefit to patient care. As such, knowledge of molecular information that does not refine classification beyond the capabilities of histomorphology, and thus essential for classification, are omitted. Although alternations such as NAB2-STAT6 fusions remains an important tool in the diagnostic work-up of solitary fibrous tumor/hemangiopericytoma therapies, this demonstration is not mandatory diagnosis of classic cases that fall along the solitary fibrous tumor/hemangiopericytoma (SFT/HPC) spectrum. The SFT/HPC spectrum also highlights the continued utility of morphologic examination. Although both these histologic variants share this similar genetic event, it is still recognized that these morphologic variants have differences in their risk of recurrence and metastatic potential despite their shared genetics.[3,20,21]

Similarly, biologically important changes that may predict response to chemotherapy (eg, MGMT promoter methylation and response to temozolomide), although extremely important, were not included in the WHO classification, because, unlike 1p19q-codeletion seen in oligodendrogliomas, MGMT methylation status does not define a distinct tumor class with substantially unique biology. Moreover, MGMT promoter methylation is heterogeneously found among different glioma subtypes (eg, found in both IDH-wildtype and IDH-mutant cases), suggesting that it is not a key biologic driver of a distinct disease. Its therapeutic relevance is currently tied to a specific agent and not in itself an independent predictor of the natural history of the disease.

INCREASED NEED FOR AN INTEGRATED MOLECULAR/HISTOMORPHOLOGIC CLASSIFICATION SYSTEM

Although resource limitations and the availability of emerging molecular technologies present challenges to some pathology departments, there is still a compelling reason to have an integrated classification scheme that incorporates both morphologic and genetic elements. Correlation with morphologic findings, rather than blind use of molecular information, provides extremely valuable information. It is clear that many alterations occur across distinct tumor entities (eg, IDH mutations are common in chondrosarcoma, cholangiocarcinoma, and acute myelogenous leukemia), and therefore the presence of an alteration such as IDH mutation needs to be placed in context with the clinical and histomorphologic findings of the specific case in question. Along similar lines, the authors recently reported a glioblastoma with a NAB2-STAT6 fusion, which is a pathognomonic hallmark of solitary fibrous tumors.[22] Histomorphology is by no means derivative or to be discarded; it is a useful tool that has served as the basis for classification for many decades. Rather than abandon histomorphology, new paradigms for brain tumor classification will aim to take such information and complement it with molecular data, where such data can increase precision and provide biologically relevant information. Similarly, tumor grading still provides valuable prognostic information based on microscopic features (eg, mitoses, necrosis, and microvascular proliferation) not fully captured by molecular studies. Until more routine genome-wide testing can differentiate these tumor types, morphology still adds significant value to the brain tumor classification scheme. At a more practical level, molecular testing is also a highly laborious process and in many cases results (eg, MGMT testing) can take many days to weeks to be completed. Morphologic features provide prompt information to help initiate early personalized care. Although technological improvement may improve turn-around times and cost,[23] it is likely that morphology will remain the primary driver leading classification in acute (eg, intra-operative) settings and when molecular testing is not feasible. Similarly, a unified classification scheme helps maintain the mission of the WHO of providing a consistent classification system that can be widely used across centers.

ADAPTING THE PRACTICALITIES OF INCORPORATING MOLECULAR INFORMATION

Tumor classification remains an important part of how tumors are clinically treated and studied. As such, dramatic revolutionary changes should follow only after a more conservative approach has allowed time and experience to guide smaller incremental evolutionary changes. It is important to stress that incorporation of any changes, especially ones requiring huge investment in new infrastructure, can be hard for many diagnostic departments. This may explain why neuropathologists are among the most conservative when it comes to nonactionable changes in brain tumor classification. For example, the authors' survey data indicated that, while 96% endorsed routine testing for 1p19q-codeletion, only 67% thought IDH mutation status was an important addition. These changes likely reflect the increased workload, cost, and infrastructure need to carry out IDH1/2-mutational analysis and the current lack of changes to management for mutated cases. It is also important to be aware of practical limitations for prompt updates.

Another practical issue that occurs in an era of histologic-molecular integration is the timing and reporting of results. A typical workflow in an anatomic pathology department that relied on routine histology and immunohistochemistry for diagnosis allowed for reporting in a matter of days. The WHO 2016 guidelines can, depending on specific testing method and tumor type, depend on methodologies that typically require additional turnaround time. For example, mutation detection, changes in chromosomal copy number, and fusion detection in many centers require additional time for assay performance and reporting, which may extend the turnaround time for compete integrated diagnosis. Practical solutions to this issue can incorporate a process of an interim or preliminary diagnosis, issued promptly following histologic/immunohistochemical interpretation, followed by a complete integrated diagnosis after completion of molecular testing. For example, at their center, the authors might issue an initial report of diffuse glioma, or diffuse glioma with oligodendroglial features, with indication of additional results/final report to follow. Once additional data are received, a final report is issued with the WHO 2016 diagnosis (eg, oligodendroglioma, IDH-mutant and 1p/19q codeleted). In this workflow, a balance is attempted to report information in a timely manner while also ensuring completeness and molecular integration.

In an era of increased molecular profiling and new technologies to enable discovery, it may not be surprising that medical oncologists are among the most keen to embrace any relevant molecular information, regardless of its relevance to classification. To meet these demands, new initiatives are emerging to provide more immediate guidance in this fast-paced molecular era. Specifically, an initiative known as cIMPACT-NOW (Consortium to Inform Molecular and Practical Approaches to CNS Tumor Taxonomy) aims to promptly consider and publish consensus recommendations to allow additional molecular discoveries to reach clinical practice and patients before they reach future iterations of the WHO updates.[2,24,25]

SUMMARY

The recent update to the 2016 CNS WHO classification scheme represents an aggregate effort of over 100 participants from 20 countries[3] and was meant to provide much needed objective, rather than subjective readouts for brain tumor classification. At large, the community has found these change a positive step toward these goals. The added classes now more faithfully recapitulate the biologically distinct groups and thus provide refined information to clinicians and researchers alike. As more centers continue to expand their molecular capabilities, it is likely that additional, perhaps superfluous molecular data will be included. For the reasons mentioned, certain diagnostically useful designations such as NOS will continue to persist. In addition to remaining inclusive, these categories allow for cases with nontraditional genetics to find refuge within the classification system. Furthermore, as molecular technologies continue to evolve, it will be a challenge to ensure appropriate and uniform implementation of criteria to define key alterations. On the 1 hand, there is a need for consistency over time of diagnostic criteria, as well as the need to ensure that changes in the classification be thoroughly validated before implementation. On the other hand, molecular advances in the understanding of CNS tumors is occurring at an increasingly rapid pace, and clearly some of this new information will conceivably be clinically relevant diagnostically useful. A balance is required that considers these and other issues as changes and updates in diagnostic criteria are considered. These issues highlight the compromises necessary to result in a practical and forward-looking classification of tumors of the CNS.

REFERENCES

1. Louis DN, Ohgaki H, Wiestler OD, et al. The 2007 WHO classification of tumours of the central nervous system. Acta Neuropathol 2007;114:97–109.
2. Louis DN, Perry A, Burger P, et al. International Society Of Neuropathology–Haarlem consensus guidelines for nervous system tumor classification and grading. Brain Pathol 2014;24:429–35.
3. Louis DN, Perry A, Reifenberger G, et al. The 2016 World Health Organization classification of tumors of the central nervous system: a summary. Acta Neuropathol 2016;131. https://doi.org/10.1007/s00401-016-1545-1.
4. Reuss DE, Sahm F, Schrimpf D, et al. ATRX and IDH1-R132H immunohistochemistry with subsequent copy number analysis and IDH sequencing as a basis for an "integrated" diagnostic approach for adult astrocytoma, oligodendroglioma and glioblastoma. Acta Neuropathol 2015;129:133–46.
5. Wiestler B, Capper D, Sill M, et al. Integrated DNA methylation and copy-number profiling identify three clinically and biologically relevant groups of anaplastic glioma. Acta Neuropathol 2014;128:561–71.
6. Pajtler KW, Witt H, Sill M, et al. Molecular classification of ependymal tumors across all CNS compartments, histopathological grades, and age groups. Cancer Cell 2015;27:728–43.
7. Labussiere M, Boisselier B, Mokhtari K, et al. Combined analysis of TERT, EGFR, and IDH status defines distinct prognostic glioblastoma classes. Neurology 2014; 83:1200–6.
8. Aldape K, Nejad R, Louis DN, et al. Integrating molecular markers into the World Health Organization classification of CNS tumors: a survey of the neuro-oncology community. Neuro Oncol 2016;19:now181.
9. Wu G, Broniscer A, McEachron TA, et al. Somatic histone H3 alterations in pediatric diffuse intrinsic pontine gliomas and non-brainstem glioblastomas. Nat Genet 2012;44:251–3.
10. Khuong-Quang D-A, Buczkowicz P, Rakopoulos P, et al. K27M mutation in histone H3.3 defines clinically and biologically distinct subgroups of pediatric diffuse intrinsic pontine gliomas. Acta Neuropathol 2012;124:439–47.
11. Giannini C, Scheithauer BW, Weaver AL, et al. Oligodendrogliomas: reproducibility and prognostic value of histologic diagnosis and grading. J Neuropathol Exp Neurol 2001;60:248–62. Available at: http://www.ncbi.nlm.nih.gov/pubmed/11245209. Accessed July 27, 2017.
12. van den Bent MJ. Interobserver variation of the histopathological diagnosis in clinical trials on glioma: a clinician's perspective. Acta Neuropathol 2010;120:297–304.

13. Cancer Genome Atlas Research Network, Brat DJ, Verhaak RGW, Aldape KD, et al. Comprehensive, integrative genomic analysis of diffuse lower-grade gliomas. N Engl J Med 2015;372:2481–98.
14. Sahm F, Reuss D, Koelsche C, et al. Farewell to oligoastrocytoma: in situ molecular genetics favor classification as either oligodendroglioma or astrocytoma. Acta Neuropathol 2014;128:551–9.
15. Huse JT, Diamond EL, Wang L, et al. Mixed glioma with molecular features of composite oligodendroglioma and astrocytoma: a true "oligoastrocytoma"? Acta Neuropathol 2015;129:151–3.
16. Wilcox P, Li CCY, Lee M, et al. Oligoastrocytomas: throwing the baby out with the bathwater? Acta Neuropathol 2015;129:147–9.
17. Taylor MD, Northcott PA, Korshunov A, et al. Molecular subgroups of medulloblastoma: the current consensus. Acta Neuropathol 2012;123:465–72.
18. Parker M, Mohankumar KM, Punchihewa C, et al. C11orf95-RELA fusions drive oncogenic NF-κB signaling in ependymoma. Nature 2014;506:451–5.
19. Pietsch T, Wohlers I, Goschzik T, et al. Supratentorial ependymomas of childhood carry C11orf95-RELA fusions leading to pathological activation of the NF-κB signaling pathway. Acta Neuropathol 2014;127:609–11.
20. Robinson DR, Wu Y-M, Kalyana-Sundaram S, et al. Identification of recurrent NAB2-STAT6 gene fusions in solitary fibrous tumor by integrative sequencing. Nat Genet 2013;45:180–5.
21. Chmielecki J, Crago AM, Rosenberg M, et al. Whole-exome sequencing identifies a recurrent NAB2-STAT6 fusion in solitary fibrous tumors. Nat Genet 2013;45:131–2.
22. Diamandis P, Ferrer-Luna R, Huang RY, et al. Case report: next generation sequencing identifies a NAB2-STAT6 fusion in Glioblastoma. Diagn Pathol 2016;11:13.
23. Diamandis P, Aldape KD. Insights from molecular profiling of adult glioma. J Clin Oncol 2017;35:2386–93.
24. Louis DN, Aldape K, Brat DJ, et al. cIMPACT-NOW (the Consortium to Inform Molecular and Practical Approaches to CNS Tumor Taxonomy): a new initiative in advancing nervous system tumor classification. Brain Pathol 2017;27(6):851–2.
25. Louis DN, Aldape K, Brat DJ, et al. Announcing cIMPACT-NOW: the Consortium to Inform Molecular and Practical Approaches to CNS Tumor Taxonomy. Acta Neuropathol 2017;133:1–3.

Neurologic and Medical Management of Brain Tumors

Kester A. Phillips, MD[a], Camilo E. Fadul, MD[b], David Schiff, MD[c],*

KEYWORDS

- Bevacizumab • Brain tumor • Chemotherapy • Cognition • Corticosteroids
- Fatigue • Mood • Seizure

KEY POINTS

- Prophylactic anticonvulsants are not recommended for patients with seizure-naive brain tumor.
- Monotherapy with a nonenzyme-inducing anticonvulsant is the preferred initial treatment for patients with tumor-related epilepsy.
- Asymptomatic patients with brain tumors do not require corticosteroids.
- Low-molecular-weight heparins are safer and more effective than oral anticoagulants for the management of venous thromboembolism in patients with brain cancer.
- Bevacizumab has steroid-sparing properties that often permits steroid taper.

INTRODUCTION

The complexity of the care of patients with neuro-oncologic disorders demands a multidisciplinary approach, where the neurologist may play a major role. An understanding of the spectrum of neurologic and systemic complications associated with brain cancer and cancer therapy is essential for guiding appropriate treatment.[1] We review aspects of relevance to the neurologist regarding the supportive care of patients with brain tumors, with attention to the management of seizures, brain edema, venous thromboembolism (VTE), fatigue and mood alterations, cognitive dysfunction, as well as the deleterious effects of antitumor and supportive therapy.

Disclosure Statement: The authors report no relevant disclosures.
[a] Department of Neuroscience, Inova Health System, Inova Fairfax Hospital, 3300 Gallows Road, Falls Church, VA 22042, USA; [b] Division of Neuro-Oncology, University of Virginia Health System, 1300 Jefferson Park Avenue, West Complex, Room 6228, Charlottesville, VA 22903-0156, USA; [c] Division of Neuro-Oncology, University of Virginia Health System, 1300 Jefferson Park Avenue, West Complex, Room 6225, Charlottesville, VA 22903-0156, USA
* Corresponding author.
E-mail address: ds4jd@virginia.edu

Neurol Clin 36 (2018) 449–466
https://doi.org/10.1016/j.ncl.2018.04.004
0733-8619/18/© 2018 Elsevier Inc. All rights reserved.

SEIZURES

Epilepsy and its treatment is a frequent cause of morbidity in patients with intracranial neoplasm. Approximately 30% to 50% of patients with brain tumor present with seizures and 30% will become intractable.[2] The incidence will vary according to the type (**Table 1**) and location of the tumor. Focal seizures occur in about 60% of the cases with secondary generalization in 40%.[3] In the pediatric and young adult population, gangliogliomas and dysembryoplastic neuroepithelial tumors are more frequently associated with intractable epilepsy.[4,5] Seizures are a common manifestation of low-grade gliomas (LGG) because of their indolent growth rate and location,[6] with cortically located oligodendrogliomas carrying a higher risk than deep midline-located tumors.[7] Furthermore, in LGG, the accumulation of 2-hydroxyglutarate in isocitrate dehydrogenase 1–mutated tumors has been postulated as a driver of epileptogenesis.[8] Only about one-third of patients with brain metastases present with seizures, but when the primary is melanoma the incidence of seizures is approximately 67% possibly related to the cortical predilection, widespread distribution, and the tendency for hemorrhage.[6]

Oncologic treatment plays an important role in the management of tumor-related epilepsy. Antitumor therapies have a favorable impact on seizure control in patients with brain tumor. In LGG, complete resection predicts favorable seizure outcome.[6] Gross total resection is the most important factor for predicting seizure freedom; however, preoperative seizure control during antiepileptic drug (AED) administration as well as the duration of seizures of $\leq$ 1 year also confers favorable seizure control.[9] Conventional radiotherapy[10] and Gamma Knife radiosurgery[11] have a positive influence on seizure control. In addition, significant seizure reduction during chemotherapy in patients with LGG has been observed.[12,13] Furthermore, seizure response during antitumor therapy has been proposed as a metric in brain tumor trials.[14]

Use of Antiepileptic Drugs

AED administration after seizure secondary to brain tumor is the standard of care. In seizure-naive patients, however, prophylactic AEDs are not recommended. A meta-analysis did not justify prophylactic AED administration,[15] and this has been corroborated in more contemporary systematic reviews.[4,15–18] In neurosurgical practice, the goal of AED prophylaxis is to prevent acute postoperative seizures, but it remains unclear whether prolonged prophylactic AED therapy reduces seizure frequency after craniotomy. Several studies have failed to demonstrate efficacy of postoperative

Table 1 Estimated seizure frequency by tumor type	
Tumor Type	**Frequency**
Glioneuronal tumor[33]	80%–100%
Oligodendroglioma[33,124]	70%–90%
Diffuse low-grade glioma[33]	60%–85%
Anaplastic astrocytoma[124]	60%–70%
Glioblastoma[33,124]	40%–60%
Meningioma[6,124]	20%–50%
Metastasis[6,29]	20%–35%
Primary CNS lymphoma[125]	10%

Abbreviation: CNS, central nervous system.

AED prophylaxis.[19–23] Despite these results, many patients without seizures are still prescribed AEDs during the perioperative period.[24] In this situation, tapering and discontinuing AEDs after the first postoperative week is recommended.[15]

There are no prospective data to guide AED withdrawal in patients with tumor-related epilepsy. The risk of seizure relapse after AED withdrawal is of concern, but the medication side effects can negatively affect the quality of life of patients with brain tumor (see later discussion). AED withdrawal has been suggested for patients with glioma with good prognosis, stable disease, and long-term seizure freedom[14,25,26]; but a consensus on the duration of seizure freedom to justify AED withdrawal remains controversial. Consideration for AED withdrawal has been suggested for those LGG patients with stable disease who have achieved greater than 2 years of seizure freedom postoperatively or after treatment with radiation and chemotherapy.[25] Nevertheless, approximately 25% of the patients will experience a seizure, although usually related to tumor progression.

Side Effects and Drug Interactions

Patients with brain tumor may have increased susceptibility to adverse AED effects.[15] In patients with tumor-related epilepsy, a higher frequency of rash was associated with carbamazepine, phenobarbital, and phenytoin.[27] Patients undergoing cranial irradiation with concurrent carbamazepine and steroid taper are at risk for developing Stevens-Johnson syndrome and toxic epidermal necrolysis.[28] Levetiracetam use in patients with brain tumor has been associated with fatigue, irritability, and depression.[29] Other common AED side effects include sedation, dizziness, tremor, weight gain, myelosuppression, and hepatotoxicity. Lamotrigine, pregabalin, zonisamide, and lacosamide have demonstrated favorable toxicity profiles.[30–33]

Drug-drug interaction between AEDs and chemotherapeutic agents is a significant concern in neuro-oncology practice. The coadministration of CYP3A4 enzyme–inducing AEDs (phenytoin, phenobarbital, oxcarbazepine, and carbamazepine) and chemotherapeutic agents metabolized by the liver should be avoided because their clearance is accelerated by the AED resulting in lower concentrations of the chemotherapy. However, temozolomide has minimal hepatic clearance, but its coadministration with levetiracetam was an independent risk factor for hepatotoxicity.[34] Furthermore, phenytoin induces hepatic metabolism and significantly reduces the half-life and bioavailability of dexamethasone, the most frequent corticosteroid prescribed to manage brain tumor edema. Meanwhile, dexamethasone induces CYP3A4 enzyme and may reduce phenytoin concentrations requiring frequent serum monitoring in patients receiving concurrent dexamethasone.[35] Although topiramate is not usually cited as an enzyme-inducing AED, clinical studies have shown clinically relevant dose-dependent induction at daily doses of 200 mg and above.[36]

Selecting an Antiepileptic Drug

The AED is selected based on patient profile, seizure type, potential drug-drug interaction, comorbidities, potential side effects, and convenience. Monotherapy with a nonenzyme-inducing anticonvulsant is the preferred initial treatment for patients with tumor-related epilepsy. Levetiracetam is the most frequently prescribed AED because it has few drug-drug interactions, has a broad-spectrum profile, does not require serum monitoring, has both oral and intravenous formulations, is well tolerated by most patients, and has generic formulations. Other first-line considerations include valproic acid (VPA), lamotrigine, oxcarbazepine, and gabapentin. VPA gained interest as the AED of choice stemming from an observed survival benefit in patients with glioblastoma treated with VPA at the start of standard radiotherapy and temozolomide in a trial.[37] However, a pooled analysis of several key studies found no difference in progression-free survival (PFS) or overall survival (OS) in patients treated with VPA or levetiracetam.[38] A small study showed that lacosamide is well tolerated and effective as add-on therapy but larger randomized trials are needed.[39] Of the new AEDs, perampanel showed an objective seizure response in 75% of patients with glioma.[40] However, the safety and efficacy of third-generation AEDs (ezogabine, clobazam, perampanel, brivaracetam, eslicarbazepine, topiramate extended-release, and oxcarbazepine extended-release) in patients with brain tumor have not been verified in randomized controlled trials. Levetiracetam is recommended as initial therapy for patients with brain tumors and seizures.[41] About 50% of the patients will have to change the AED because of lack of seizure control and/or side effects.[3]

BRAIN EDEMA

Symptoms related to vasogenic brain edema frequently herald the presence of an intracranial neoplasm.[42,43] Edema is the result of several interrelated pathogenic mechanisms, including changes in the endothelial tight junctions, abnormalities in aquaporin-4, and secretion of vascular endothelial growth factor (VEGF) and leukotrienes.[42,43] Uncontrolled brain edema may have dire consequences including permanent neurologic impairment and death. Meanwhile, antiedema agents may also have untoward effects, and finding a balanced therapeutic ratio may be challenging.

Corticosteroid Use

Corticosteroids improve symptomatic brain tumor–related edema and, in the case of brain lymphoma, they are also oncolytic.[44] There are no guidelines for corticosteroid dose and schedule for brain tumors, but there is agreement that higher doses are associated with more adverse effects. In fact, in patients with glioblastoma, a study showed that dexamethasone use correlated with shorter survival.[45] Dexamethasone is preferred given its lack of mineralocorticoid activity and extended biological half-life (34–54 h), allowing for a once or twice daily dosing schedule.[46] A starting dose of 16 mg daily has been suggested, but a study showed equal efficacy of 4 mg and 16 mg dexamethasone for the treatment of symptomatic edema from brain metastases.[47] Patients typically achieve symptomatic relief within 24 to 72 hours. The duration of corticosteroid use is associated with the appearance of side effects; therefore, dexamethasone should be tapered once symptoms begin to improve. A slow stepwise decrease in the dose or dosing interval over a period of 2 to 4 weeks with longer periods for symptomatic patients is recommended.[48] Only about 20% of the patients with glioblastoma are able to discontinue steroids immediately after surgery.[49] Steroid taper during radiation is frequently associated with recrudescence of symptoms that require dose escalation. Asymptomatic patients with brain tumor do not require corticosteroids. Chronic high-dose steroids will suppress the hypothalamic-pituitary-adrenal axis function and may result in symptoms of adrenal insufficiency after abrupt withdrawal. If an early morning serum cortisol level is low, replacement is recommended with 20 mg of hydrocortisone in the morning and 10 mg in the afternoon.[50] The hydrocortisone can be slowly tapered on a weekly schedule and can be stopped according to the morning cortisol concentration.[51]

Corticosteroid Complications

Adverse effects of dexamethasone are more common with the prolonged use of high doses with any organ system potentially affected (**Table 2**). Although all side effects

Table 2
Neurologic and systemic complications of corticosteroids

Side Effects	Symptoms
Cushing syndrome	Weight gain
	Obesity
	Hypertension
	Hyperglycemia
	Fatigue
	Striae
	Easy bruising
Osteoporosis	Pain
	Fracture
Myopathy	Proximal muscle weakness/atrophy
Immunosuppression	Opportunistic infections
Psychiatric disorders	Psychosis
	Insomnia
	Mood disorders
Vision blurring	
Hiccups	

can be clinically significant, only those most relevant in neuro-oncology practice are described in this article.

Glucocorticoid-induced myopathy is common and disproportionately produces symmetric proximal lower extremity weakness. Patients typically present with weakness of the proximal lower extremities followed by atrophy that negatively affects activities of daily living and quality of life.[52] In severe cases, the myopathy may compromise respiratory function.[53] The frequency of clinically significant steroid-induced myopathy is about 10% in adults with brain tumors receiving more than 2 weeks of daily dexamethasone.[52] Serum muscle enzymes and electromyography are usually normal—the diagnosis is based on clinical features. Treatment involves tapering or discontinuing steroids along with rehabilitation.

Peptic ulcer disease (PUD) is a rare complication of corticosteroid therapy. A meta-analysis reported the development of PUD in 0.4% of patients treated with steroids.[54] In a study, gastrointestinal (GI) bleeding occurred in 1.9% and 3.5% of patients receiving 16 mg and 100 mg of dexamethasone, respectively.[55] GI prophylaxis using a proton pump inhibitor or H2 antagonist during high-dose corticosteroid treatment alone has not been proved to be effective. GI perforation is a less well-recognized complication of steroid therapy in neuro-oncology, being difficult to diagnose because the classic symptoms of peritonitis may be absent.[55] The perforation in these patients occurs more frequently in the rectosigmoid and is frequently associated with constipation. Therefore, aggressive treatment of constipation during high-dose corticosteroid administration is advised.

Chronic glucocorticoid therapy also predisposes patients to osteoporosis, leading to fractures of the spine and hip. In general, prophylactic calcium and vitamin D supplementation at standard doses are recommended for those patients receiving chronic steroid therapy.[56] Oral bisphosphonates can be considered, but there is an increased risk of PUD, especially in conjunction with corticosteroids. Osteonecrosis should be considered in patients with hip pain during chronic steroids use.[57] Dexamethasone-induced hiccup is a burdensome underrecognized symptom that usually responds to dose reduction or agents such as phenothiazines and baclofen.[58]

Furthermore, mood disorders (eg, emotional lability, depression, hypomania, mania, anxiety, and suicidality) are known side effects of corticosteroids but psychiatric or metabolic disorders should be ruled out. Occasionally, patients may require neuroleptics, lithium, or VPA. Tricyclic antidepressants are not recommended.

Other Drugs

The burden of corticosteroid-related side effects may be relieved by steroid-sparing agents. VEGF-A plays an essential role in the pathogenesis of tumor-related edema. An assessment of corticosteroid use in a study showed that most patients required reduced corticosteroid doses during treatment with the anti-VEGF agent, bevacizumab.[59] In clinical practice, bevacizumab administration (**Fig. 1**) often permits steroid

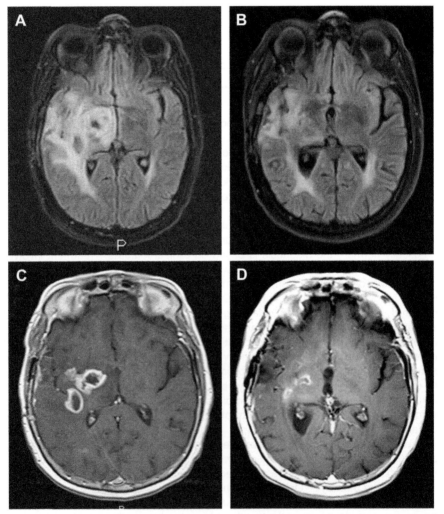

Fig. 1. Patient with glioblastoma. Axial FLAIR images before (*A*) and after bevacizumab (*B*). Axial T1 with contrast before (*C*) and after four doses of bevacizumab (*D*). FLAIR, fluid-attenuated inversion recovery.

taper in patients with glioma. Clinical trials illustrated the steroid-sparing effects of tyrosine kinase inhibitors targeting VEGF receptor 2, but these agents have not been repurposed. Corticorelin acetate,[60] angiotensin-II receptor blockers (ARBs),[61] celecoxib,[62] and boswellia[63] have been credited with antivasogenic edema property but await further evaluation.

VENOUS THROMBOEMBOLISM

Patients with brain tumor are at increased risk for VTE during and beyond the perioperative period. An estimated 3% to 20% of patients with high-grade glioma develop perioperative deep venous thrombosis (DVT) or pulmonary embolism (PE).[64] Leg paresis, age greater than 60 years, large tumor size, glioblastoma histology, and use of chemotherapy have been identified as risk factors for VTE.[65] The risk of VTE persists beyond the perioperative period, with about 24% of the patients with newly diagnosed glioma developing a VTE.[66] The median time between surgery and diagnosis of VTE is 14 weeks. The pathogenesis includes the production of procoagulants (eg, tissue factor, proinflammatory cytokines) by tumor cells, thereby activating the clotting cascade. A recent study reported isocitrate dehydrogenase 1 wild-type status as the most powerful predictive marker for VTE in patients with glioma possibly as a result of tissue factor expression[67]; however, this has not been validated by other studies. Antiangiogenic therapy, such as bevacizumab, is also associated with an increased risk for thrombosis and will be discussed later. In patients with glioma, there should be a low clinical threshold for requesting diagnostic studies to exclude VTE.

Anticoagulation is safe and effective in the treatment of VTE in patients with brain tumor despite the perceived risk for intracranial hemorrhage.[68] The standard of care for the management of cancer-related VTE is low-molecular-weight heparin (LMWH) for at least 6 months.[69,70] In general, a minimum duration of 3 to 6 months of anticoagulation is recommended for the treatment of VTE in patients with brain tumor.[68,71] LMWH is the preferred initial treatment, whereas unfractionated heparin is generally reserved for symptomatic PE, renal insufficiency, or patients at high risk for bleeding.[72] Fondaparinux has shown efficacy in preventing VTE; however, its use in patients with cancer is limited by its long half-life (17–21 h) and lack of an antidote.[73] Inferior vena cava (IVC) filter placement is an alternative to anticoagulation, but in patients with brain tumor its use was associated with a 12% incidence of recurrent PE along with a 57% incidence of postphlebitic syndrome, recurrent DVT, or IVC filter thrombosis.[74] Given the risk of procedure-associated morbidity, IVC filter is offered to those patients with VTE and contraindications to anticoagulation. Evidence supporting IVC filter use with concurrent anticoagulation is limited.[75] Lifelong anticoagulation with LMWH has been recommended for patients with cancer with documented VTE and risk factors for recurrence. LMWH, such as enoxaparin, dalteparin, or tinzaparin, with warfarin as a backup, are potential treatment options.[72] New oral anticoagulants, factor Xa inhibitors (eg, rivaroxaban, apixaban and edoxaban) and direct thrombin inhibitors (eg, dabigatran), have shown efficacy for the management of VTE in non–cancer patients. However, in the absence of data, an ongoing trial is expected to clarify the efficacy and safety of these agents for the prevention of recurrent cancer-associated VTE (NCT02744092).

Mechanical approaches to VTE prophylaxis during the immediate postoperative period include early ambulation, compression stockings, and intermittent external pneumatic compression devices. In neurosurgical patients, mechanical prophylaxis showed up to a 50% reduction in VTE compared with controls with pneumatic compression yielding the greatest effect.[76] Subcutaneous LMWH combined with compression stockings is more effective than compression stockings alone in postoperative VTE prevention without an increase in the risk of bleeding.[77,78]

ADVERSE EVENTS WITH VASCULAR ENDOTHELIAL GROWTH FACTOR/VEGFR TARGETING AGENTS

Bevacizumab targets VEGF-A and has demonstrated improved PFS but not OS in patients with primary or recurrent glioblastoma.[79,80] Bevacizumab therapy has shown promising results in the management of vestibular schwannoma and neurofibromatosis type 2,[81] meningioma,[82] ependymoma,[83] hemangioblastoma,[84] some metastatic central nervous system (CNS) tumors,[85–87] and symptomatic radiation necrosis.[88] Despite the improved patient outcome, bevacizumab administration is associated with deleterious side effects. Fatigue is the most common adverse event associated with anti-VEGF therapy. Fatigue of any grade was experienced in 45% of the patients with recurrent glioblastoma in the BRAIN study.[59] Grade ≥ 3 fatigue developed in 34% of patients in another study.[89] Hypertension is also common during bevacizumab therapy and occurs in about 39% of patients with glioblastoma during treatment.[89] Management paradigm includes the initiation of angiotensin-converting enzyme (ACE) inhibitors, ARBs, calcium channel blockers, or thiazide diuretics with the goal of maintaining blood pressure less than 140/90 mm Hg.[90] VEGF inhibition has been implicated in thrombotic microangiopathy of the glomerular microvasculature, leading to proteinuria. Proteinuria of any grade developed in 16% of patients with glioblastoma, with 5% developing grade ≥ 3 proteinuria.[89] Thus periodic monitoring of urinary protein is recommended. The administration of ACE inhibitors and ARBs has a demonstrable antiproteinuric effect. Bevacizumab-induced dysphonia is also common, but improvement can be achieved with the discontinuation of treatment.[91,92]

Less common and often severe adverse events associated with anti-VEGF/VEGFR (vascular endothelial growth factor receptor) therapy include increased risk for hypercoagulability,[93] hemorrhage,[94] ischemic stroke,[95] posterior reversible encephalopathy syndrome (PRES),[96] and gastrointestinal perforation.[97] The diagnosis of atherothromboembolism, intracranial hemorrhage, and PRES precludes further bevacizumab therapy, but treatment may be continued in VTE patients who are adequately anticoagulated. Bevacizumab is associated with wound-healing complications; therefore, a four-week minimum window is recommended between bevacizumab and surgery both before and following craniotomy. In patients with perforated bowel, medical management is the initial treatment of choice, but surgical intervention may be warranted in severe cases.

HEMATOLOGICAL TOXICITY FROM CHEMOTHERAPY

Chemotherapy-induced hematotoxicity is common during brain tumor therapy. Common chemotherapeutic offenders include lomustine, cisplatin, carboplatin, procarbazine, temozolomide, and cyclophosphamide. Methotrexate and cytarabine may cause myelosuppression. Profound anemia and neutropenia is rare with temozolomide but slightly more common with nitrosoureas. Temozolomide-induced thrombocytopenia is common and may warrant the discontinuation of chemotherapy and/or platelet administration. In a study, temozolomide was associated with grade 3 to 4 thrombocytopenia in 19% of patients with high-grade glioma.[98] As a rule, a complete hemogram with differential is routinely monitored during chemotherapy. In the face of abnormal laboratory values, the offending agent is held until counts recover. A platelet count of at least 100,000/mm^3 is the threshold for restarting temozolomide. Management guidelines for acute hematotoxicity, including decisions regarding the administration of blood products and colony-stimulating factors in patients with brain tumor, were adopted from medical oncology.

INFECTIONS

Immunosuppression predisposes patients with brain tumor to infection. Prolonged corticosteroid administration increases the risk for opportunistic infections such as *Pneumocystis jirovecii* pneumonia (PJP) warranting prophylactic antibiotics.[99] Generally, prophylaxis against PJP is initiated when the lymphocyte count is less than 500 cell/µl or a CD4+ cell count is less than 200 cells/µl and should continue until CD4+ and lymphocyte counts return to normal.[100] Reduced CD4+ cell and lymphocyte counts have been observed in patients with glioblastoma receiving chemoradiation or dose-dense temozolomide.[101–104] Therefore, some advocate the monitoring of CD4+ and lymphocyte counts during temozolomide administration to guide the decision of whether to discontinue PJP prophylaxis.[100] Trimethoprim/sulfamethoxazole (TMP/SMX) is the recommended first-line agent, but pentamidine inhalations, atovaquone, or dapsone are alternatives for those patients with contraindications to TMP/SMX. Oral candidiasis is common during brain tumor treatment; however, prophylactic antifungal is not justified.[105] Several temozolomide-related infections include herpes zoster, cytomegalovirus, aspergillus, Bordetella bronchiseptica, *Cryptococcus*, hepatitis B reactivation, and tuberculosis.[106] Ibrutinib monotherapy in patients with primary CNS lymphoma has been associated with aspergillosis.[107] Rituximab is associated with reactivation of hepatitis B virus and progressive multifocal leukoencephalopathy.[108] Hepatitis B virus screening is recommended before the initiation of immunosuppressive or chemotherapy.[109] Antiviral prophylaxis during chemotherapy administration is recommended for hepatitis B surface antigen carriers.[110] For patients with infections or symptoms suspicious for infection, a consultation by an infectious diseases specialist should be solicited.

FATIGUE

Fatigue is one of the most common and vexing symptoms afflicting patients with gliomas independent of tumor grade and oncologic treatment.[111] In this population, fatigue does not occur in isolation but is associated with other symptoms such as pain, depression, and sleep disturbances.[112] An analysis of published clinical trials revealed that there was no evidence of the effectiveness of any pharmacologic and nonpharmacologic interventions for the management of fatigue in patients with primary brain tumor.[113] Recommendations for the management of cancer-related fatigue and insomnia, in general, have been extrapolated to patients with brain tumors, but again the efficacy of these interventions in this patient population is unknown.[114] Evaluating secondary causes of fatigue, including medications, emotional distress, sleep disturbance, and anemia, may be helpful.

MOOD DISORDERS

Patients with brain tumor frequently experience mood disorders that affect the quality of life and survival. Approximately 20% of all patients with glioma developed major depressive disorder in the first 6 months after starting radiotherapy.[115] Depression was the most common postoperative complication after surgery for high-grade glioma, with a correlation between more extensive resection and less depression.[116] In a prospective study, depression was more frequent in brain tumor patients with anteriorly located tumors, and the depression level decreased after tumor resection.[117] Deregulation of the hypothalamic–pituitary–adrenal axis and changes in cytokine levels have been implicated in the pathogenesis.[118] There is discordance between physician-reported recognition of depression and patient-reported symptoms of depression; thus, depression is frequently underdiagnosed.[116] Furthermore, aggressive treatment of depression improved not only quality of life but also survival. Therefore, screening for depression and adequate treatment should be part of the comprehensive management of the patient diagnosed with glioma. The optimal treatment of depression in patients with brain tumor is unclear, but there is evidence for psychological (eg, cognitive behavioral therapy or interpersonal therapy) and pharmacologic approaches (eg, selective serotonin reuptake inhibitors, serotonin norepinephrine reuptake inhibitors, anxiolytics).[119] It is uncertain which antidepressant is more effective and better tolerated in patients with cancer-related depression.[120]

NEUROCOGNITIVE IMPAIRMENT

Patients with brain tumors are prone to cognitive impairment secondary to the neoplasm and its treatment, and this is the major determinant of quality of life in long-term survivors.[50] Late radiation neurotoxicity remains the most significant risk factor for progressive cognitive impairment after treatment of brain tumor. The pathogenesis underlying radiation-induced cognitive impairment remains unknown, although vascular injury, neuroinflammation, and impaired neurogenesis have been postulated.[121] Several drugs have been evaluated for potential prevention or improvement of cognitive impairment in patients with brain tumors. Donepezil demonstrated significant improvement in cognition.[122] However, in a follow-up study neurocognitive composite score (primary outcome) was not improved, but a modest benefit was observed in patients with greater baseline neurocognitive impairment.[123] Small pilot studies suggested a benefit from methylphenidate and modafinil.[124,125] Memantine showed a delay in time to cognitive decline and a reduced rate of decline in memory, executive function, and processing speed in patients receiving whole-brain radiotherapy for brain metastases, although the results were not statistically significant.[126] Because memantine is usually well tolerated and there was a trend in improvement, it is recommended for patients being treated with whole-brain radiation.

Intensity-modulated radiation therapy, proton beam therapy, and hippocampus-sparing whole-brain radiotherapy may limit radiation-induced neurotoxicity. There is the perception by patients and families that cognitive rehabilitation is beneficial.[127] A randomized trial showed that the addition of cognitive training to rehabilitation results in a significant improvement in cognitive function in patients admitted to a rehabilitation facility within 2 weeks from brain tumor surgery.[128] Communicating hydrocephalus is an uncommon sequela of radiotherapy in patients with glioblastoma. In symptomatic patients with hydrocephalus, shunt placement may provide clinical improvement.[129]

SUMMARY

Patients with brain tumor experience a myriad of both tumor and treatment-related complications during their disease course that significantly affects quality of life. The effective management of tumor-related epilepsy, brain edema, thromboembolic complications, neurocognitive impairment, depression, and fatigue is of paramount importance for improving patient well-being and perhaps, overall survival. Although this review provides practical recommendations for the neurologist, the balancing act of limited treatment options and associated adverse effects for symptomatic management remains a challenge in neuro-oncologic practice. Studies evaluating the optimal management strategy for these complications are urgently needed.

REFERENCES

1. Clouston PD, DeAngelis LM, Posner JB. The spectrum of neurological disease in patients with systemic cancer. Ann Neurol 1992;31(3):268–73.
2. You G, Sha Z, Jiang T. The pathogenesis of tumor-related epilepsy and its implications for clinical treatment. Seizure 2012;21:153–9. England: A 2012 British Epilepsy Association. Published by Elsevier Ltd.
3. Maschio M, Beghi E, Casazza MML, et al. Patterns of care of brain tumor-related epilepsy. A cohort study done in Italian Epilepsy Center. PLoS One 2017;12(7): e0180470.
4. Morris HH, Matkovic Z, Estes ML, et al. Ganglioglioma and intractable epilepsy: clinical and neurophysiologic features and predictors of outcome after surgery. Epilepsia 1998;39(3):307–13.
5. Daumas-Duport C, Scheithauer BW, Chodkiewicz JP, et al. Dysembryoplastic neuroepithelial tumor: a surgically curable tumor of young patients with intractable partial seizures. Report of thirty-nine cases. Neurosurgery 1988;23(5): 545–56.
6. Englot DJ, Chang EF, Vecht CJ. Epilepsy and brain tumors. Handb Clin Neurol 2016;134:267–85.
7. Ruda R, Bello L, Duffau H, et al. Seizures in low-grade gliomas: natural history, pathogenesis, and outcome after treatments. Neuro Oncol 2012;14(Suppl 4): iv55–64.
8. Liubinas SV, D'Abaco GM, Moffat BM, et al. IDH1 mutation is associated with seizures and protoplasmic subtype in patients with low-grade gliomas. Epilepsia 2014;55(9):1438–43.
9. Englot DJ, Berger MS, Barbaro NM, et al. Predictors of seizure freedom after resection of supratentorial low-grade gliomas. A review. J Neurosurg 2011; 115(2):240–4.
10. Ruda R, Magliola U, Bertero L, et al. Seizure control following radiotherapy in patients with diffuse gliomas: a retrospective study. Neuro Oncol 2013;15(12): 1739–49.
11. Schrottner O, Unger F, Eder HG, et al. Gamma-Knife radiosurgery of mesiotemporal tumour epilepsy observations and long-term results. Acta Neurochir Suppl 2002;84:49–55.
12. Sherman JH, Moldovan K, Yeoh HK, et al. Impact of temozolomide chemotherapy on seizure frequency in patients with low-grade gliomas. J Neurosurg 2011;114(6):1617–21.
13. Soffietti R, Ruda R, Bradac GB, et al. PCV chemotherapy for recurrent oligodendrogliomas and oligoastrocytomas. Neurosurgery 1998;43(5):1066–73.
14. Avila EK, Chamberlain M, Schiff D, et al. Seizure control as a new metric in assessing efficacy of tumor treatment in low-grade glioma trials. Neuro Oncol 2017;19(1):12–21.
15. Glantz MJ, Cole BF, Forsyth PA, et al. Practice parameter: anticonvulsant prophylaxis in patients with newly diagnosed brain tumors. Report of the quality standards subcommittee of the American Academy of Neurology. Neurology 2000;54(10):1886–93.

16. Mikkelsen T, Paleologos NA, Robinson PD, et al. The role of prophylactic anti-convulsants in the management of brain metastases: a systematic review and evidence-based clinical practice guideline. J Neurooncol 2010;96(1):97–102.

17. Perry J, Zinman L, Chambers A, et al. The use of prophylactic anticonvulsants in patients with brain tumours-a systematic review. Curr Oncol 2006;13(6):222–9.

18. Kong X, Guan J, Yang Y, et al. A meta-analysis: do prophylactic antiepileptic drugs in patients with brain tumors decrease the incidence of seizures? Clin Neurol Neurosurg 2015;134:98–103. Netherlands: 2015; Elsevier B.V.

19. Wu AS, Trinh VT, Suki D, et al. A prospective randomized trial of perioperative seizure prophylaxis in patients with intraparenchymal brain tumors. J Neurosurg 2013;118(4):873–83.

20. Lockney DT, Vaziri S, Walch F, et al. Prophylactic antiepileptic drug use in patients with brain tumors undergoing craniotomy. World Neurosurg 2017;98:28–33. United States: 2016 Elsevier Inc.

21. Foy PM, Copeland GP, Shaw MD. The incidence of postoperative seizures. Acta Neurochir (Wien) 1981;55(3–4):253–64.

22. Kuijlen JM, Teernstra OP, Kessels AG, et al. Effectiveness of antiepileptic prophylaxis used with supratentorial craniotomies: a meta-analysis. Seizure 1996;5(4):291–8.

23. Pulman J, Greenhalgh J, Marson AG. Antiepileptic drugs as prophylaxis for post-craniotomy seizures. Cochrane Database Syst Rev 2013;(2):CD007286.

24. Chang SM, Parney IF, Huang W, et al. Patterns of care for adults with newly diagnosed malignant glioma. JAMA 2005;293:557–64. United States.

25. Kahlenberg CA, Fadul CE, Roberts DW, et al. Seizure prognosis of patients with low-grade tumors. Seizure 2012;21(7):540–5.

26. Koekkoek JA, Dirven L, Taphoorn MJ. The withdrawal of antiepileptic drugs in patients with low-grade and anaplastic glioma. Expert Rev Neurother 2017;17(2):193–202.

27. Mamon HJ, Wen PY, Burns AC, et al. Allergic skin reactions to anticonvulsant medications in patients receiving cranial radiation therapy. Epilepsia 1999;40(3):341–4.

28. Hoang-Xuan K, Delattre JY, Poisson M. Stevens-Johnson syndrome in a patient receiving cranial irradiation and carbamazepine. Neurology 1990;40(7):1144–5.

29. Lynam LM, Lyons MK, Drazkowski JF, et al. Frequency of seizures in patients with newly diagnosed brain tumors: a retrospective review. Clin Neurol Neurosurg 2007;109:634–8. Netherlands.

30. Maschio M, Dinapoli L, Zarabla A, et al. Zonisamide in brain tumor-related epilepsy: an observational pilot study. Clin Neuropharmacol 2017;40(3):113–9.

31. Villanueva V, Saiz-Diaz R, Toledo M, et al. NEOPLASM study: real-life use of lacosamide in patients with brain tumor-related epilepsy. Epilepsy Behav 2016;65:25–32. United States: 2016 Elsevier Inc.

32. Rossetti AO, Jeckelmann S, Novy J, et al. Levetiracetam and pregabalin for antiepileptic monotherapy in patients with primary brain tumors. A phase II randomized study. Neuro Oncol 2014;16(4):584–8.

33. Vecht CJ, Kerkhof M, Duran-Pena A. Seizure prognosis in brain tumors: new insights and evidence-based management. Oncologist 2014;19(7):751–9.

34. Khoury T, Chen S, Abu Rmeileh A, et al. Acute liver injury induced by levetiracetam and temozolomide co-treatment. Dig Liver Dis 2017;49:297–300. Netherlands: 2016 Editrice Gastroenterologica Italiana S.r.l. Published by Elsevier Ltd.

35. Liddle C, Goodwin BJ, George J, et al. Separate and interactive regulation of cytochrome P450 3A4 by triiodothyronine, dexamethasone, and growth hormone in cultured hepatocytes. J Clin Endocrinol Metab 1998;83(7):2411–6.
36. Brodie MJ, Mintzer S, Pack AM, et al. Enzyme induction with antiepileptic drugs: cause for concern? Epilepsia 2013;54(1):11–27.
37. Weller M, Gorlia T, Cairncross JG, et al. Prolonged survival with valproic acid use in the EORTC/NCIC temozolomide trial for glioblastoma. Neurology 2011; 77(12):1156–64.
38. Happold C, Gorlia T, Chinot O, et al. Does valproic acid or levetiracetam improve survival in glioblastoma? A pooled analysis of prospective clinical trials in newly diagnosed glioblastoma. J Clin Oncol 2016;34(7):731–9.
39. Sepulveda-Sanchez JM, Conde-Moreno A, Baron M, et al. Efficacy and tolerability of lacosamide for secondary epileptic seizures in patients with brain tumor: a multicenter, observational retrospective study. Oncol Lett 2017;13(6): 4093–100.
40. Vecht C, Duran-Pena A, Houillier C, et al. Seizure response to perampanel in drug-resistant epilepsy with gliomas: early observations. J Neurooncol 2017; 133:603–7.
41. Nasr ZG, Paravattil B, Wilby KJ. Levetiracetam for seizure prevention in brain tumor patients: a systematic review. J Neurooncol 2016;129(1):1–13.
42. Wick W, Kuker W. Brain edema in neurooncology: radiological assessment and management. Onkologie 2004;27(3):261–6.
43. Papadopoulos MC, Saadoun S, Binder DK, et al. Molecular mechanisms of brain tumor edema. Neuroscience 2004;129(4):1011–20.
44. Inaba H, Pui CH. Glucocorticoid use in acute lymphoblastic leukaemia. Lancet Oncol 2010;11(11):1096–106.
45. Pitter KL, Tamagno I, Alikhanyan K, et al. Corticosteroids compromise survival in glioblastoma. Brain 2016;139(Pt 5):1458–71.
46. Weissman DE, Janjan NA, Erickson B, et al. Twice-daily tapering dexamethasone treatment during cranial radiation for newly diagnosed brain metastases. J Neurooncol 1991;11(3):235–9.
47. Vecht CJ, Hovestadt A, Verbiest HB, et al. Dose-effect relationship of dexamethasone on Karnofsky performance in metastatic brain tumors: a randomized study of doses of 4, 8, and 16 mg per day. Neurology 1994;44(4):675–80.
48. Sturdza A, Millar BA, Bana N, et al. The use and toxicity of steroids in the management of patients with brain metastases. Support Care Cancer 2008;16(9): 1041–8.
49. Deutsch MB, Panageas KS, Lassman AB, et al. Steroid management in newly diagnosed glioblastoma. J Neurooncol 2013;113(1):111–6.
50. Pruitt AA. Medical management of patients with brain tumors. Continuum (Minneap Minn) 2015;21(2 Neuro-oncology):314–31.
51. Byyny RL. Withdrawal from glucocorticoid therapy. N Engl J Med 1976;295(1): 30–2.
52. Dropcho EJ, Soong SJ. Steroid-induced weakness in patients with primary brain tumors. Neurology 1991;41(8):1235–9.
53. Batchelor TT, Taylor LP, Thaler HT, et al. Steroid myopathy in cancer patients. Neurology 1997;48(5):1234–8.
54. Conn HO, Poynard T. Corticosteroids and peptic ulcer: meta-analysis of adverse events during steroid therapy. J Intern Med 1994;236(6):619–32.

55. Fadul CE, Lemann W, Thaler HT, et al. Perforation of the gastrointestinal tract in patients receiving steroids for neurologic disease. Neurology 1988;38(3): 348–52.

56. Grossman JM, Gordon R, Ranganath VK, et al. American College of Rheumatology 2010 recommendations for the prevention and treatment of glucocorticoid-induced osteoporosis. Arthritis Care Res (Hoboken) 2010;62(11):1515–26.

57. Da Silva AN, Heras-Herzig A, Schiff D. Bone health in patients with brain tumors. Surg Neurol 2007;68:525–33 [discussion: 533].

58. Kang JH, Hui D, Kim MJ, et al. Corticosteroid rotation to alleviate dexamethasone-induced hiccup: a case series at a single institution. J Pain Symptom Manage 2012;43:625–30. United States: A 2011 U.S. Cancer Pain Relief Committee. Published by Elsevier Inc.

59. Vredenburgh JJ, Cloughesy T, Samant M, et al. Corticosteroid use in patients with glioblastoma at first or second relapse treated with bevacizumab in the BRAIN study. The oncologist 2010;15(12):1329–34.

60. Batchelor TT, Duda DG, di Tomaso E, et al. Phase II study of cediranib, an oral pan-vascular endothelial growth factor receptor tyrosine kinase inhibitor, in patients with recurrent glioblastoma. J Clin Oncol 2010;28(17):2817–23.

61. Kourilsky A, Bertrand G, Ursu R, et al. Impact of Angiotensin-II receptor blockers on vasogenic edema in glioblastoma patients. J Neurol 2016;263: 524–30. Germany.

62. Rutz HP, Hofer S, Peghini PE, et al. Avoiding glucocorticoid administration in a neurooncological case. Cancer Biol Ther 2005;4:1186–9. United States.

63. Kirste S, Treier M, Wehrle SJ, et al. Boswellia serrata acts on cerebral edema in patients irradiated for brain tumors: a prospective, randomized, placebo-controlled, double-blind pilot trial. Cancer 2011;117(16):3788–95.

64. Perry JR. Thromboembolic disease in patients with high-grade glioma. Neuro Oncol 2012;14(Suppl 4):iv73–80.

65. Brandes AA, Scelzi E, Salmistraro G, et al. Incidence of risk of thromboembolism during treatment high-grade gliomas: a prospective study. Eur J Cancer 1997; 33:1592–6. England.

66. Streiff MB, Ye X, Kickler TS, et al. A prospective multicenter study of venous thromboembolism in patients with newly-diagnosed high-grade glioma: hazard rate and risk factors. J Neurooncol 2015;124(2):299–305.

67. Unruh D, Schwarze S, Khoury L. Mutant IDH1 and thrombosis in gliomas. Acta Neuropathol 2016;132:917–30.

68. Jenkins EO, Schiff D, Mackman N, et al. Venous thromboembolism in malignant gliomas. J Thromb Haemost 2010;8(2):221–7.

69. Louzada ML, Majeed H, Wells PS. Efficacy of low- molecular- weight- heparin versus vitamin K antagonists for long term treatment of cancer-associated venous thromboembolism in adults: a systematic review of randomized controlled trials. Thromb Res 2009;123:837–44.

70. Lee AY. Treatment of established thrombotic events in patients with cancer. Thromb Res 2012;129(Suppl 1):S146–53. United States: 2012 Elsevier Ltd.

71. Lyman G, Bohlke K, Khorana A. American Society of Clinical Oncology Venous thromboembolism prophylaxis and treatment in patients with cancer: American Society of Clinical Oncology clinical practice guideline update. J Clin Oncol 2015;33(6):654–6.

72. Jo J, Schiff D, Perry J. Thrombosis in brain tumors. Semin Thromb Hemost 2014; 40(3):325–31.

73. Ikushima S, Ono R, Fukuda K, et al. Trousseau's syndrome: cancer-associated thrombosis. Jpn J Clin Oncol 2016;46(3):204–8.
74. Levin JM, Schiff D, Loeffler JS, et al. Complications of therapy for venous thromboembolic disease in patients with brain tumors. Neurology 1993;43(6):1111–4.
75. Decousus H, Leizorovicz A, Parent F, et al. A clinical trial of vena caval filters in the prevention of pulmonary embolism in patients with proximal deep-vein thrombosis. Prevention du Risque d'Embolie Pulmonaire par Interruption Cave Study Group. N Engl J Med 1998;338(7):409–15.
76. Turpie AG, Hirsh J, Gent M, et al. Prevention of deep vein thrombosis in potential neurosurgical patients. A randomized trial comparing graduated compression stockings alone or graduated compression stockings plus intermittent pneumatic compression with control. Arch Intern Med 1989;149(3):679–81.
77. Agnelli G, Piovella F, Buoncristiani P, et al. Enoxaparin plus compression stockings compared with compression stockings alone in the prevention of venous thromboembolism after elective neurosurgery. N Engl J Med 1998;339(2):80–5.
78. Nurmohamed MT, van Riel AM, Henkens CM, et al. Low molecular weight heparin and compression stockings in the prevention of venous thromboembolism in neurosurgery. Thromb Haemost 1996;75(2):233–8.
79. Kreisl TN, Kim L, Moore K, et al. Phase II trial of single-agent bevacizumab followed by bevacizumab plus irinotecan at tumor progression in recurrent glioblastoma. J Clin Oncol 2009;27(5):740–5.
80. Gilbert MR, Dignam JJ, Armstrong TS, et al. A randomized trial of bevacizumab for newly diagnosed glioblastoma. N Engl J Med 2014;370(8):699–708.
81. Plotkin SR, Stemmer-Rachamimov AO, Barker FG 2nd, et al. Hearing improvement after bevacizumab in patients with neurofibromatosis type 2. N Engl J Med 2009;361(4):358–67.
82. Nayak L, Iwamoto FM, Rudnick JD, et al. Atypical and anaplastic meningiomas treated with bevacizumab. J Neurooncol 2012;109(1):187–93.
83. Green RM, Cloughesy TF, Stupp R, et al. Bevacizumab for recurrent ependymoma. Neurology 2009;73(20):1677–80.
84. Omar AI. Bevacizumab for the treatment of surgically unresectable cervical cord hemangioblastoma: a case report. J Med Case Rep 2012;6(1):238.
85. Bhaskara A, Eng C. Bevacizumab in the treatment of a patient with metastatic colorectal carcinoma with brain metastases. Clin Colorectal Cancer 2008;7:65–8. United States.
86. De Braganca KC, Janjigian YY, Azzoli CG, et al. Efficacy and safety of bevacizumab in active brain metastases from non-small cell lung cancer. J Neurooncol 2010;100(3):443–7.
87. Kountourakis P, Dokou A, Kardara E, et al. Bevacizumab therapy may contribute to irradiation deferral in patients with breast cancer and with central nervous system metastases: findings of a case series. Clin Breast Cancer 2012;12:282–6. United States.
88. Levin VA, Bidaut L, Hou P, et al. Randomized double-blind placebo-controlled trial of bevacizumab therapy for radiation necrosis of the central nervous system. Int J Radiat Oncol Biol Phys 2011;79(5):1487–95.
89. Chinot OL, Wick W, Mason W, et al. Bevacizumab plus radiotherapy-temozolomide for newly diagnosed glioblastoma. N Engl J Med 2014;370(8):709–22.
90. Maitland ML, Bakris GL, Black HR, et al. Initial assessment, surveillance, and management of blood pressure in patients receiving vascular endothelial growth factor signaling pathway inhibitors. J Natl Cancer Inst 2010;102(9):596–604.

91. Saavedra E, Hollebecque A, Soria JC, et al. Dysphonia induced by anti-angiogenic compounds. Invest New Drugs 2014;32(4):774–82.
92. Carter CA, Caroen SZ, Oronsky AL, et al. Dysphonia after bevacizumab rechallenge: a case report. Case Rep Oncol 2015;8(3):423–5.
93. Nalluri SR, Chu D, Keresztes R, et al. Risk of venous thromboembolism with the angiogenesis inhibitor bevacizumab in cancer patients: a meta-analysis. JAMA 2008;300:2277–85. United States.
94. Letarte N, Bressler LR, Villano JL. Bevacizumab and central nervous system (CNS) hemorrhage. Cancer Chemother Pharmacol 2013;71(6):1561–5.
95. Seidel C, Hentschel B, Simon M, et al. A comprehensive analysis of vascular complications in 3,889 glioma patients from the German Glioma Network. J Neurol 2013;260(3):847–55.
96. Tlemsani C, Mir O, Boudou-Rouquette P, et al. Posterior reversible encephalopathy syndrome induced by anti-VEGF agents. Target Oncol 2011;6(4):253–8.
97. Abu-Hejleh T, Mezhir JJ, Goodheart MJ, et al. Incidence and management of gastrointestinal perforation from bevacizumab in advanced cancers. Curr Oncol Rep 2012;14(4):277–84.
98. Gerber DE, Grossman SA, Zeltzman M, et al. The impact of thrombocytopenia from temozolomide and radiation in newly diagnosed adults with high-grade gliomas. Neuro Oncol 2007;9(1):47–52.
99. Schiff D. Pneumocystis pneumonia in brain tumor patients: risk factors and clinical features. J Neurooncol 1996;27(3):235–40.
100. De Vos FY, Gijtenbeek JM, Bleeker-Rovers CP, et al. Pneumocystis jirovecii pneumonia prophylaxis during temozolomide treatment for high-grade gliomas. Crit Rev Oncol Hematol 2013;85:373–82. Netherlands: 2012 Elsevier Ireland Ltd.
101. Stupp R, Dietrich PY, Ostermann Kraljevic S, et al. Promising survival for patients with newly diagnosed glioblastoma multiforme treated with concomitant radiation plus temozolomide followed by adjuvant temozolomide. J Clin Oncol 2002;20(5):1375–82.
102. Grossman SA, Ye X, Lesser G, et al. Immunosuppression in patients with high-grade gliomas treated with radiation and temozolomide. Clin Cancer Res 2011;17(16):5473–80.
103. Wick A, Felsberg J, Steinbach JP, et al. Efficacy and tolerability of temozolomide in an alternating weekly regimen in patients with recurrent glioma. J Clin Oncol 2007;25:3357–61. United States.
104. Berrocal A, Perez Segura P, Gil M, et al. Extended-schedule dose-dense temozolomide in refractory gliomas. J Neurooncol 2010;96(3):417–22.
105. Hansen RM, Reinerio N, Sohnle PG, et al. Ketoconazole in the prevention of candidiasis in patients with cancer. A prospective, randomized, controlled, double-blind study. Arch Intern Med 1987;147(4):710–2.
106. Kizilarslanoglu MC, Aksoy S, Yildirim NO, et al. Temozolomide-related infections: review of the literature. J BUON 2011;16(3):547–50.
107. Lionakis MS, Dunleavy K, Roschewski M, et al. Inhibition of B cell receptor signaling by ibrutinib in primary CNS lymphoma. Cancer Cell 2017;31:833–43.e5. United States: Published by Elsevier Inc.
108. Carson KR, Evens AM, Richey EA, et al. Progressive multifocal leukoencephalopathy after rituximab therapy in HIV-negative patients: a report of 57 cases from the research on adverse drug events and reports project. Blood 2009;113(20):4834–40.

109. Ohishi W, Chayama K. Prevention of hepatitis B virus reactivation in immunosuppressive therapy or chemotherapy. Clin Exp Nephrol 2011;15(5):634–40.
110. Kohrt HE, Ouyang DL, Keeffe EB. Systematic review: lamivudine prophylaxis for chemotherapy-induced reactivation of chronic hepatitis B virus infection. Aliment Pharmacol Ther 2006;24:1003–16. England.
111. Valko PO, Siddique A, Linsenmeier C, et al. Prevalence and predictors of fatigue in glioblastoma: a prospective study. Neuro Oncol 2015;17(2):274–81.
112. Armstrong TS, Cron SG, Bolanos EV, et al. Risk factors for fatigue severity in primary brain tumor patients. Cancer 2010;116(11):2707–15.
113. Day J, Yust-Katz S, Cachia D, et al. Interventions for the management of fatigue in adults with a primary brain tumour. Cochrane Database Syst Rev 2016;(4):CD011376.
114. Armstrong TS, Gilbert MR. Practical strategies for management of fatigue and sleep disorders in people with brain tumors. Neuro Oncol 2012;14(Suppl 4): iv65–72.
115. Rooney AG, McNamara S, Mackinnon M, et al. Frequency, clinical associations, and longitudinal course of major depressive disorder in adults with cerebral glioma. J Clin Oncol 2011;29(32):4307–12.
116. Litofsky NS, Farace E, Anderson F Jr, et al. Depression in patients with high-grade glioma: results of the glioma outcomes project. Neurosurgery 2004; 54(2):358–66 [discussion: 366–7].
117. Seddighi A, Seddighi AS, Nikouei A, et al. Psychological aspects in brain tumor patients: a prospective study. Hell J Nucl Med 2015;18(Suppl 1):63–7.
118. Spiegel D. Cancer and depression. Br J Psychiatry Suppl 1996;(30):109–16.
119. Hart SL, Hoyt MA, Diefenbach M, et al. Meta-analysis of efficacy of interventions for elevated depressive symptoms in adults diagnosed with cancer. J Natl Cancer Inst 2012;104(13):990–1004.
120. Riblet N, Larson R, Watts BV, et al. Reevaluating the role of antidepressants in cancer-related depression: a systematic review and meta-analysis. Gen Hosp Psychiatry 2014;36(5):466–73.
121. Greene-Schloesser D, Moore E, Robbins ME. Molecular pathways: radiation-induced cognitive impairment. Clin Cancer Res 2013;19(9):2294–300.
122. Shaw EG, Rosdhal R, D'Agostino RB Jr, et al. Phase II study of donepezil in irradiated brain tumor patients: effect on cognitive function, mood, and quality of life. J Clin Oncol 2006;24(9):1415–20.
123. Rapp SR, Case LD, Peiffer A, et al. Donepezil for irradiated brain tumor survivors: a phase III randomized placebo-controlled clinical trial. J Clin Oncol 2015;33(15):1653–9.
124. Gehring K, Patwardhan SY, Collins R, et al. A randomized trial on the efficacy of methylphenidate and modafinil for improving cognitive functioning and symptoms in patients with a primary brain tumor. J Neurooncol 2012;107(1):165–74.
125. Meyers CA, Weitzner MA, Valentine AD, et al. Methylphenidate therapy improves cognition, mood, and function of brain tumor patients. J Clin Oncol 1998;16(7):2522–7.
126. Brown PD, Pugh S, Laack NN, et al. Memantine for the prevention of cognitive dysfunction in patients receiving whole-brain radiotherapy: a randomized, double-blind, placebo-controlled trial. Neuro Oncol 2013;15(10):1429–37.
127. Bergo E, Lombardi G, Pambuku A, et al. Cognitive rehabilitation in patients with gliomas and other brain tumors: state of the art. Biomed Res Int 2016;2016: 3041824.

128. Zucchella C, Capone A, Codella V, et al. Cognitive rehabilitation for early post-surgery inpatients affected by primary brain tumor: a randomized, controlled trial. J Neurooncol 2013;114(1):93–100.

129. Montano N, D'Alessandris QG, Bianchi F, et al. Communicating hydrocephalus following surgery and adjuvant radiochemotherapy for glioblastoma. J Neurosurg 2011;115(6):1126–30.

Grade II and III Oligodendroglioma and Astrocytoma

Martin J. van den Bent, MD[a],*, Susan M. Chang, MD[b]

KEYWORDS

- Astrocytoma • Oligodendroglioma • Anaplastic • *IDH* • 1p/19q codeletion • PCV
- Temozolomide • Bevacizumab

KEY POINTS

- The World Health Organization classification of glioma is now based on molecular criteria, in particular, based on the presence or absence of *IDH* mutations and 1p/19q codeletion. *IDH*-mutated gliomas have a more favorable outcome, especially if combined with 1p/19q codeletion.
- If an extensive resection is safely possible, early surgery should be considered in patients presenting with seizures only and a nonenhancing lesion on MRI presumed to represent a low-grade glioma.
- Delayed effects of radiotherapy on cognition warrant postponing adjuvant radiotherapy if safely possible.
- Adjuvant chemotherapy given immediately after radiotherapy improves survival in grade II and III glioma.
- Upfront treatment with chemotherapy alone as opposed to radiotherapy followed by adjuvant chemotherapy may jeopardize survival.

INTRODUCTION

With its emphasis on molecular tumor characteristics, the 2016 World Health Organization (WHO) Classification of Tumors of the Central Nervous System has radically changed the diagnostics of diffuse glioma.[1] Traditionally, diffuse grade II and III gliomas were separated into 2 basic morphologic subtypes: oligodendroglioma and astrocytoma, with a third "mixed" category of oligoastrocytoma for those cases in which histologic examination showed elements of both. Today, to make the diagnosis

Disclosures: M.J. van den Bent received honoraria from MSD.
[a] Brain Tumor Center, Erasmus MC Cancer Institute, Groene Hilledijk 301, Rotterdam 3075EA, The Netherlands; [b] Department of Neurosurgery, University of California, San Francisco, Box 0112, 505 Parnassus Avenue M779, San Francisco, CA 94143, USA
* Corresponding author.
E-mail address: m.vandenbent@erasmusmc.nl

Neurol Clin 36 (2018) 467–484
https://doi.org/10.1016/j.ncl.2018.04.005   **neurologic.theclinics.com**

of an (anaplastic) oligodendroglioma, the presence of both codeletion of chromosome arms 1p and19q and mutation (mt) of the isocitrate dehydrogenase gene (*IDH1* or *IDH2*) is required; for (anaplastic) astrocytoma, both an *IDHmt* and an *IDH* wild-type (wt) exist. This revised classification of diffuse gliomas is far more robust and much more informative prognostically than the classic histopathological approach. Clinicians must now incorporate these revisions into their everyday diagnostics and treatment of diffuse glioma.[2]

CLINICAL PRESENTATION

Each year, 4500 to 5000 patients in the United States are diagnosed with a grade II (low-grade) or III (anaplastic) astrocytoma or oligodendroglioma.[3] Low-grade glioma (LGG) usually presents in patients between 25 and 45 years of age; patients with anaplastic tumors tend to be somewhat older (30–50 years). Occasionally, *IDHmt* astrocytomas are diagnosed in older children and adolescents (even those younger than 15), whereas some 1/19q codeleted *IDHmt* oligodendrogliomas are first diagnosed in patients older than 60 to 65 years. In general, the chance of diagnosing an *IDH* mutation in grade II and III glioma decreases in patients who are older than 50 to 55 years. The clinical presentation of brain tumors is nonspecific and depends on tumor localization and rate of growth. Most low-grade and anaplastic tumors first present with seizures; focal deficits are less common at the time of first diagnosis. Typically, LGGs are slow-growing lesions with an annual growth rate of 4 to 6 mm if left untreated.[4] Clinical prognostic factors include age of the patient, size of the tumor, frontal location, and performance status of the patient; favorable factors are in general associated with the presence of *IDH* mutations.[5,6]

MOLECULAR BACKGROUND

In 2008, genetic analysis of a series of glioblastomas discovered mutations in the gene encoding for *IDH1* and *IDH2*, which were subsequently shown to be present in 70% to 80% of grade II and III glioma.[7] Tumors with *IDH* mutations are associated with an increased survival compared with histologically similar tumors without *IDH* mutations.[7–9] *IDH* mutations represent early mutations and may very well represent the driving mutation in *IDHmt* glioma. The mutations in the *IDH1* and *IDH2* genes are somatic, missense, heterozygous, and involve either codon 132 (*IDH1*) or codon 172 (*IDH2*). *IDH* mutations induce an altered substrate affinity of the *IDH* enzyme resulting in increased levels of 2-hydroxyglutarate and lower levels of α-ketoglutarate and nicotinamide adenine dinucleotide phosphate (NADPH).[10] This can induce the development of a global methylation of CpG islands, which often includes the *MGMT* promoter region.[10,11] This may at least partially explain the sensitivity to chemotherapy of *IDHmt* tumors. Another plausible explanation is that resistance mechanisms to alkylating chemotherapy are dependent on the level of α-ketoglutarate.[12] Similarly, the lower levels of NADPH production by *IDHmt* cells have been correlated to increased sensitivity to radiotherapy.[13] There is preliminary evidence that *IDHmt* induces a defective homologous recombination and in vitro studies suggest this may render them sensitive to poly ADP ribose polymerase (PARP) inhibitors.[14,15] Previously, genetic analysis demonstrated that combined loss of 1p/19q is a typical molecular feature for (anaplastic) oligodendroglioma and is associated with increased responsiveness to procarbazine, CCNU (lomustine), vincristine (PCV) chemotherapy and temozolomide chemotherapy.[16–18] This 1p/19q codeletion is an early event that remains present at the time of tumor progression. More recent studies indicate that 1p/19q codeletion develops in tumors in which an *IDH* mutation has already occurred.[19]

Diagnosis According to the World Health Organization 2016 Classification

The clinical utility of the prior histopathological WHO classification was limited, in part, because of major interobserver and intraobserver variability and because of the heterogeneous clinical outcome among histologically similar tumors.[20,21] A multitude of recent studies have shown the superior prognostic and predictive significance of a molecular glioma classification, based on the presence or absence of 1p/19q codeletion and *IDH* mutations (**Fig. 1**).[19,22,23] These observations resulted in the revised WHO 2016 classification for astrocytoma and oligodendroglioma (**Box 1**).[1,24] Regardless of the histopathological findings, the presence of 1p/19q codeletion and an *IDH* mutation leads to the diagnosis of an oligodendroglioma; the presence of only *IDH* mutation but no 1p/19q codeletion results in the diagnosis of an astrocytoma. Only in those cases with glioma histology in which molecular testing was not possible or remained inconclusive, the phrase "Not Otherwise Specified" (NOS) is to be used. Because of this change, mixed oligoastrocytomas have ceased to exist, as they typically have both 1p/19q codeletion and an *IDH* mutation (now reclassified as an oligodendroglioma) or only an *IDH* mutation (now reclassified as an astrocytoma) or neither (suggestive of a glioblastomalike genotype); the exceptional case report with confusing molecular data does not negate the general classification scheme.[25] **Table 1** summarizes the overall survival (OS) and progression-free survival (PFS) reported in molecular subtypes observed in prospective trials on diffuse grade II and III glioma. Taken together, median OS in *IDHmt* astrocytoma is in the 9 to 10 years range, and in *IDHmt* 1p/19q codeleted tumors more than 14 years.[26] Survival in *IDHwt* (anaplastic) astrocytoma is significantly less.[26]

Remarks on the Assessment of Molecular Lesions and of the Tumor Grade

Ninety percent of all *IDH* mutations affect the *IDH1* R132H position, which can be diagnosed with a sensitive and reliable immunohistochemistry (IHC) assay. If IHC is used for *IDH* mutation analysis, this should be followed in negative cases by sequencing of

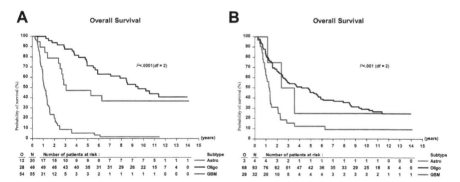

Fig. 1. Kaplan-Meier OS curves of 133 patients with locally diagnosed anaplastic oligodendroglial tumors treated on the EORTC 26951 study (*A*) according to different histologic subtypes as diagnosed by the central study pathologist and (*B*) according to the 3 molecularly defined diffuse glioma classes, demonstrating the much more powerful discrimination of tumor types by genetic analysis. Nine patients remained unclassified with this approach, including 2 patients with H3F3A-mutated tumors. Astro, astrocytoma; GBM, glioblastoma; Oligo, oligodendroglioma. (*From* Dubbink HJ, Atmodimedjo PN, Kros JM, et al, Molecular classification of anaplastic oligodendroglioma using next generation sequencing. A report of the prospective randomized EORTC Brain Tumor Group 26951 phase III trial. Neuro Oncol 2016;18:388–400; with permission of Oxford University Press/Society for Neuro-Oncology.)

Box 1
The revised World Health Organization 2016 classification for astrocytoma and oligodendroglioma

Diffuse astrocytoma and oligodendroglial tumors
    Diffuse astrocytoma, *IDH* mutant
    Gemistocytic astrocytoma, *IDH* mutant
    Diffuse astrocytoma, *IDH* wild-type
    Diffuse astrocytoma, not otherwise specified (NOS)
    Anaplastic astrocytoma, *IDH* mutant
    Anaplastic astrocytoma, *IDH* wild-type
    Anaplastic astrocytoma, NOS
    Diffuse midline glioma, H3 K27M-mutant
    Oligodendroglioma, *IDH* mutant and 1p/19q codeleted
    Oligodendroglioma, NOS
    Anaplastic oligodendroglioma, *IDH* mutant and 1p/19q codeleted
    Anaplastic oligodendroglioma, NOS
    Oligoastrocytoma, NOS
    Anaplastic oligoastrocytoma, NOS

---

both the *IDH1* and *IDH2*, as IHC will miss 10% of all *IDH* mutations. The 1p/19q code-letion is in fact a balanced t(1;19) (q10;p10) translocation resulting in the loss of both the entire 1p and 19q arm.[27] Therefore, the diagnostic assay for 1p and 19q should cover the entire length of these chromosomal arms; a shortcoming of the used

Table 1
Median survival regardless of assigned treatment in *IDHwt*, *IDHmt* and 1p/19q codeleted tumors in prospective trials with retrospective molecular analysis

Histology/Molecular Subgroup	Treatment	n	Median PFS	Median OS
Low-grade glioma[62]				
IDH R132Hmt	RT ± PCV	71	—	13.1 y
IDHwt		42	—	5.1 y
Low-grade glioma[67]				
IDHmt 1p/19q codeleted	RT or TMZ	104	5.2 y	NS
IDHmt		165	4 y	
IDHwt		49	1.7 y	
Anaplastic astrocytoma[69]				
IDH R132H mutated	RT/TMZ, BCNU or CCNU	49	—	7.9 y
IDHwt		54	—	2.8 y
Anaplastic oligodendroglioma[a,22]				
IDHmt 1p/19q codeleted	RT ± PCV	49	—	9.5 y
IDH mt		20	—	3.1 y
IDHwt		55	—	1.1 y
Anaplastic oligodendroglioma[a,64]				
IDHmt 1p/19q codeleted	RT/PCV	42	—	14.7 y
IDH mt		37	—	5.5 y
IDHwt		26	—	1.3 y
Anaplastic glioma[66,91]				
IDHmt, 1p/19q codeleted	RT, PCV, or TMZ	69	7.5–8.7 y	NR
IDHmt		83	2.1–3.0 y	7.0–7.3 y
IDHwt		58	0.8 y	3.1–4.7 y

Abbreviations: BCNU, carmustine, CCNU (lomustine); OS, overall survival; PCV, procarbazine, CCNA, and vincristine; NA, not stated; NR, not reported; PFS, progression-free survival; RT, radiotherapy; TMZ, temozolomide.
[a] Next generation sequencing (NGS) data on a subset of patients.

fluorescence in situ hybridization assays is that they only assess loss at the end of 1p and 19q.[28] The grading of diffuse glioma is based on certain rather subjective characteristics, such as the presence or absence of nuclear atypia, high cellularity, mitosis, endothelial proliferation, and necrosis. The clinical significance of grading of the diffuse gliomas within the WHO 2016 warrants reevaluation, as the histologic grade of *IDHmt* tumors is clinically less important compared with that of *IDHwt* tumors.[26,29,30]

Other Mutations and IDHwt Tumors

Most (approximately 95%) of the *IDHmt* astrocytomas also have a *TP53* mutation, and in 70% to 90%, inactivating alterations of *ATRX* are present. In 50% to 70% of the molecularly defined oligodendroglioma (*IDHmt* 1p/19 codel), inactivating mutations of *CIC* are present, and 15% to 30% of tumors have mutations in *FUBP* located on 1p.[31] Their clinical significance remains unclear. 1p/19q codeleted tumors also have mutations in the telomerase reverse transcriptase (*TERT*) promoter (*TERTp*) region, which are typically mutually exclusive with the *ATRX* mutations found in *IDHmt* astrocytoma.[26] *IDHwt* astrocytoma are heterogeneous and merit further molecular testing. In particular, *IDHwt* astrocytoma often show mutations in the epidermal growth factor receptor (EGFR) and phosphatase and tensin homolog (PTEN) gene, and those that show polysomy of chromosome 7, loss of heterozygosity of chromosome 10q, and *TERTp* mutations have a poor prognosis.[19,26,32–34] However, subsets of *IDHwt* astrocytoma may have entirely different and clinically relevant mutations, like *BRAF* mutations, or mutations in the histone *H3F3A* and *HIST1H3B* genes, which are found in clinically aggressive midline tumor (eg, pontine or thalamic gliomas) of adolescents and young adults. Thus, *IDHwt* gliomas are not to be considered a single entity, and further molecular diagnostics of these cases need to be pursued to better segregate this subgroup into different subtypes with different prognosis and response to treatment.

IMAGING

IDH-mutated tumors are more often located in the frontal lobes.[35,36] On non–contrast-enhanced computed tomography (NECT), both oligodendroglioma and astrocytoma typically appear as low-density lesions, and on MRI, they are hypointense on T1-weighted and hyperintense on T2-weighted images. Other typical radiological features of oligodendroglioma include a cortical-subcortical location, a rather heterogeneous signal intensity on T2-weighted images, and an indistinct border (**Fig. 2**). Coarse calcifications, which can be poorly visible on MRI and are best visible on NECT, are present in up to 90% of cases of oligodendroglioma. In contrast, astrocytomas typically do not calcify, do not involve the cortex, have a homogeneous signal intensity on T2-weighted images, and usually have a more distinct border (**Fig. 3**A).[37] Recently a typical pattern of *IDH*-mutated astrocytoma was described, in which the inner area of the fluid-attenuated inversion recover (FLAIR) images show low signal intensity despite a high signal intensity on T2-weighted images ("T2-FLAIR mismatch").[38] This appears to be quite specific for *IDHmt* astrocytoma, but is likely of limited sensitivity (**Fig. 4**). After contrast administration, low-grade astrocytomas do not enhance (**Fig. 3**B), whereas minimal to moderate patchy and multifocal enhancement with a dotlike or lacy pattern is present in up to 50% of low-grade oligodendroglioma. This makes differentiation with MR from anaplastic oligodendroglioma challenging. Although contrast enhancement is typically considered a feature of high-grade tumor, this has only 63% sensitivity and 50% specificity for differentiating high-grade from low-grade oligodendroglioma.[39] Anaplastic astrocytomas often do not show contrast

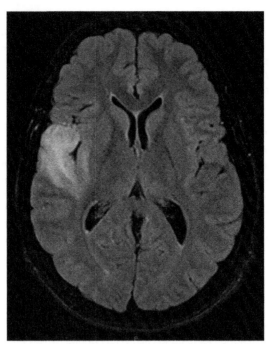

Fig. 2. Typical axial T2-weighted MRIs of an oligodendroglioma, *IDHmt* and 1p/19q code-leted, showing a hyperintense signal intensity lesion. Note the heterogeneous signal intensity, cortical involvement, and indistinct border of the tumor.

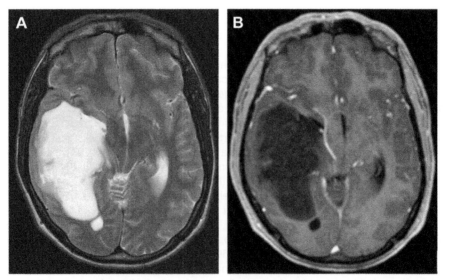

Fig. 3. Typical T2-weighted (*A*) and postcontrast T1-weighted (*B*) images of an astrocytoma, *IDHmt*. There is homogeneous signal intensity, a sharp border, and no involvement of the cortex in the astrocytoma, and no indication of enhancement.

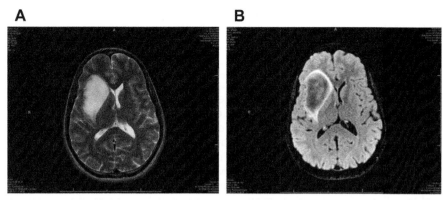

Fig. 4. T2-weighted (*A*) and FLAIR (*B*) MRIs of an *IDHmt* astrocytoma with T2-FLAIR mismatch. On T2 images, a homogeneously increased signal intensity of a sharply delineated tumor is visible without involvement of cortex. Despite an outer rim of increased signal intensity on FLAIR images, the central part of the tumor shows an area with decreased signal intensity.

enhancement, and if present it usually has a patchy, focal, or nodular appearance (in contrast to glioblastomas, that usually show extensive, intense, and commonly ringlike contrast enhancement). Perfusion MRI has reported high accuracy (>90%) in distinguishing high-grade from low-grade astrocytoma, with relative tumor blood volume being increased in high-grade astrocytoma.[40] In oligodendroglioma, perfusion is also commonly increased, and therefore is not useful in differentiating low-grade from high-grade tumor. Importantly, the appearance of new enhancement in a previously nonenhancing, untreated tumor is suggestive of malignant transformation. The same holds true of an increased growth rate.[41] Grade II gliomas are slow-growing tumors and often continue to follow a nonenhancing slow-growth pattern even when progressing after initial treatment (**Fig. 5**). Because of minimal changes from scan to

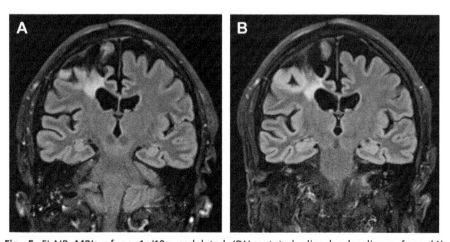

Fig. 5. FLAIR MRIs of an 1p/19q codeleted *IDH*-mutated oligodendroglioma from (*A*) February 2015 and (*B*) June 2017 when the patient returned with increased frequency of focal seizures. On initial review, the June 2017 MRI appeared stable compared with recent imaging; however, when compared with MRI from February 2015, tumor progression is clear.

scan, follow-up images must be compared with older images and not only with the most recent follow-up.

TREATMENT
Surgery

Surgery in diffuse glioma has 3 major objectives: (1) obtaining tissue diagnosis, (2) improving quality of life by relieving focal deficits and/or improving seizure control, and (2) increasing PFS and OS. The role of early surgery in nonenhancing, (presumed) LGG remains poorly understood, particularly in cases of incidentally discovered or relatively small lesions. There are no randomized trials examining the benefit of extensive surgery in LGG; data suggesting survival benefit with more extensive resections are from uncontrolled series that typically show the greatest survival benefit with (near) total resection.[6,42] A second question regarding surgical management concerns the timing of surgery in nonenhancing tumors. A retrospective study from 2 centers in Norway reported improved survival in the center that advocated early extensive surgery as opposed to the center that was inclined to biopsy only.[43] An update of this series shows that most of these patients had *IDH*-mutated tumors, but patient characteristics (eg, age, performance status, presence of enhancement) of this series do not reflect those of patients with favorable LGG.[44] A similar series failed to show convincing benefit from early surgery, leaving the question open if close surveillance of presumed LGG is a reasonable option.[45] Surgery should never be delayed in clearly enhancing or growing tumors, as they are likely to behave more aggressively.[46]

Nonetheless, with many retrospective series showing favorable survival after near total resection, it has become standard of care to operate early on suspected and well-defined "LGG-like" lesions if an extensive resection is expected to be safely possible. A variety of intraoperative monitoring techniques may allow a more extensive resection without increasing morbidity, especially in tumors located in eloquent areas.[47] In a prospective study of patients with favorable prognosis LGG, residual disease postoperatively, astrocytic histology, and large preoperative tumor size were negative prognostic factors for PFS.[48] Several studies of grade III glioma have confirmed the major impact of the extent of resection, which may be even more significant for *IDHmt* non-1p/19q codeleted tumors.[6,49,50] Resection should include the nonenhancing tumor part if safely possible.[51]

Radiotherapy

Three older trials have studied the dosage and timing of radiotherapy in histologically defined LGG. In controlled trials, no survival difference was observed between 45.0-Gy and 59.4-Gy radiotherapy or between 54.0-Gy and 65.0-Gy radiotherapy, with a tendency to fewer side effects after a lower dosage of radiotherapy.[52,53] Current trials in LGG typically use 50.4 Gy (54.0 in fractions of 1.8 Gy). A third trial reported no difference in OS between early radiotherapy (postoperatively) versus delayed radiotherapy (at the time of progression), but the clear increase in PFS shows that the timing is of less relevance as long as radiotherapy is given.[54] No radiotherapy dose-finding trials have been performed in grade III glioma or in *IDHmt* glioma, leaving the optimal radiotherapy dosage for grade III *IDHmt* glioma unexplored. Based on an older series, it has become standard practice to treat anaplastic gliomas with 33 fractions of 1.8 Gy to a total dose of 59.4 Gy, but whether indeed *IDHmt* 1p/19q codeleted anaplastic oligodendrogliomas require a dosage as high as 59.4 Gy for optimal management is unknown. This question is highly relevant when confronted with a patient with a large anaplastic oligodendroglioma in the which the radiation field may be large and the risk to neurocognition may be greater. With newer radiation therapy techniques (eg, proton therapy), the radiotherapy dosage to structures at risk (eg, hippocampal area) can be decreased, but whether that will decrease the risk of delayed radiation toxicities while maintaining the same survival benefit remains to be demonstrated.[55]

Chemotherapy

The sensitivity of grade II and III gliomas to PCV (procarbazine, CCNU or lomustine, and vincristine) and temozolomide chemotherapy was initially established in trials on recurrent (anaplastic) oligodendroglioma and astrocytoma.[18,56–59] These trials showed higher response rates of longer duration in oligodendroglioma (particularly those with combined 1p/19q loss) compared with astrocytoma. Randomized controlled trials have now established the efficacy of adding chemotherapy to radiotherapy in newly diagnosed grade II and III gliomas (**Table 2**). Three trials studied PCV: 2 in anaplastic oligodendroglioma[60,61] and 1 in LGG.[62] A fourth trial investigated temozolomide in 1p/19 non-codeleted anaplastic glioma.[63] In all these trials, outcome was improved with the addition of chemotherapy to radiotherapy, despite high crossover rates to chemotherapy (56%–79%) in the radiotherapy-only arm at tumor progression.[60–63] The trials on PCV chemotherapy in anaplastic oligodendroglioma showed more pronounced survival benefit in patients with 1p/19q codeleted tumors.[64,65] Within these trials, 3 related candidate predictive markers for benefit to adjuvant PCV have been proposed: *IDH* mutational status, CpG Island Methylated Phenotype (CIMP), and *MGMT* promoter methylation. In one study, *MGMT* promoter methylation assessed by a genomic-wide methylation assay was found to be the best predictor for benefit to chemotherapy. Another study identified *IDH* mutational status as a predictive factor.[64,65]

Two trials compared chemotherapy versus radiotherapy, either temozolomide or PCV versus radiotherapy, in a German anaplastic glioma trial and temozolomide versus radiotherapy in a European trial on LGG.[66,67] Neither study demonstrated improvement of outcome in patients initially treated with chemotherapy alone. In the European study on LGG, patients with *IDH* non-codeleted tumors treated with

Table 2
Hazard ratios (HRs) and 95% confidence intervals (CIs) reported in trials of adjuvant chemotherapy in grade II and III glioma

Histology	Trial Question	n	HR [95% CI] for OS
Anaplastic oligodendroglioma[61]	RT/PCV vs RT	368	0.75 [0.60–0.95]
Anaplastic oligodendroglioma[60]	RT/PCV-i vs RT	291	0.79 [0.60–1.04]
Low-grade glioma[62]	RT/PCV vs RT	251	0.59 [0.42–0.83]
Anaplastic astrocytoma[92]	RT/carmustine + DBD vs RT	193	0.77 [0.56–1.06]
Anaplastic glioma, 1p/19q intact[63]	RT vs RT/TMZ	745	0.65[a] [0.45–0.93]
Anaplastic glioma[66]	TMZ or PCV vs RT	318	1.11 [0.8–1.55]
Low-grade glioma[b,67]	RT vs TMZ	447	1.16 [0.9–1.5]
Anaplastic astrocytoma[69]	RT/TMZ vs RT/lomustine or carmustine	197	0.94 [0.67–1.32]

Abbreviations: DBD, dibromodulciterol; PCV, procarbazine, CCNU (lomustine), and vincristine; RT, radiotherapy; TMZ, temozolomide.
[a] 99.145% confidence interval.
[b] Primary endpoint: PFS.

radiotherapy had a longer PFS than those treated with temozolomide.[67] An uncontrolled study on initial treatment with temozolomide only reported an OS of 9.7 to 11.2 years in *IDHmt* tumors, with or without 1p/19q codeletion.[50] In the absence of a formal comparison of chemotherapy versus chemotherapy plus radiotherapy, it is prudent to assume that combination therapy will increase survival compared with any single-modality treatment (either radiotherapy alone or chemotherapy alone). A major consideration in favor of chemotherapy alone is that this may avoid or delay radiotherapy-induced delayed cognitive effects, but the current data suggest this may also jeopardize OS. Although better tolerated than PCV, the use of temozolomide has been associated with the development of a hypermutated tumor phenotype at progression through temozolomide-induced mutations of mismatch repair pathway genes.[68] Although this indicates resistance to temozolomide, from a clinical perspective, the DNA pattern at progression is less relevant than the duration of treatment response and OS.

Improved survival in newly diagnosed grade II and III tumors was first demonstrated in trials that investigated adjuvant PCV chemotherapy. The results of the Concurrent and Adjuvant Temozolomide Chemotherapy in Non-1p/19q Deleted Anaplastic Glioma (CATNON) trial show that adjuvant temozolomide is associated with a prolonged survival benefit for patients with grade III 1p/19q non-codeleted tumors, and it seems reasonable to assume this is also the case for grade II 1p/19q non-codeleted tumors. Another trial on anaplastic astrocytoma compared adjuvant temozolomide to adjuvant BCNU (carmustine) or CCNU in addition to radiotherapy, and observed no survival difference between these 2 treatments, but more myelosuppression in the nitrosourea-treated patients leading to more frequent early treatment discontinuation.[69] Some retrospective reports and subgroup analyses of larger studies have suggested a better outcome after PCV treatment compared with temozolomide treatment in 1p/19q codeleted tumors.[66,70,71] The ongoing CODEL study (NCT00887146) that compares radiation plus PCV chemotherapy versus radiation plus temozolomide in codeleted grade II and III tumors is designed to answer this question, but will take many years to conclude.

Postsurgical Treatment: Timing of Treatment

Because of the potential (delayed) side effects of surgery and radiotherapy, some advocate a wait-and-see policy for patients presenting with LGG, especially in those patients with favorable prognostic factors or in those who have undergone a (near) total resection. Data on the incidence of these delayed side effects and on the development of cognitive decline after radiotherapy in the absence of tumor progression are, however, limited. Randomized studies did not reveal a significant decline of the mini-mental status examination (MMSE) in patients with radiotherapy-treated LGG or a difference between patients treated with radiotherapy and chemotherapy, but the MMSE is of very limited sensitivity for detecting mild cognitive decline.[72,73] A study in long-term survivors of LGG after more than 10 years follow-up showed that patients who did not receive radiotherapy had stable radiological and cognitive status, but patients treated with radiotherapy showed a progressive decline in attentional functioning (even if treated with fraction doses that are regarded as safe; ie, 2 Gy or less).[74] A cohort study of long-term anaplastic oligodendroglioma survivors who received radiotherapy followed by adjuvant PCV showed that, among patients who remained progression free, 26% had no cognitive impairment, 44% had mild to moderate impairment, and 30% were severely impaired; 41% were employed and 81% could live independently.[75] The few patients in this cohort who had progressed during follow-up appeared to be doing worse. Of note, delayed cognitive complications are relevant only for patients who achieve long-term survivorship. Taken together, these data on cognitive deficits in long-term glioma survivors have been used as a rationale to delay radiotherapy and treat first with chemotherapy only; the current randomized trials, however, suggest that chemotherapy alone may jeopardize survival and tumor growth is also likely to affect cognitive functioning.

Because the pivotal PCV trial in LGG used incomplete resections and/or age older than 40 as inclusion criteria, it is routinely assumed these are the clinical factors that dictate which patients with LGG should receive adjuvant treatment.[62] These criteria have, however, a limited clinical rationale and incorporate no molecular or clinical features of treatment sensitivity.[76] For example, there is no clinical justification for a strict age cutoff, and other prognostic factors should be considered in clinical decision making. Delaying postoperative treatment is particularly relevant if prognostic factors suggest that a delay of several years is likely without jeopardizing the outcome of the patient. There are no data from trials on early versus delayed adjuvant treatment with radiotherapy and chemotherapy; many centers delay adjuvant treatment in patients with (near) totally resected LGG until further progression. For patients with 1p/19q codeleted *IDH*-mutated tumors, the age limit to follow them after a resection may be higher. Importantly, the presence of uncontrolled seizures after surgery is an important reason for postoperative treatment, as both chemotherapy and radiotherapy may improve seizure control.[54,77] The use of antiepileptics (AEDs) is associated with decreased cognitive functioning, and lowering the AED dosage once better seizure control is achieved also may improve cognitive functioning and reduce other side effects.[74]

Bevacizumab

In the past decade, bevacizumab has been extensively evaluated in patients with glioma, both at first diagnosis and at progression, predominantly in glioblastoma. However, several uncontrolled studies have reported outcomes in recurrent grade II and III tumors.[78–81] Response rates vary between 50% and 70%, 6-month PFS (PFS6) between 40% and 70%, and OS between 9 and 15 months. Despite its impact on PFS, bevacizumab does not improve OS in glioblastoma, neither in first-line treatment nor when given at progression as a single agent or in combination with lomustine. Similarly, in a randomized phase II trial in patients with recurrent 1p/19q non-codeleted grade II and III glioma and enhancing disease, the addition of bevacizumab to lomustine failed to increase PFS and OS.[82] Taken together, the role of bevacizumab in recurrent grade II and III tumors seems limited to the palliative care setting (edema reduction, symptom improvement), as a true antitumor effect is unlikely.

Treatment at Progression After Prior Chemotherapy

Past trials in patients with recurrent grade II and III glioma have documented responsiveness predominantly to regimens that are now used as first-line treatment following radiotherapy: PCV and temozolomide.[57,59,83,84] The treatment of tumors relapsing after prior chemotherapy (either given adjuvant or after first progression) is less clear. Data on second-line treatment with nitrosoureas or temozolomide are limited, but suggest lesser activity. Studies on second-line treatment in oligodendroglial tumors showed some activity of PCV after prior temozolomide or vice versa; but outcome was no longer associated with 1p/19q loss.[17,85,86] Similarly, single-agent lomustine was shown to have some activity after prior radiotherapy and temozolomide, with a

PFS6 rate of 40%.[87] Obviously, treatment options for progression after prior chemo-therapy is a high-priority, unmet clinical need.

FUTURE PERSPECTIVES

Future directions include the development of personalized therapies that target the metabolic and cytogenetic characteristics of astrocytic and oligodendroglial tu-mors. The PI3K/Akt/mammalian target of rapamycin (mTOR) pathway regulates cellular proliferation and is often activated in LGGs. A recent trial evaluated ever-olimus, an inhibitor of mTOR, in recurrent LGG,[88] and there are ongoing studies evaluating this pathway in high-risk LGG. The mutated *IDH* complex has been tar-geted with *IDH* inhibitors in clinical trials.[89] The use of these agents in combination with classic chemotherapy or radiotherapy may not be very promising, as in vitro studies suggest that the metabolic changes induced by *IDH* mutations may actu-ally sensitize cells for radiotherapy and chemotherapy.[12,13] In vitro studies also suggest that PARP inhibitors may be beneficial in *IDH* mutant tumors.[14,15] Several immunotherapy studies are being developed for grade II glioma. Examples are vaccine therapies that target the *IDH* mutation, and peptide vaccines (such as GBM6-AD-poly-ICLC, a vaccine created from autologous dendritic cells pulsed with autologous tumor lysate).[90]

SUMMARY AND TREATMENT RECOMMENDATIONS

The WHO classification of diffuse grade II/III glioma is now based on molecular characteristics. This new classification has significant clinical implications, both with respect to prognosis and treatment selection. Patients with grade II/III gli-oma with an *IDH* mutation have a better prognosis, even more so if their tumor is also 1p/19q codeleted. *IDHwt* gliomas are a heterogeneous group of tumors, but the presence of *TERTp* mutations or trisomy of 7 and loss of heterozygosity (LOH) of 10q indicate poor outcome. An early and extensive resection (if safe) is standard of care in patients with presumed LGGs. If extensive resection is not possible and treatment is not immediately indicated, an alternative approach is to wait until growth has been documented on follow-up imaging. At that time, a biopsy should be performed if a resection is still not feasible. Physiologic imaging, such as perfusion, may direct the biopsy to the most aggressive component. If a favorable prognosis patient with a grade II *IDHmt* tumor has undergone an exten-sive resection, further treatment can be postponed until tumor progression. It re-mains unclear what amount of growth amounts to progression; this must be decided on a case-by-case basis. At the time of progression, a reoperation also should be considered.

Combined chemo-radiation with temozolomide should be considered in *IDHwt* grade II and III glioma, especially in the presence of other alterations that suggest a glioblastomalike outcome (*TERTp* mutations, or 7+/10q LOH). The best postsurgical treatment for patients with grade II and III *IDHmt* glioma is a combination of radiotherapy and chemotherapy. For *IDHmt* non-codeleted tumors, the use of temozolomide is now evidence based; whether PCV (over temozolomide) is indeed the regimen of choice in 1p/19q codeleted tumors re-mains unresolved. Chemotherapy-only treatment should be limited to patients in whom radiotherapy would require a very large treatment volume, with increased risks of delayed cognitive effects. The possibility of a decreased survival with an initial chemotherapy-only approach must be discussed with the patient. Last, of-fering patients with glioma access to a rehabilitation program is important; with longer survival possible in many patients, cognitive dysfunction will affect quality of life.

REFERENCES

1. Louis DN, Ohgaki H, Wiestler OD, et al. WHO classification of tumours of the central nervous sytem. 4th edition. Lyon (France): International Agency for Research on Cancer; 2016.
2. van den Bent MJ, Smits M, Kros JM, et al. Diffuse infiltrating oligodendroglioma and astrocytoma. J Clin Oncol 2017;35(21):2394–401.
3. Ostrom QT, Gittleman H, Xu J, et al. CBTRUS statistical report: primary brain and central nervous system tumors diagnosed in the United States in 2009-2013. Neuro Oncol 2016;18(Suppl 5):iv1–62.
4. Mandonnet E, Delattre JY, Tanguy ML, et al. Continuous growth of mean tumor diameter in a subset of grade II gliomas. Ann Neurol 2003;53:524–8.
5. Gorlia T, Wu W, Wang M, et al. New validated prognostic models and prognostic calculators in patients with low-grade gliomas diagnosed by central pathology review: a pooled analysis of EORTC/RTOG/NCCTG phase III clinical trials. Neuro Oncol 2013;15:1568–79.
6. Gorlia T, Delattre JY, Brandes AA, et al. New clinical, pathological and molecular prognostic models and calculators in patients with locally diagnosed anaplastic oligodendroglioma or oligoastrocytoma. A prognostic factor analysis of European Organisation for Research and Treatment of Cancer Brain Tumour Group Study 26951. Eur J Cancer 2013;49:3477–85.
7. Parsons DW, Jones S, Zhang X, et al. An integrated genomic analysis of human glioblastoma multiforme. Science 2008;321:1807–12.
8. van den Bent MJ, Dubbink HJ, Marie Y, et al. IDH1 and IDH2 mutations are prognostic but not predictive for outcome in anaplastic oligodendroglial tumors: a report of the European Organization for Research and Treatment of Cancer Brain Tumor Group. Clin Cancer Res 2010;16:1597–604.
9. Metellus P, Coulibaly B, Colin C, et al. Absence of IDH mutation identifies a novel radiologic and molecular subtype of WHO grade II gliomas with dismal prognosis. Acta Neuropathol 2010;120:719–29.
10. Lu C, Ward PS, Kapoor GS, et al. IDH mutation impairs histone demethylation and results in a block to cell differentiation. Nature 2012;483(7390):474–8.
11. Turcan S, Rohle D, Goenka A, et al. IDH1 mutation is sufficient to establish the glioma hypermethylator phenotype. Nature 2012;483:479–83.
12. Wang P, Wu J, Ma S, et al. Oncometabolite D-2-hydroxyglutarate inhibits ALKBH DNA repair enzymes and sensitizes IDH mutant cells to alkylating agents. Cell Rep 2015;13:2353–61.
13. Molenaar RJ, Botman D, Smits MA, et al. Radioprotection of IDH1-mutated cancer cells by the IDH1-mutant inhibitor AGI-5198. Cancer Res 2015;75:4790–802.
14. Sulkowski PL, Corso CD, Robinson ND, et al. 2-Hydroxyglutarate produced by neomorphic IDH mutations suppresses homologous recombination and induces PARP inhibitor sensitivity. Sci Transl Med 2017;9 [pii:eaal2463].
15. Lu Y, Kwintkiewicz J, Liu Y, et al. Chemosensitivity of IDH1-mutated gliomas due to an impairment in PARP1-mediated DNA repair. Cancer Res 2017;77:1709–18.
16. Reifenberger J, Reifenberger G, Liu L, et al. Molecular genetic analysis of oligodendroglial tumors shows preferential allelic deletions on 19q and 1p. Am J Pathol 1994;145:1175–90.

17. Kouwenhoven MC, Kros JM, French PJ, et al. 1p/19q loss within oligodendro-glioma is predictive for response to first line temozolomide but not to salvage treatment. Eur J Cancer 2006;42:2499–503.
18. Cairncross JG, Ueki K, Zlatescu MC, et al. Specific genetic predictors of chemo-therapeutic response and survival in patients with anaplastic oligodendroglio-mas. J Natl Cancer Inst 1998;90:1473–9.
19. Brat DJ, Verhaak RG, Aldape KD, et al. Comprehensive, integrative genomic analysis of diffuse lower-grade gliomas. N Engl J Med 2015;372:2481–98.
20. Louis DN, Ohgaki H, Wiestler OD, et al. WHO classification of tumours of the cen-tral nervous system. Lyon (France): International Agency for Research on Cancer (IARC); 2007.
21. van den Bent MJ. Interobserver variation of the histopathological diagnosis in clinical trials on glioma: a clinician's perspective. Acta Neuropathol 2010;120: 297–304.
22. Dubbink HJ, Atmodimedjo PN, Kros JM, et al. Molecular classification of anaplastic oligodendroglioma using next generation sequencing. A report of the prospective randomized EORTC Brain Tumor Group 26951 phase III trial. Neuro Oncol 2016;18:388–400.
23. Wiestler B, Capper D, Sill M, et al. Integrated DNA methylation and copy-number profiling identify three clinically and biologically relevant groups of anaplastic glioma. Acta Neuropathol 2014;128:561–71.
24. Louis DN, Perry A, Reifenberger G, et al. The 2016 World Health Organization classification of tumors of the central nervous system: a summary. Acta Neuropa-thol 2016;131:803–20.
25. Sahm F, Reuss D, Koelsche C, et al. Farewell to oligoastrocytoma: in situ molec-ular genetics favor classification as either oligodendroglioma or astrocytoma. Acta Neuropathol 2014;128:551–9.
26. Pekmezci M, Rice T, Molinaro AM, et al. Adult infiltrating gliomas with WHO 2016 integrated diagnosis: additional prognostic roles of ATRX and TERT. Acta Neuro-pathol 2017;133:1001–16.
27. Jenkins RB, Blair H, Ballman KV, et al. A t(1;19)(q10;p10) mediates the combined deletions of 1p and 19q and predicts a better prognosis of patients with oligoden-droglioma. Cancer Res 2006;66:9852–61.
28. Idbaih A, Marie Y, Pierron G, et al. Two types of chromosome 1p losses with opposite significance in gliomas. Ann Neurol 2005;58:483–7.
29. Reuss DE, Mamatjan Y, Schrimpf D, et al. IDH mutant diffuse and anaplastic astrocytomas have similar age at presentation and little difference in survival: a grading problem for WHO. Acta Neuropathol 2015;129:867–73.
30. Olar A, Wani KM, Alfaro-Munoz KD, et al. IDH mutation status and role of WHO grade and mitotic index in overall survival in grade II-III diffuse gliomas. Acta Neuropathol 2015;129:585–96.
31. Yip S, Butterfield YS, Morozova O, et al. Concurrent CIC mutations, IDH muta-tions, and 1p/19q loss distinguish oligodendrogliomas from other cancers. J Pathol 2012;226:7–16.
32. Weller M, Weber RG, Willscher E, et al. Molecular classification of diffuse cerebral WHO grade II/III gliomas using genome- and transcriptome-wide profiling im-proves stratification of prognostically distinct patient groups. Acta Neuropathol 2015;129:679–93.
33. Weller M, Sommer N, Stevnes A, et al. Increased intrathecal synthesis of fibro-nectin in bacterial and carcinomatous meningitis. Acta Neurol Scand 1990;82: 138–42.

34. Ceccarelli M, Barthel FP, Malta TM, et al. Molecular profiling reveals biologically discrete subsets and pathways of progression in diffuse glioma. Cell 2016;164: 550–63.

35. Lai A, Kharbanda S, Pope WB, et al. Evidence for sequenced molecular evolution of IDH1 mutant glioblastoma from a distinct cell of origin. J Clin Oncol 2011;29: 4482–90.

36. Smits M, van den Bent MJ. Imaging correlates of adult glioma genotypes. Radiology 2017;284(2):316–31.

37. Smits M. Imaging of oligodendroglioma. Br J Radiol 2016;89:20150857.

38. Patel SH, Poisson LM, Brat DJ, et al. T2-FLAIR mismatch, an imaging biomarker for IDH and 1p/19q status in lower grade gliomas: a TCGA/TCIA project. Clin Cancer Res 2017;23(20):6078–85.

39. White ML, Zhang Y, Kirby P, et al. Can tumor contrast enhancement be used as a criterion for differentiating tumor grades of oligodendrogliomas? AJNR Am J Neuroradiol 2005;26:784–90.

40. Morita N, Wang S, Chawla S, et al. Dynamic susceptibility contrast perfusion weighted imaging in grading of nonenhancing astrocytomas. J Magn Reson Imaging 2010;32:803–8.

41. Rees J, Watt H, Jager HR, et al. Volumes and growth rates of untreated adult low-grade gliomas indicate risk of early malignant transformation. Eur J Radiol 2009; 72(1):54–64.

42. Smith JS, Chang EF, Lamborn KR, et al. Role of extent of resection in the long-term outcome of low-grade hemispheric gliomas. J Clin Oncol 2008;26:1338–45.

43. Jakola AS, Myrmel KS, Kloster R, et al. Comparison of a strategy favoring early surgical resection vs a strategy favoring watchful waiting in low-grade gliomas. JAMA 2012;308:1881–8.

44. Jakola AS, Skjulsvik AJ, Myrmel KS, et al. Surgical resection versus watchful waiting in low-grade gliomas. Ann Oncol 2017;28(8):1942–8.

45. Wijnenga MMJ, Mattni T, French PJ, et al. Does early resection of presumed low-grade glioma improve survival? A clinical perspective. J Neurooncol 2017;133: 137–46.

46. Pallud J, Capelle L, Taillandier L, et al. Prognostic significance of imaging contrast enhancement for WHO grade II gliomas. Neuro Oncol 2009;11:176–82.

47. Duffau H, Lopes M, Arthuis F, et al. Contribution of intraoperative electrical stimulations in surgery of low grade gliomas: a comparative study between two series without (1985-96) and with (1996-2003) functional mapping in the same institution. J Neurol Neurosurg Psychiatry 2005;76:845–51.

48. Shaw EG, Berkey B, Coons SW, et al. Recurrence following neurosurgeon-determined gross-total resection of adult supratentorial low-grade glioma: results of a prospective clinical trial. J Neurosurg 2008;109:835–41.

49. Kawaguchi T, Sonoda Y, Shibahara I, et al. Impact of gross total resection in patients with WHO grade III glioma harboring the IDH 1/2 mutation without the 1p/19q co-deletion. J Neurooncol 2016;129:505–14.

50. Wahl M, Phillips JJ, Molinaro AM, et al. Chemotherapy for adult low-grade gliomas: clinical outcomes by molecular subtype in a phase II study of adjuvant temozolomide. Neuro Oncol 2017;19:242–51.

51. Beiko J, Suki D, Hess KR, et al. IDH1 mutant malignant astrocytomas are more amenable to surgical resection and have a survival benefit associated with maximal surgical resection. Neuro Oncol 2014;16:81–91.

52. Shaw E, Arusell RM, Scheithauer B, et al. A prospective randomized trial of low versus high dose radiation in adults with a supratentorial low grade glioma: initial report of a NCCTG-RTOG-ECOG study. J Clin Oncol 2002;20:2267–76.
53. Karim ABMF, Maat B, Hatlevoll R, et al. A randomized trial on dose-response in radiation therapy of low grade cerebral glioma: European Organization for Research and Treatment of Cancer (EORTC) study 2284. Int J Radiat Oncol Biol Phys 1996;36:549–56.
54. van den Bent MJ, Afra D, De Witte O, et al. Long term results of EORTC study 22845: a randomized trial on the efficacy of early versus delayed radiation therapy of low-grade astrocytoma and oligodendroglioma in the adult. Lancet 2005;366:985–90.
55. Harrabi SB, Bougatf N, Mohr A, et al. Dosimetric advantages of proton therapy over conventional radiotherapy with photons in young patients and adults with low-grade glioma. Strahlenther Onkol 2016;192:759–69.
56. Cairncross G, Macdonald D, Ludwin S, et al. Chemotherapy for anaplastic oligodendroglioma. J Clin Oncol 1994;12:2013–21.
57. Yung WKA, Prados M, Yaya-Tur R, et al. Multicenter phase II trial of temozolomide in patients with anaplastic astrocytoma or anaplastic oligoastrocytoma at first relapse. J Clin Oncol 1999;17:2762–71.
58. van den Bent MJ, Taphoorn MJ, Brandes AA, et al. Phase II study of first-line chemotherapy with temozolomide in recurrent oligodendroglioma: the European Organisation of Research and Treatment of Cancer Brain Tumor Group study 26971. J Clin Oncol 2003;21:2525–8.
59. Taal W, Dubbink HJ, Zonnenberg CB, et al. First-line temozolomide chemotherapy in progressive low-grade astrocytomas after radiotherapy: molecular characteristics in relation to response. Neuro Oncol 2011;13:235–41.
60. Cairncross G, Wang M, Shaw E, et al. Phase III trial of chemoradiotherapy for anaplastic oligodendroglioma: long-term results of RTOG 9402. J Clin Oncol 2013;31:337–43.
61. van den Bent MJ, Brandes AA, Taphoorn MJ, et al. Adjuvant procarbazine, lomustine, and vincristine chemotherapy in newly diagnosed anaplastic oligodendroglioma: long-term follow-up of EORTC Brain Tumor Group Study 26951. J Clin Oncol 2013;31:344–50.
62. Buckner JC, Shaw EG, Pugh SL, et al. Radiation plus procarbazine, CCNU, and vincristine in low-grade glioma. N Engl J Med 2016;374:1344–55.
63. van den Bent MJ, Baumert B, Erridge SC, et al. Interim results from the CATNON trial (EORTC study 26053–22054) of treatment with concurrent and adjuvant temozolomide for 1p/19q non-co-deleted anaplastic glioma: a phase 3, randomised, open-label intergroup study. Lancet 2017;390(10103):1645–53.
64. Cairncross JG, Wang M, Jenkins RB, et al. Benefit from procarbazine, lomustine, and vincristine in oligodendroglial tumors is associated with mutation of IDH. J Clin Oncol 2014;32:783–90.
65. van den Bent MJ, Erdem-Eraslan L, Idbaih A, et al. MGMT-STP27 methylation status as predictive marker for response to PCV in anaplastic oligodendrogliomas and oligoastrocytomas. A report from EORTC study 26951. Clin Cancer Res 2013;19:5513–22.
66. Wick W, Roth P, Hartmann C, et al. Long-term analysis of the NOA-04 randomized phase III trial of sequential radiochemotherapy of anaplastic glioma with PCV or temozolomide. Neuro Oncol 2016;18(11):1529–37.
67. Baumert BG, Hegi ME, van den Bent MJ, et al. Temozolomide chemotherapy versus radiotherapy in high-risk low-grade glioma (EORTC 22033-26033): a

randomised, open-label, phase 3 intergroup study. Lancet Oncol 2016;17(11): 1521–32.

68. Johnson BE, Mazor T, Hong C, et al. Mutational analysis reveals the origin and therapy-driven evolution of recurrent glioma. Science 2014;343:189–93.

69. Chang S, Zhang P, Cairncross JG, et al. Phase III randomized study of radiation and temozolomide versus radiation and nitrosourea therapy for anaplastic astrocytoma: results of NRG Oncology RTOG 9813. Neuro Oncol 2017;19(2):252–8.

70. Lassman AB, Iwamoto FM, Cloughesy TF, et al. International retrospective study of over 1000 adults with anaplastic oligodendroglial tumors. Neuro Oncol 2011; 13:649–59.

71. Figarella-Branger D, Mokhtari K, Dehais C, et al. Mitotic index, microvascular proliferation, and necrosis define 3 groups of 1p/19q codeleted anaplastic oligodendrogliomas associated with different genomic alterations. Neuro Oncol 2014;16: 1244–54.

72. Prabhu RS, Won M, Shaw EG, et al. Effect of the addition of chemotherapy to radiotherapy on cognitive function in patients with low-grade glioma: secondary analysis of RTOG 98-02. J Clin Oncol 2014;32:535–41.

73. Reijneveld JC, Taphoorn MJ, Coens C, et al. Health-related quality of life in patients with high-risk low-grade glioma (EORTC 22033-26033): a randomised, open-label, phase 3 intergroup study. Lancet Oncol 2016;17:1533–42.

74. Douw L, Klein M, Fagel SS, et al. Cognitive and radiological effects of radiotherapy in patients with low-grade glioma: long-term follow-up. Lancet Neurol 2009;8:810–8.

75. Habets EJ, Taphoorn MJ, Nederend S, et al. Health-related quality of life and cognitive functioning in long-term anaplastic oligodendroglioma and oligoastrocytoma survivors. J Neurooncol 2014;116:161–8.

76. van den Bent MJ. Practice changing mature results of RTOG study 9802: another positive PCV trial makes adjuvant chemotherapy part of standard of care in low-grade glioma. Neuro Oncol 2014;16:1570–4.

77. Koekkoek JA, Kerkhof M, Dirven L, et al. Seizure outcome after radiotherapy and chemotherapy in low-grade glioma patients: a systematic review. Neuro Oncol 2015;17:924–34.

78. Desjardins A, Reardon DA, Herndon JE, et al. Bevacizumab plus irinotecan in recurrent WHO grade 3 malignant gliomas. Clin Cancer Res 2008;14:7068–73.

79. Chamberlain MC, Johnston S. Bevacizumab for recurrent alkylator-refractory anaplastic oligodendroglioma. Cancer 2009;115:1734–43.

80. Chamberlain MC, Johnston S. Salvage chemotherapy with bevacizumab for recurrent alkylator-refractory anaplastic astrocytoma. J Neurooncol 2009;91: 359–67.

81. Taillibert S, Vincent LA, Granger B, et al. Bevacizumab and irinotecan for recurrent oligodendroglial tumors. Neurology 2009;72:1601–6.

82. Van Den Bent MJ, Klein M, Smits M, et al. Final results of the EORTC Brain Tumor Group randomized phase II TAVAREC trial on temozolomide with or without bevacizumab in 1st recurrence grade II/III glioma without 1p/19q co-deletion. J Clin Oncol 2017;35:2009.

83. Cairncross JG, Macdonald DR. Successful chemotherapy for recurrent oligodendroglioma. Ann Neurol 1988;23:360–4.

84. van den Bent MJ, Kros JM, Schellens JHM, et al. PCV-chemotherapy in anaplastic oligodendroglioma: time for a prospective, randomised study [abstract]. J Neurooncol 1996;30:130.

85. van den Bent MJ, Chinot O, Boogerd W, et al. Second line chemotherapy with Temozolomide in recurrent oligodendroglioma after PCV (procarbazine, lomustine and vincristine) chemotherapy: EORTC Brain Tumor Group phase II study 26972. Ann Oncol 2003;14:599–602.

86. Triebels V, Taphoorn MJB, Brandes AA, et al. Response to 2nd line PCV chemotherapy in recurrent oligodendroglioma after 1st line temozolomide. Neurology 2004;63:904–6.

87. Chamberlain MC. Salvage therapy with lomustine for temozolomide refractory recurrent anaplastic astrocytoma: a retrospective study. J Neurooncol 2015; 122:329–38.

88. McBride SM, Perez DA, Polley MY, et al. Activation of PI3K/mTOR pathway occurs in most adult low-grade gliomas and predicts patient survival. J Neurooncol 2010;97(1):33–40.

89. Clark O, Yen K, Mellinghoff IK. Molecular pathways: isocitrate dehydrogenase mutations in cancer. Clin Cancer Res 2016;22:1837–42.

90. Schumacher T, Bunse L, Pusch S, et al. A vaccine targeting mutant IDH1 induces antitumour immunity. Nature 2014;512:324–7.

91. Wick W, Roth P, Hartmann C, et al. Long-term analysis of the NOA-04 randomized phase III trial of sequential radiochemotherapy of anaplastic glioma with PCV or temozolomide. Neuro Oncol 2016;18:1529–37.

92. Hildebrand J, Gorlia T, Kros JM, et al. Adjuvant dibromodulcitol and BCNU chemotherapy in anaplastic astrocytoma: results of a randomised European Organisation for Research and Treatment of Cancer phase III study (EORTC study 26882). Eur J Cancer 2008;44:1210–6.

Understanding and Treating Glioblastoma

Wolfgang Wick, MD[a,b,]*, Michael Platten, MD[c,d]

KEYWORDS

- Glioblastoma • MGMT • Repositioning of drugs • Precision medicine • Biomarker
- Radiomics • Treatment resistance • Immunotherapy

KEY POINTS

- Molecular biomarkers are entering diagnostics in neurooncology; current efforts aim at developing biomarkers-based treatment concepts.
- Understanding and overcoming resistance at multiple levels is the key challenge in glioblastoma; reviewing the failure of past concept-driven approaches such as antiangiogenic therapies or trials of unselected populations is necessary.
- The failure of recent immunotherapy trials should provide lessons for future development.
- Despite limited options to molecularly stratify glioblastoma into different age groups, patient functional status and age are key factors to consider for treatment decisions.

INTRODUCTION

The natural disease course in glioblastoma (GB) is invariably grim. A clinical event (eg, a seizure) or a cerebral image incidentally triggers clinical workup, commonly resulting in a maximal safe surgery. Diagnosis is made by careful neuropathological assessment of the tissue, including immunohistochemistry and selected molecular tests. Adjuvant treatments include radiotherapy (RT) to an area of the brain defined by the contrast-enhancing volume plus a safety margin, as well as alkylating chemotherapy with temozolomide (TMZ).[1] Variation at this stage is limited and may include modification of RT (and sometimes chemotherapy) according to age,[2] and the intensification or omission of alkylating chemotherapy according to the methylation status of the promotor region of the O^6-methylguanine DNA-methyltransferase (MGMT) gene[1,3,4] and

[a] Neurology Clinic, University of Heidelberg, INF 400, 69120 Heidelberg, Germany; [b] Clinical Cooperation Unit (CCU) Neurooncology, German Cancer Consortium (DKTK), German Cancer Research Center (DKFZ), Heidelberg, Germany; [c] Department of Neurology, Universitätsmedizin Mannheim, Medical Faculty Mannheim, Heidelberg University, Theodor-Kutzer-Ufer 1-3, 68167 Mannheim, Germany; [d] Clinical Cooperation Unit Neuroimmunology and Brain Tumor Immunology, German Cancer Consortium (DKTK), German Cancer Research Center (DKFZ), Heidelberg, Germany
* Corresponding author. Neurology Clinic, University of Heidelberg, INF 400, 69120 Heidelberg, Germany.
E-mail address: wolfgang.wick@med.uni-heidelberg.de

Neurol Clin 36 (2018) 485–499
https://doi.org/10.1016/j.ncl.2018.04.006
0733-8619/18/© 2018 Elsevier Inc. All rights reserved.
neurologic.theclinics.com

potentially point mutations in the promoter of the *telomerase reverse transcriptase* (*TERT*) gene, resulting in increased telomerase expression.[5]

Currently available GB treatments are not curative but there are subgroups of patients who derive greater benefit from current treatments, radiation, and alkylating chemotherapy, as well as experimental targeted or immune therapies. Features hampering treatment efficacy across many cancers are prominently present in GB: rapid and infiltrative growth, most likely imitating features of normal brain development[6]; clonal heterogeneity with a component of primitive (or stem-like) features, varying over time with treatment selection[7]; and pathologic angiogenesis, resulting in a hypoxic and immunosuppressive microenvironment.[8]

Whereas the concept of molecular subclassification defined by gene expression and DNA methylation has been spearheaded[9] and further refined[10,11] in GB, the immediate clinical impact on the diagnostic classification,[12] treatment, or even trial development has remained limited. Consequently, trials to date do not use epigenetic or genetic criteria to biologically subdivide GB. *MGMT* promoter hypermethylation (despite its relevance as a predictive marker for response to alkylating chemotherapy) has almost no impact on clinical decision-making, except perhaps in elderly patients.

Understanding of molecular characteristics and cell intrinsic mechanisms of GB pathogenesis has evolved in the last decade.[6,9–11,13] The updated 2016 World Health Organization classification of central nervous system tumors[12] integrates genotypic and phenotypic parameters to GB diagnostics, notably the presence or absence of *isocitrate dehydrogenase* (*IDH*) mutations. These and other mutated drivers in GB are putative targets for treatment. Recent studies in colon cancer revealed that subjects with mismatch repair deficiency (dMMR) respond better to anti-programmed death (PD)-1 therapy.[14] Additional studies indicate that other solid tumors with MMR deficiency, including GB, are sensitive to anti-PD1 therapy.[15,16] There is increasing effort to integrate molecularly informed diagnoses into therapy decision-making.[17–19] Although precision medicine in cancer proposes that genomic characterization of tumors can inform personalized targeted therapies, this proposition is complicated in GB by spatial and temporal heterogeneity.[20]

In parallel with the generation of increasingly complex molecular models for ex vivo data analysis, advanced MRI and data analysis (eg, radiomics) are being developed to decipher information about tumors noninvasively.[21]

Despite all efforts and successes in other solid tumors and the enormous power of basic science in neurooncology, a lack of stringent integration of the existing knowledge into clinical (research) practices has left GB lagging behind the current evolution of modern oncology. The focus to date on traditional all-comers trials, as well as the dearth of widely accepted molecular tests and subsequent enrichment strategies, are important obstacles. An example of concepts in which selection might have made a difference includes the antiangiogenic studies with bevacizumab. Despite the post hoc development of a predictive RNA expression signature favoring bevacizumab treatment in proneural subtypes,[22] the proof-of-concept study has still not been planned. Other examples of putative biomarkers that can be used for subject selection include methylation levels for CpG2 in the region of the *CD95 ligand* (*CD95L*) gene promotor as a predictive biomarker for the CD95L inhibitory recombinant protein asunercept combined with reirradiation in recurrent GB[23] and mechanistic target of rapamycin (mTOR) Ser2448 phosphorylation as a predictive biomarker for the mTOR inhibitor temsirolimus in newly diagnosed GB.[24]

In GB, which harms patients by locally destructive brain growth as opposed to systemic metastases, immunosuppression has been extensively studied. Multiple pathways are proposed to mediate GB-associated immunosuppression.

Among these are transforming growth factor beta (TGF-ß) and CD95 signaling; checkpoint receptors, such as cytotoxic T cell antigen-4 and PD-1; and intracellular signaling involving tryptophan metabolism and enzymes, such as indoleamine-2,3-dioxygenase (IDO) or tryptophan-2,3-dioxygenase (TDO).[25,26] Although trials to inhibit TGF-ß have largely failed to date,[27] the success story of checkpoint inhibition in melanoma and other cancers awaits confirmation in GB. Again, current clinical trial data do not support the efficacy of checkpoint inhibitor in all-comers, unselected population trials in GB. However, there is already a path for GB patients harboring microsatellite instability-high (MSI-H) or dMMR to be treated with the PD-1 inhibitor pembrolizumab. The US Food and Drug Administration granted accelerated approval to pembrolizumab for adult and pediatric patients with unresectable or metastatic MSI-H or dMMR solid tumors who have progressed following prior treatment and who have no satisfactory alternative treatment options.

Vaccine-based immunotherapies vary in design with respect to target selection and vaccine generation. Targets selected for vaccine development in GB include monogenic approaches, such as epidermal growth factor receptor variant III (EGFRvIII),[28] IDH1 (R132H),[29,30] or H3.3K27 M[31]; predefined multiepitope approaches, such as in IMA950[32]; profiling-based selection of a limited number of targets (eg, glioma actively personalized vaccine [GAPVAC]); unbiased approaches with undefined tumor-derived peptides (eg, HSPPC-96); or whole tumor cell lysates (eg, DCVax). To date, well-conducted phase 3 randomized controlled trials, such as ACT IV (examining the addition of rindopepimut, a vaccine against epidermal growth factor receptor variant III (EGFRvIII), to standard of care in newly diagnosed EGFRvIII mutant GB) have not demonstrated efficacy for glioma vaccines.[28,33] The failures in these trials should not distract investigators from developing further vaccine trials in glioma subjects. Instead, important questions, such as target and subject selection, vaccine vehicle, and combination strategies should be addressed upfront in any vaccine trial. This will require innovative, well-designed clinical trials, including assessment of posttreatment tumor tissue. Only then can the magnitude and nature of the intratumoral immune response in response to treatment, and the mechanisms of response and resistance in correlation to peripheral immune biomarkers, imaging parameters, and outcome, be understood.

CURRENT CHALLENGES AND OPPORTUNITIES

Several groups have proposed that GB is a widespread disease of the brain and not a focal malignant growth. The efficacy of currently available therapies is likely limited by GB's propensity for rapid and infiltrative growth. GB cells interconnect via a functional tumor cell network composed of thin and very long membrane tubes called tumor microtubes (TMs),[6] most likely imitating features of brain development. Growth associated protein 43 (Gap43) and tweety-homolog 1 (Tthy1), 2 already known molecular drivers of TM formation in GB, also play an important role in neurodevelopment.[34] Given the prominent role of TMs, discovering and exploring functional candidates to target and disrupt the network will be a challenge but also an opportunity for the future.

Improving Standard Therapies

Maximal safe surgery has shown to be beneficial for subjects in several trials and the extent of surgical resection is often among the most important prognostic factors in trials. Despite the conceptual challenges of further improving a local treatment, surgery is key for tissue sampling from different areas of the tumor, thus allowing spatial annotation of samples to model heterogeneity in GB. Therefore, it seems plausible to adapt and refine surgical techniques with the addition of fluorescence to dissect GB cell compartments with lower or higher oxygen levels and differential stem cell content,[35] or with intraoperative MRI to optimize macroscopic tumor removal.[36]

RT to a limited part of the brain (despite the conceptual shortcomings of focal treatments) can likewise further improve radiation target definition (ie, using metabolic imaging[37]) and avoid neurotoxicity (eg, with protons by reducing nontarget tissue dose), although the overall clinical benefit of dosimetric advantages in GB patients remains to be determined.[38] Also, the claimed differential DNA repair pathway choice following proton versus photon radiation[39] needs clinical substantiation.

Tumor-treating fields (TTFields) use alternating electrical fields to inhibit mitoses via disruption of the spindle apparatus.[40] In a randomized trial, the addition of TTFields to standard RT and TMZ in newly diagnosed GB extended overall survival (OS) (hazard ratio [HR] 0.64, 99.4% CI 0.42–0.98, $P = .004$).[40] Whether the magnitude of OS benefit justifies the individual burden and the societal cost is yet to be determined. The long-term relevance of these fields will be determined by whether they are routinely integrated into daily practice and the success (or not) of other concepts (see later discussion).

Other recent data regarding improving the standard of care treatment concern the intensity or duration of TMZ. There is no clear benefit to extending TMZ maintenance therapy beyond 6 cycles.[41] In contrast, results from the CeTeG/NOA-09 phase III trial in subjects with newly diagnosed hypermethylated *MGMT* GB suggest an OS benefit for the combination of RT with lomustine (CCNU) and TMZ[4] (see later discussion).

UPDATE ON THE ELDERLY

According to the Central Brain Tumor Registry of the United States (CBTRUS) statistical report, which comprises data on subjects with malignant primary central nervous system tumors diagnosed between 2006 and 2010, the median age at GB diagnosis is 64 years.[42] This means that almost half of all patients diagnosed in the United States with GB are elderly (age ≥65–70 years) as defined in GB clinical trials. Treatment principles should be the same for both elderly and young GB patients, with a focus on maximizing benefit and minimizing risk from every intervention. However, a more detailed assessment of the risks and benefits are needed for elderly patients because the benefit is generally not as great in elderly compared with younger patients. Based on a variety of trials in elderly subjects, options could include standard RT and alkylating chemotherapy as per standard of care in younger patients, hypofractionated RT and TMZ, RT alone (either standard or hypofractionated schemes), or TMZ alone (**Table 1**).

In patients with good Karnofsky Performance Status (KPS) greater than or equal to 70, aged 65 to 70 years, and with hypermethylated *MGMT* promoter, combined hypofractionated RT and TMZ is recommended based on randomized data from CCTG CE.6/EORTC 26062 (Canadian Clinical Trial Group (CCTG) CE.6/European Organization for Research and Treatment of Cancer (EORTC) 26062).[43] As long as randomized data on TMZ monotherapy (or the previous CETEG regimen) versus chemoradiation are lacking, TMZ alone seems reasonable in MGMT-methylated elderly patients when poor KPS or patient preference suggests that combined treatment may be too toxic.

In patients with KPS 70 years and older, and age 65 to 70 years and older, unmethylated *MGMT*, hypofractionated RT and TMZ is also recommended, recognizing that the benefit of adding TMZ is less in the unmethylated MGMT population.[43] Similarly, RT alone seems reasonable in unmethylated MGMT elderly patients when poor KPS or patient preference suggests that combined treatment may be too toxic. Further research on patients with unmethylated *MGMT* is needed.

Table 1
Compilation of therapy options and recommendations for patients with glioblastoma in different age groups according to Karnofsky Performance Status[a]

MGMT	Age (y)	Karnofsky Performance Status	First Choice	Second Choice
Hypermethylated or undetermined	>70	50–70	TMZ	Hypofractionated (Hypo) RT or TMZ
	>70	>70	Hypo RT or TMZ	TMZ
	<70	<70	Hypo RT or TMZ	(TMZ)
	<70	>70	RT or TMZ	—
Unmethylated	>70	50–70	Hypo RT	(Hypo RT or TMZ)
	>70	>70	Hypo RT	Hypo RT or TMZ
	<70	<70	Hypo RT	Hypo RT or TMZ
	<70	>70	RT or trial	RT or (TMZ)

[a] Regimens are depicted as hypofractionated RT-TMZ[43] or RT-TMZ.[68]

RECENT TRIALS

CCTG CE.6/EORTC 26062 (the aforementioned randomized phase III trial in elderly subjects comparing hypofractionated RT alone or in combination with TMZ) clearly has an impact on practice and provides evidence for shorter chemoradiation schedules for select subjects and advocates for TMZ use in these subjects, although the authors of this review question the utility of testing for *MGMT* in subjects with good KPS because combined chemoradiation is recommended regardless of MGMT. In contrast, other recent trials also aimed to change practice but largely failed. Lessons may or may not be gleaned from these negative trials.

ACT IV was a randomized, double-blind, phase III trial, which recruited adult subjects with newly diagnosed GB with centrally assessed EGFRvIII expression from 165 hospitals in 22 countries. Subjects were required to have undergone a maximal surgical resection and completion of standard RT and concurrent TMZ without progression. During TMZ maintenance therapy (6–12 cycles), subjects were randomized the EGFRvIII vaccine rindopepimut (500 μg admixed with 150 μg GM-CSF) or control (100 μg keyhole limpet hemocyanin), administered via monthly intradermal injection until progression or intolerance. The addition of rindopepimut failed to improve OS with a median OS of 20.1 months (95% CI 18.5–22.1) in the rindopepimut group versus 20.0 (95% CI 18.1–21.9) months in the control group resulting to a HR of 1.01 (95% CI 0.79–1.30, $P = .93$).[28] Because ACT IV followed a promising small, uncontrolled trial of rindopepimut, the lessons learned should include an even higher skepticism concerning small, uncontrolled trial data.[33] This earlier trial also demonstrated an absence of EGFRvIII in rindopepimut-treated tumor specimens and was considered a proof of benefit from rindopepimut.[44,45] However, analysis of posttreatment tumor specimens from ACT IV reveal that a variable percentage of subjects lose EGFRvIII (based on RT-PCR) regardless of treatment arm, raising suspicion of the limited relevance of the EGFRvIII mutation in general. Such information could have been detected earlier with a control in the earlier study.[28,46] Interestingly, contrasting data from 106 subjects demonstrated that EGFRvIII status was unchanged at recurrence in 35 of 40 subjects with EGFR-amplified primary tumors (87.5%).[47] Four subjects lost and 1 subject gained EGFRvIII positivity at recurrence.[47] Agreement on methodological discrepancies for defining EGFR amplification and EGFRvIII positivity may solve the issue. Despite this negative phase III trial of EGFRvIII-directed immunotherapy,[28] the target may still be relevant for precision approaches; for example, with the drug-antibody conjugate composed of the humanized chimeric EGFR-targeted monoclonal antibody ABT-806 conjugated via a stable maleimidocaproyl linker to the tubulin inhibitor, monomethylauristatin.[48]

After the failure of bevacizumab to demonstrate an OS benefit when added to standard of care in the newly diagnosed setting, the Bevacizumab, Lomustine, or Both (BELOB) trial provided a promising survival signal in recurrent GB, which prompted the EORTC 26101 phase II trial to be transformed into a full phase III study. BELOB demonstrated improved OS at 9 and 12 months for combined bevacizumab and lomustine versus either agent alone. Of note, bevacizumab was not accessible in the Netherlands, where the BELOB study was performed, thus restricting crossover to bevacizumab in the control group (n = 1).[49] The subsequent randomized, phase III EORTC 26101 compared lomustine with or without bevacizumab. Despite prolonging progression-free survival (PFS) (HR 0.49, 95% CI 0.39–0.61), combined lomustine and bevacizumab treatment does not confer an OS advantage (HR 0.95, 95% CI 0.74–1.21, P = .650) compared with treatment with lomustine alone in subjects with progressive GB.[50] In this study, crossover to bevacizumab occurred in 35.5% of subjects in the control arm; whereas 18.7% of subjects in the combination arm continued bevacizumab at progression.

Large-scale clinical trials are currently evaluating the efficacy of immune checkpoint inhibitors, namely nivolumab, in newly diagnosed and recurrent GB. Whereas the trials in newly diagnosed subjects separated according to *MGMT* promoter methylation status are ongoing, results from the study in progressive GB comparing nivolumab and bevacizumab have been reported. This trial randomized 369 subjects at first progression after standard of care to nivolumab 3 mg/kg every 2 weeks (n = 184) or bevacizumab 10 mg/kg every 2 weeks (n = 185). The most common adverse events leading to discontinuation (>2 subjects in either the nivolumab or bevacizumab arm) were cerebrovascular accident (0% and 2%, respectively) and pulmonary embolism (<1% and 2%, respectively). PFS favored bevacizumab (HR = 1.97, 95% CI 1.57–2.48) with median PFS 3.5 months (2.9–4.6) for bevacizumab and 1.5 months (1.5–1.6) for nivolumab. OS was similar in this unselected subject population (HR = 1.04, 95% CI 0.83–1.30, P = .76) with median OS 10.0 months (9.0–11.8) for bevacizumab and 9.8 months (8.2–11.8) for nivolumab.[51] CheckMate 498 (nivolumab or TMZ in combination with RT in newly diagnosed subjects with *MGMT*-unmethylated GB) and CheckMate 548 (nivolumab or placebo in combination with RT plus TMZ in newly diagnosed subjects with *MGMT*-methylated or indeterminate GB) are ongoing. These trials also do not enrich for subjects more likely to benefit from the immune intervention.[16]

As previously mentioned, the CETEG trial used *MGMT* promoter hypermethylation to identify subjects most likely to benefit from alkylating chemotherapy. Newly diagnosed GB subjects harboring a hypermethylated MGMT promoter were randomized (1:1) to standard chemoradiation with TMZ concurrent and adjuvant for 6 cycles versus experimental therapy with RT and CCNU/TMZ. The experimental chemotherapy was given as 6 42-day courses of CCNU at 100 mg/m^2 on day 1 and TMZ 100 mg/m^2 on days 2 to 6. The first cycle of alkylating chemotherapy was dosed to coincide with days 1 to 6 of RT, replacing continuous concomitant TMZ. The TMZ dose was adapted according to tolerance. The trial randomized 141 subjects (63 TMZ, 66 CCNU/TMZ) with 129 subjects in the modified intention-to-treat (mITT) population of subjects receiving at least 1 dose of study drug. OS was superior in the CCNU/TMZ arm as compared with the TMZ arm (P = .049) after stratification for recursive partitioning class and center. In the mITT population, median OS trended toward benefit in the CCNU/TMZ arm at 37.9 months (95% CI 29.2–51.4 months) compared with 31.4 months (95% CI 27.0–44.8 months) in the TMZ arm (HR 0.60, 95% CI 0.35–1.03, $P = .064$).[4] This trial constitutes an advantage in the group of GB subjects sensitive to alkylating chemotherapy. Due to its limited size, adaption for unevenly distributed risk factors was necessary. Whether a desired confirmatory trial is feasible, given the wide availability of the drugs and the reasonable costs, needs to be discussed.

The sheer number of negative GB trials over the past years despite concepts or compounds that work well in other diseases should trigger appraisal of potential factors contributing to these failures:

- More than in other solid malignancies, residual tumor after surgery may harbor yet unknown properties that limit treatment efficacy. An argument for this is the newly discovered network of TMs.[6]
- There is a failure to conceptually understand that the overarching principle to be tackled is the heterogeneity of the disease[20] and there is a lack of smart, tolerable combination approaches that appropriately tackle this issue.
- Molecular diagnostics, wherever possible, should be used to improve accuracy of patient selection.
- There was failure to decide if standard of care for all GB subjects should include TMZ[1] (and/or TTFields[40]) or if treatment should be better individualized.
- A rush to pivotal, phase III trials driven by the rules of the market and regulatory bodies for approval prevents step-wise understanding, building on controlled early-phase data, as well as prudent use of scientifically sound biomarkers, for determining subsets of patients who benefit.
- Trials at recurrence are largely built on information of the newly diagnosed disease.
- The measures to determine treatment response or resistance are largely MRI-based, which, despite all standardization,[52] may be insufficient compared with liquid biopsies or radiomic integration of data.[21]
- Currently, trials of targeted therapies and immunotherapies in GB are mainly in unselected subject groups.

In the following sections, some of these concepts are discussed.

PRECISION MEDICINE APPROACHES

Precision neurooncology relies on the existence of biomarkers that predict response and ultimately benefit from a given therapy. The most prominent example for a predictive biomarker in gliomas so far is *MGMT*.[1,3] However, some investigators suggest that predicting response to TMZ is more complex than just MGMT methylation status and defining the right subgroups that do not benefit from TMZ may also involve global methylation profiles and TERT status.[5]

Examples of putative predictive biomarkers exist. Patients with newly diagnosed GB harboring a proneural subtype based on expression analyses[53] may derive benefit from the addition of VEGF antibody bevacizumab to standard treatment. If independently confirmed, this would make the proneural subtype a predictive lesion for response to bevacizumab.[22] Similarly, lower levels of methylation of the CpG2 in the promoter of the CD95L were predictive for an improved OS with the CD95 inhibitory treatment with asunercept (APG101) in combination with reirradiation compared with reirradiation alone. Interestingly, patients with lower methylation of the promoter treated with reirradiation alone (ie, not treated with the CD95 inhibitory therapy) did worse.[23] Also, based on retrospective analysis, mTOR Ser2448 phosphorylation is an interesting putative predictive biomarker for the response to the mTOR inhibitor temsirolimus plus radiation in patients with newly diagnosed GB without *MGMT* promoter methylation.[24] This seems even more important because, without population preselection, mTOR inhibition is not only ineffective but may even confer a survival disadvantage compared with the standard of care. The addition of a different mTOR inhibitor, everolimus, in a recent controlled study did not provide any advantage in an unselected group of subjects with newly diagnosed GB irrespective of *MGMT* status.[54] In some GBs, B-raf proto-oncogene (BRAF) mutations may indicate response to BRAF inhibitory treatments.[55] Only recently, an association between a reduced capacity of the tumor cells to repair DNA lesions (MMR deficiency) and positive response to immune checkpoint inhibition has been proposed for lung cancer.[14]

Therefore, well-considered allocation of subjects to clinical trials based on the molecular characteristics of the tumor, as well as necessary retrospective validation of potential biomarkers, is essential in a clinical setting. Current concepts prospectively using biomarkers to enrich for potentially benefitting patients are the Individualized Therapy for Relapsed Malignancies in Childhood (INFORM) trial[56] and the Nationale Centrum für Tumorerkrankungen (NCT) Neuro Master Match (N^{2}M^2), a trial of molecularly matched targeted therapies plus RT in subjects with newly diagnosed GB without MGMT promoter methylation.[19] The GB Adaptive, Global, Innovative Learning Environment (AGILE) consortium is planning to take a differential approach by reassessing potential biomarkers from an unselected cohort with given therapies first and integrating this information via adaptive processes to enrich while the trial accrues.[57]

Similar concepts are also being developed for the recurrent disease. One example is that subjects with progressive GB undergo reresection for extensive biomarker analysis to allow selection of appropriate treatments from a large set of agents.[18] The concept and potential candidate drugs are outlined in **Fig. 1**.

IMMUNOTHERAPY

Immunotherapy may represent the next big step for patients with GB (**Fig. 2**). In addition to the successes in other malignancies, this optimism is fueled by single cases and attractive concepts. Independent of the approach (eg, checkpoint inhibition, targeted vaccine, or adoptive T-cell transfer), the clonal representation of the target antigen and the immunosuppressive microenvironment must be taken into account for clinical development. For instance, EGFRvIII is a subclonal antigen with heterogeneous expression in the tumor tissue, which may, in theory, be subjected to immune evasion. The early founder mutations IDH1R132H[29] and H3.3K27M[31] represent clonal antigens.

Several chimeric antigen receptors (CARs) are in clinical development for GB-targeting tumor antigens, such as interleukin 13 receptor-α2, EGFRvIII, and human epidermal growth factor receptor 2. A proof-of-concept report in a patient with recurrent, multifocal GB validates a robust antitumor killing capability of CAR T cells in general.[58] In a series of 10 subjects, intravenous delivery of a single dose of autologous T cells redirected to the EGFRvIII mutation by a CAR showed feasibility of manufacturing and intravenous delivery of CAR T–EGFRvIII cells.[59] There was no evidence of a cytokine release syndrome and CAR T–EGFRvIII cells transiently expanded in the peripheral blood.[59]

- Concepts to enhance activity of drugs and prevent development of resistance deserve exploration of strategies against immune inhibitory pathways, potentially

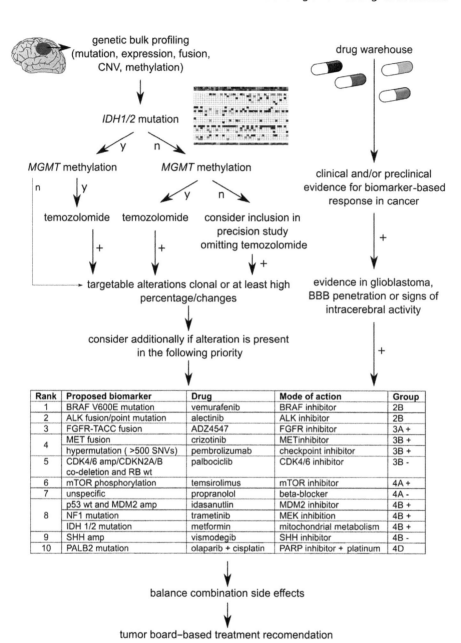

Fig. 1. Path toward precision. Paradigmatic work flow from a recurrent GB tissue sample is outlined. ALK, anaplastic lymphoma receptor tyrosine kinase; amp, amplification; BBB, blood-brain barrier; CDK, cyclin-dependent kinase; CDKN 2A/B, cyclin-dependent kinase inhibitor; CNV, copy-number variation; FGFR, fibroblast growth factor receptor; MDM 2, mouse double minute; MEK, mitogen-activated protein kinase; MET, hepatocyte growth factor receptor; n, no; NF1, neurofibromin; PALB 2, partner and localizer of BRCA; poly (ADP-ribose)-polymerase; RB, retinoblastoma; SHH, sonic hedgehog; SNV, small nucleotide variants; TACC, transforming acidic coiled-coil; wt, wild-type; y, yes.

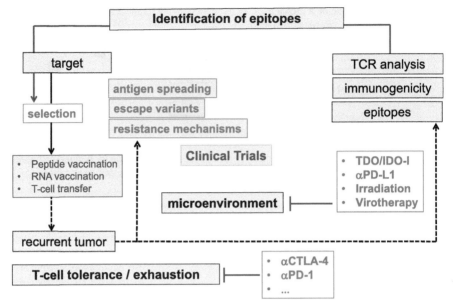

Fig. 2. Algorithm for rational development of immunotherapy trials in GB. TCR, T cell receptor.

with a focus on indoleamine-pyrrole 2,3-dioxygenase 1 (*IDO1*) and forkhead box P3 (*FoxP3*), as well as tandem CAR T cells designed to target multiple tumor antigens.[60]

- GAPVAC initiated a phase I trial on integration of tumor-associated and tumor-specific peptides into upfront chemoradiation. Peptides with the highest tumor association and (at the same time) most immunogenic peptides are selected for each subject to maximize the number of effective antitumor immune responses. Mutated peptides identified by next-generation sequencing and mass spectrometry may not be used for peptide vaccination but serve as a platform for personalized immunotherapies with potentially more aggressive treatments such as CAR T cells.
- Viral therapies may serve as another mode to generate a local immune response and potentially result in neoantigen formation.[61,62]
- Checkpoint inhibitors in GB may work only with a specific immunogenic background, potentially to be defined by MSI-H or dMMR, or with associated treatment; for example, vaccination.
- The most prominent checkpoints in other malignancies may not be the most relevant in GB.[63] Other factors, such as the CD95 system TDO[25] or PD family members,[64] may be of greater importance.

SUMMARY

Current research on imaging and molecular diagnostics focuses on more objective markers and features.[12,21] Only a few GB patients benefit (sometimes for years) from currently approved and experimental therapies. A much larger proportion of patients, however, do not benefit at all. Essentially, all GB patients relapse, even those with initial benefit and less aggressive disease course. Despite these observations, treatment concepts for GB mostly have not changed, and trials to date have failed to learn from successes and defeats. Neurosurgical and standard chemoradiation approaches may have reached their boundaries; yet, the most and least benefitting patients, as well as the mechanisms of secondary resistance, are not understood.

Concepts currently explored in radiation oncology focus on target definition and use of alternative radiation qualities. After many years of focusing on targeting angiogenesis,[50,65,66] the field has shifted to immunotherapies, mainly checkpoint inhibition but also targeted (vaccination) approaches. Pathway inhibition has maintained momentum, with the biggest change in the last decade being appropriate preselection of subjects based on the proposed mechanism of action.[67] There is a need for academically driven drug development and design of trials with the focus on understanding the mechanisms of response or resistance rather than striving for short-term approval. Similarly, immunotherapy trials should also focus on getting as much information about response and resistance from each subject to inform subsequent steps (backwards translation) and rapid evolution of concepts to trials.

REFERENCES

1. Weller M, van den Bent M, Tonn JC, et al, for the European Association for Neuro-Oncology (EANO) Task Force on Gliomas. European Association for Neuro-Oncology guideline on the diagnosis and treatment of adult astrocytic and oligodendroglial gliomas. Lancet Oncol 2017;18(6):e315–29.

2. Wick A, Kessler T, Elia AEH, et al. Glioblastoma in the elderly: solid conclusions built on shifting sand? Neuro Oncol 2017. https://doi.org/10.1093/neuonc/nox133.

3. Wick W, Weller M, van den Bent M, et al. MGMT testing in neurooncology - a paradigm for prospects and challenges of biomarker-based treatment decisions. Nat Rev Neurol 2014;10:372–85.

4. Herrlinger U, Tzaridis T, Mack F, et al. Phase III trial of CCNU/temozolomide (TMZ) combination therapy vs. standard TMZ therapy for newly diagnosed MGMT-methylated glioblastoma patients: the CeTeG/NOA-09 trial. Neuro Oncol 2017;19(suppl. 6):vii13.

5. Kessler T, Sahm F, Sadik A, et al. Molecular differences in IDH wildtype glioblastoma according to MGMT promoter methylation. Neuro Oncol 2017. https://doi.org/10.1093/neuonc/nox160.

6. Osswald M, Jung E, Sahm F, et al. Brain tumour cells interconnect to a functional and resistant network. Nature 2015;528:93–8.

7. Zhu Z, Khan MA, Weiler M, et al. Targeting self-renewal in high-grade brain tumors leads to loss of brain tumor stem cells and prolonged survival. Cell Stem Cell 2014;15(2):185–98.

8. Platten M, Bunse L, Wick W, et al. Concepts in glioma immunotherapy. Cancer Immunol Immunother 2016;65(10):1269–75.

9. Sturm D, Witt H, Hovestadt V, et al. Hotspot mutations in H3F3A and IDH1 define distinct epigenetic and biological subgroups of glioblastoma. Cancer Cell 2012;22(4):425–37.

10. Brennan CW, Verhaak RG, McKenna A, et al. The somatic genomic landscape of glioblastoma. Cell 2013;155:462–77.

11. Patel AP, Tirosh I, Trombetta JJ, et al. Single-cell RNA-seq highlights intratumoral heterogeneity in primary glioblastoma. Science 2014;344:1396–401.

12. Louis DN, Perry A, Reifenberger G, et al. The 2016 World Health Organization Classification of tumors of the central nervous system: a summary. Acta Neuropathol 2016;131(6):803–20.
13. Parsons DW, Jones S, Zhang X, et al. An integrated genomic analysis of human glioblastoma multiforme. Science 2008;321:1807–12.
14. Le DT, Uram JN, Wang H, et al. PD-1 blockade in tumors with mismatch-repair deficiency. N Engl J Med 2015;372:2509–20.
15. Le DT, Durham JN, Smith KN, et al. Mismatch-repair deficiency predicts response of solid tumors to PD-1 blockade. Science 2017;357:409–13.
16. Bouffet E, Larouche V, Campbell BB, et al. Immune checkpoint inhibition for hypermutant glioblastoma multiforme resulting from germline biallelic mismatch repair deficiency. J Clin Oncol 2016;34:2206–11.
17. Wick W, Kessler T. Drug repositioning meets precision in glioblastoma. Clin Cancer Res 2017;24(2):256–8.
18. Byron SA, Tran NL, Halperin RF, et al. Prospective feasibility trial for genomics-informed treatment in recurrent and progressive glioblastoma. Clin Cancer Res 2017;24(2):295–305.
19. Pfaff E, Kessler T, Balasubramanian GP, et al. Feasibility of real-time molecular profiling for patients with newly diagnosed glioblastoma without MGMT promoter-hypermethylation - the NCT Neuro Master Match (N2M2) pilot study. Neuro Oncol 2018;20(6):826–37.
20. Lee JK, Wang J, Sa JK, et al. Spatiotemporal genomic architecture informs precision oncology in glioblastoma. Nat Genet 2017;49:594–9.
21. Kickingereder P, Götz M, Muschelli J, et al. Large-scale radiomic profiling of recurrent glioblastoma identifies an imaging predictor for stratifying anti-angiogenic treatment response. Clin Cancer Res 2016;22:5765–71.
22. Sandmann T, Bourgon R, Garcia J, et al. Patients with proneural glioblastoma may derive overall survival benefit from the addition of bevacizumab to first-line radiotherapy and temozolomide: retrospective analysis of the AVAglio trial. J Clin Oncol 2015;33:2735–44.
23. Wick W, Fricke H, Junge K, et al. A phase II, randomised, study of weekly APG101 + reirradiation versus reirradiation in progressive glioblastoma. Clin Cancer Res 2014;20:6304–13.
24. Wick W, Gorlia T, Bady P, et al. Phase II study of radiotherapy and temsirolimus versus radiochemotherapy with temozolomide in patients with newly diagnosed glioblastoma without MGMT promoter hypermethylation (EORTC 26082). Clin Cancer Res 2016;22:4797–806.
25. Opitz CA, Litzenburger UM, Sahm F, et al. An endogenous ligand of the human aryl hydrocarbon receptor promotes tumor formation. Nature 2011;478:197–203.
26. Platten M, Wick W, Van den Eynde BJ. Tryptophan catabolism in cancer: beyond IDO and tryptophan depletion. Cancer Res 2012;72:5435–40.
27. Brandes AA, Carpentier AF, Kesari S, et al. A Phase II randomized study of galunisertib monotherapy or galunisertib plus lomustine compared with lomustine monotherapy in patients with recurrent glioblastoma. Neuro Oncol 2016;18(8):1146–56.
28. Weller M, Butowski N, Tran DD, et al, ACT IV trial investigators. Rindopepimut with temozolomide for patients with newly diagnosed, EGFRvIII- expressing glioblastoma (ACT IV): a randomised, double-blind, international phase 3 trial. Lancet Oncol 2017;18:1373–85.
29. Schumacher T, Bunse L, Pusch S, et al. A vaccine targeting mutant IDH1 induces antitumor immunity. Nature 2014;512:324–7.

30. Platten M, Schilling D, Bunse T, et al. A mutation-specific peptide vaccine targeting *IDH1R132H* in patients with newly diagnosed malignant astrocytomas: a first-in-man multicenter phase I clinical trial of the German Neurooncology Working Group (NOA-16). J Clin Oncol 2016;34(suppl) [abstract: TPS2082].

31. Ochs K, Ott M, Bunse T, et al. K27M-mutant histone-3 as a novel target for glioma immunotherapy. Oncoimmunology 2017;6(7):e1328340.

32. Rampling R, Peoples S, Mulholland PJ, et al. A cancer research UK first time in human phase I trial of IMA950 (novel multipeptide therapeutic vaccine) in patients with newly diagnosed glioblastoma. Clin Cancer Res 2016;22:4776–85.

33. Platten M. EGFRvIII vaccine in glioblastoma-InACT-IVe or not ReACTive enough? Neuro Oncol 2017;19:1425–6.

34. Jung E, Osswald M, Blaes J, et al. Tweety-homologue 1 drives brain colonization of gliomas. J Neurosci 2017;37:6837–50.

35. Piccirillo SG, Dietz S, Madhu B, et al. Fluorescence-guided surgical sampling of glioblastoma identifies phenotypically distinct tumour-initiating cell populations in the tumour mass and margin. Br J Cancer 2012;107:462–8.

36. Hauser SB, Kockro RA, Actor B, et al. Combining 5-Aminolevulinic acid fluorescence and intraoperative magnetic resonance imaging in glioblastoma surgery: a histology-based evaluation. Neurosurgery 2016;78:475–83.

37. Oehlke O, Mix M, Graf E, et al. Amino-acid PET versus MRI guided re-irradiation in patients with recurrent glioblastoma multiforme (GLIAA) - protocol of a randomized phase II trial (NOA 10/ARO 2013-1). BMC Cancer 2016;16(1):769.

38. Ramakrishna NR, Harper B, Burkavage R, et al. A comparison of brain and hippocampal dosimetry with protons or intensity modulated radiation therapy planning for unilateral glioblastoma. Int J Radiat Oncol Biol Phys 2016;96:E134–5.

39. Fontana AO, Augsburger MA, Grosse N, et al. Differential DNA repair pathway choice in cancer cells after proton- and photon-irradiation. Radiother Oncol 2015;116:374–80.

40. Stupp R, Taillibert S, Kanner AA, et al. Maintenance therapy with tumor-treating fields plus temozolomide vs temozolomide alone for glioblastoma: a randomized clinical trial. JAMA 2015;314(23):2535–43.

41. Gramatzki D, Kickingereder P, Hentschel B, et al. Limited role for extended maintenance temozolomide for newly diagnosed glioblastoma. Neurology 2017;88: 1422–30.

42. Ostrom QT, Gittleman H, Farah P, et al. CBTRUS statistical report: primary brain and central nervous system tumors diagnosed in the United States in 2006-2010. Neuro Oncol 2013;15(Suppl 2):ii1–56.

43. Perry JR, Laperierre N, O'Callaghan CJ, et al. Short-course radiation plus temozolomide in elderly patients with glioblastoma. N Engl J Med 2017;376:1027–37.

44. Sampson JH, Heimberger AB, Archer GE, et al. Immunologic escape after prolonged progression-free survival with epidermal growth factor receptor variant III peptide vaccination in patients with newly diagnosed glioblastoma. J Clin Oncol 2010;28:4722–9.

45. Schuster J, Lai RK, Recht LD, et al. A phase II, multicenter trial of rindopepimut (CDX-110) in newly diagnosed glioblastoma: the ACT III study. Neuro Oncol 2015;17:854–61.

46. van den Bent MJ, Gao Y, Kerkhof M, et al. Changes in the EGFR amplification and EGFRvIII expression between paired primary and recurrent glioblastomas. Neuro Oncol 2015;17:935–41.

47. Felsberg J, Hentschel B, Kaulich K, et al, German Glioma Network. Epidermal growth factor receptor variant III (EGFRvIII) positivity in EGFR-amplified

Wick & Platten

glioblastomas: Prognostic role and comparison between primary and recurrent tumors. Clin Cancer Res 2017;23:6846–55.
48. van den Bent M, Eoli M, Sepulveda J, et al. First results from the randomized phase II study on depatux-m alone, depatux-m in combination with temozolomide and either temozolomide or lomustine in recurrent EGFR amplified glioblastoma: first report from INTELLANCE 2/EORTC trial 1410. Neurooncol 2017; 19(suppl. 6):vii13.
49. Taal W, Oosterkamp HM, Walenkamp AM, et al. Single-agent bevacizumab or lomustine versus a combination of bevacizumab plus lomustine in patients with recurrent glioblastoma (BELOB trial): a randomised controlled phase 2 trial. Lancet Oncol 2014;15:943–53.
50. Wick W, Gorlia T, Bendszus M, et al. Lomustine and bevacizumab in progressive glioblastoma. N Engl J Med 2017;377(20):1954–63.
51. Reardon DA, Omuro A, Brandes AA, et al. Randomized phase 3 study evaluating the efficacy and safety of nivolumab vs bevacizumab in patients with recurrent glioblastoma: checkmate 143. Neuro-Oncology 19:iii21. https://doi.org/10.1093/neuonc/nox036.071.
52. Wen PY, Macdonald DA, Reardon DA, et al. Updated response assessment criteria for high-grade gliomas: response assessment in neuro-oncology (RANO) working group. J Clin Oncol 2010;28:1963–72.
53. Phillips HS, Kharbanda S, Chen RH, et al. Molecular subclasses of high-grade glioma predict prognosis, delineate a pattern of disease progression, and resemble stages in neurogenesis. Cancer Cell 2006;9:157–73.
54. Chinnaiyan P, Won M, Wen PY, et al. A randomized phase II study of everolimus in combination with chemoradiation in newly diagnosed glioblastoma: results of NRG Oncology RTOG 0913. Neuro Oncol 2018;20(5):666–73.
55. Robinson GW, Orr BA, Gajjar A. Complete clinical regression of a BRAF V600E-mutant pediatric glioblastoma multiforme after BRAF inhibitor therapy. BMC Cancer 2014;14:258.
56. Worst BC, van Tilburg CM, Balasubramanian GP, et al. Next-generation personalised medicine for high-risk paediatric cancer patients - the INFORM pilot study. Eur J Cancer 2016;65:91–101.
57. Alexander BM, Ba S, Berger MS, et al, GBM AGILE Network. Adaptive Global Innovative Learning Environment for Glioblastoma: GBM AGILE. Clin Cancer Res 2017. https://doi.org/10.1158/1078-0432.CCR-17-0764.
58. Brown CE, Alizadeh D, Starr R, et al. Regression of glioblastoma after chimeric antigen receptor T-cell therapy. N Engl J Med 2016;375(26):2561–9.
59. O'Rourke DM, Nasrallah MP, Desai A, et al. A single dose of peripherally infused EGFRvIII-directed CAR T cells mediates antigen loss and induces adaptive resistance in patients with recurrent glioblastoma. Sci Transl Med 2017;9(399) [pii: eaaa0984].
60. Hegde M, Mukherjee M, Grada Z, et al. Tandem CAR T cells targeting HER2 and IL13Ralpha2 mitigate tumor antigen escape. J Clin Invest 2016;126:3036–52.
61. Geletneky K, Hajda J, Angelova AL, et al. Oncolytic H-1 parvovirus shows safety and signs of immunogenic activity in a first phase I/IIa glioblastoma trial. Mol Ther 2017;25(12):2620–34.
62. Cloughesy TF, Landolfi J, Hogan DJ, et al. Phase 1 trial of vocimagene amiretrorepvec and 5-fluorocytosine for recurrent high-grade glioma. Sci Transl Med 2016; 8(341):341ra75.

63. Hodges TR, Ott M, Xiu J, et al. Mutational burden, immune checkpoint expression, and mismatch repair in glioma: implications for immune checkpoint immunotherapy. Neuro Oncol 2017;19:1047–57.
64. Lemke D, Pfenning PN, Sahm F, et al. Costimulatory protein 4IgB7H3 drives the malignant phenotype of glioblastoma by mediating immune escape and invasiveness. Clin Cancer Res 2012;18:105–17.
65. Batchelor TT, Mulholland P, Neyns B, et al. Phase III randomized trial comparing the efficacy of cediranib as monotherapy, and in combination with lomustine, versus lomustine alone in patients with recurrent glioblastoma. J Clin Oncol 2013;31:3212–8.
66. Chinot OL, Wick W, Mason W, et al. Bevacizumab plus adiotherapy/temozolomide for newly diagnosed glioblastoma. N Engl J Med 2014;370:709–22.
67. Pearl LH, Schierz AC, Ward SE, et al. Therapeutic opportunities within the DNA damage response. Nat Rev Cancer 2015;15:166–80.
68. Stupp R, Hegi ME, Mason WP, et al. Effects of radiotherapy with concomitant and adjuvant temozolomide versus radiotherapy alone on survival in glioblastoma in a randomised phase III study: 5-year analysis of the EORTC-NCIC trial. Lancet Oncol 2009;10:459–66.

Benign Intracranial Tumors

Justin T. Jordan, MD, MPH, Scott R. Plotkin, MD, PhD*

KEYWORDS

- Benign intracranial tumors • Meningioma • Schwannoma • Neurofibromatosis
- Schwannomatosis

KEY POINTS

- Meningiomas and schwannomas account for almost all incident benign intracranial tumors.
- Risk factors for meningiomas and schwannomas include exposure to ionizing radiation, as well as various genetic diseases and gene mutations.
- Although most benign intracranial tumors are primarily treated with surgery or radiation, ongoing research has identified an increasing number of effective or promising systemic therapies.

INTRODUCTION

Although there are many types of histologically benign primary intracranial tumors, the incidence of meningiomas and schwannomas in the general population accounts for the almost all such benign tumors. Although surgery is often curative for benign tumors, meningiomas and schwannomas are variably associated with unique challenges that limit the curability of individual tumors. Among these, 3 primary considerations include anatomically limited surgical accessibility of certain tumors; risk of recurrence, which is especially high after incomplete resection; and the relatively ineffective nature of traditional types of chemotherapy. Epidemiologic and genetic information for both meningiomas and schwannomas are presented, as well as therapeutic advances and considerations.

MENINGIOMA
Key Points

- Meningiomas are the most common primary intracranial tumor in adults.
- More than 80% of incident meningiomas are World Health Organization (WHO) grade I (benign meningiomas).

Disclosure Statement: J.T. Jordan and S.R. Plotkin have no disclosures related to this work.
Department of Neurology and Cancer Center, Massachusetts General Hospital, Harvard Medical School, 55 Fruit Street, Yawkey 9E, Boston, MA 02114, USA
* Corresponding author.
E-mail address: splotkin@mgh.harvard.edu

Neurol Clin 36 (2018) 501–516
https://doi.org/10.1016/j.ncl.2018.04.007
0733-8619/18/© 2018 Elsevier Inc. All rights reserved.

- Most meningiomas occur sporadically, though risk is increased with exposure to ionizing radiation and with germline mutations in the *NF2, SMARCB1, LZTR1,* or *SMARCE1* genes.

Epidemiology

Meningiomas are the most common primary intracranial tumor in adults, accounting for more than one-third of all primary central nervous system tumors.[1] The annual incidence of meningiomas is 8.3 per 100,000 population[1] and generally increases with age. Patients older than 70 years of age have a 3.5-fold increased risk of meningioma development compared with those younger than 70 years old.[2] The incidence rate in women is 56% higher than in men.[1]

Although almost all meningiomas occur sporadically (eg, without an identifiable risk factor) and as a single tumor, the risk of single or multiple such tumors is increased with exposure to ionizing radiation.[3,4] Among childhood cancer survivors, the average risk of meningioma development is increased nearly 10-fold by exposure to radiation for cancer treatment, and the median time to meningioma diagnosis in this cohort is 17 years.[3] In another systematic review of cases of radiation-associated meningiomas, the average time from radiation to meningioma development was 22.9 years, and 11.9% of reported cases had multiple meningiomas, with greater risk among patients who received higher doses of radiation.[5] Among those reported cases, 68% of radiation-induced meningiomas were WHO grade I, 27% were WHO grade II, and 5% were WHO grade III.[5]

Correlations have also been shown between meningioma development and prior head trauma or various viral infections (eg, adenovirus), although reports for these are inconsistent and the true association with tumor risk remains unknown.[6–8] Finally, excessive hormone exposure has been correlated with meningioma development and, in fact, progesterone receptors are expressed on more than 70% of meningiomas, and estrogen receptors on nearly 30%.[8,9] However, whether hormones are drivers of tumor development remains unknown.

In addition to extrinsic risk factors, 2 genetic diseases are associated with a high rate of meningioma development. Neurofibromatosis 2 (NF2) is an autosomal dominant tumor predisposition syndrome associated with loss of function mutations in the *NF2* gene on chromosome 22, leading to cell growth signaling dysregulation and constitutive activation of various pathways, including mammalian target of rapamycin complex (mTORC)-1 and mTORC2 signaling.[10,11] Although the hallmark of NF2 is bilateral vestibular schwannomas, up to 80% of patients also develop 1 or more meningiomas by the age of 70 years.[12–14] In fact, meningiomas are often the symptomatic tumor in children diagnosed with NF2, whereas adults are more commonly diagnosed after developing symptoms of vestibular schwannomas.[15]

Schwannomatosis, a separate autosomal dominant tumor predisposition syndrome, is associated with multiple schwannomas, which are usually not on the vestibular nerve (although unilateral vestibular schwannomas have been described).[16–19] Additionally, about 5% of patients with schwannomatosis will develop 1 or more meningiomas.[20] Although schwannomatosis is inherited in an autosomal dominant pattern, the disease arises from multiple genetic loci and up to 85% of cases are nonfamilial.[20] SWItch/Sucrose NonFermentable (SWI/SNF)-related matrix-associated actin-dependent regulator of chromatin subfamily B member 1 (*SMARCB1*), a gene encoding part of a nucleosome remodeling complex, is on chromosome 22q11 adjacent to the *NF2* gene, and mutations therein are responsible for 40% to 50% of familial schwannomatosis cases and about 10% of sporadic cases.[21,22] Germline mutations in Leucine Zipper-Like Transcription Regulator 1 (*LZTR1*), also located on chromosome 22q11, belonging to the Broad-Complex, Tramtrack and Bric à brac/Poxvirus and Zinc finger (*BTB/POZ*) superfamily, and contributing to chromatin regulation, have been described in roughly 40% of familial cases and 20% of sporadic cases that test negative for germline mutations in *NF2* and *SMARCB1*.[23] In another study, *LZTR1* mutations were found in the germline of 80% of schwannomatosis patients lacking evidence of germline *SMARCB1* mutation but with somatic 22q loss.[24]

Finally, more recent publications have shown recurrent mutations in SWI/SNF Related, Matrix-Associated, Actin-Dependent Regulator of Chromatin, Subfamily E, Member 1 (*SMARCE1*) in familial cases of meningioma, primarily with clear cell histology,[25,26] whereas mutations in Breast Cancer (*BRCA*) 1-Associated Protein-1 (*BAP1*) have been described in a subset of high-grade rhabdoid meningiomas.[27] In the latter case, 2 patients were reported with multiple spatially distinct recurrent tumors, though there are no reports to date of familial meningiomas associated with *BAP1* mutations.

Imaging

Imaging characteristics for meningiomas are quite specific; as such, imaging is a significant aid in the diagnosis and treatment planning for these tumors. Computerized tomography (CT) offers rapid imaging of the neuraxis and is often used as a first-line examination for neurologic complaints. CT images are often the first indication of a new meningioma, and generally show an isodense or hyperdense extraaxial lesion with a broad attachment to underlying dura, often with a cerebrospinal fluid cleft at the interface between tumor and brain. Bony remodeling is a common effect of meningiomas in the form of hyperostosis (suggestive of low-grade lesion) or osseous destruction (suggestive of high-grade lesion), and CT images are well suited to visualize these. Finally, approximately 25% of meningiomas demonstrate psammomatous calcifications, which are apparent on CT. **Fig. 1** shows an exemplary case of meningioma on CT.

MRI offers higher resolution of intracranial visualization, and is often performed as a follow-up to CT for additional lesion characterization. Characteristically, meningiomas appear isointense to parenchyma on T1-weighted and T2-weighted images, with bright, homogeneous enhancement on postcontrast images. Peritumoral edema is occasionally present, particularly with certain histologic subtypes, including secretory meningiomas. **Fig. 2** shows an exemplary case of meningioma on MRI.

Pathology

Meningiomas arise from the arachnoid cap cells.[28] The WHO grading system for meningiomas includes 3 grades: grade I (benign meningioma) accounts for 81% of cases, grade II (atypical meningioma) accounts for 17% of cases, and grade III (malignant meningioma) accounts for about 2% of cases.[1] Although there is a wide array of histologic meningioma subtypes described, the most common subtypes are meningothelial, fibrous, and transitional meningiomas.[28] Most histologic subtypes are WHO grade I and, therefore, have a low risk of recurrence after complete surgical resection, though clear cell meningiomas and choroid meningiomas are classified as WHO grade II, and papillary meningioma and rhabdoid meningioma are classified as WHO grade III. As such, these 4 histologic subtypes have a higher likelihood of recurrence than WHO grade I tumors.[29] Aside from the aforementioned subtypes, additional histologic features that may increase the grade of a meningioma to atypical (WHO grade II) or malignant (WHO grade III) include increased mitotic rate, brain invasion, hypercellularity, neoplastic-appearing cells, sheeting of cells, and foci of spontaneous necrosis.[28]

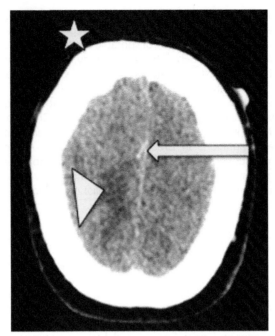

Fig. 1. CT image showing right frontal meningioma, which is mostly isodense to adjacent parenchyma with an area of hyperdensity (*arrow*) likely representing calcification, adjacent hypodensity (*arrowhead*) representing peritumoral edema, and overlying hyperostosis (*star*).

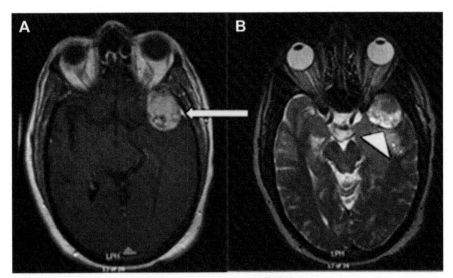

Fig. 2. MRI showing left anterior temporal fossa meningioma, which is brightly enhancing on postgadolinium imaging (*A*) with a dural tail (*arrow*) and (*B*) an adjacent hyperintense cleft of cerebrospinal fluid (*arrowhead*) visible on T2 imaging.

Genetics

In recent years there have been increasing efforts to sequence sporadic (nonfamilial) meningiomas to uncover driver mutations. Chief among these, driver mutations are found in the NF2 gene in about 50% to 60% of sporadic meningiomas and 100% of meningiomas associated with the NF2 disease.[30,31] More recent work exploring non-NF2 mutant tumors identified mutually exclusive mutations in v-akt murine thymoma viral oncogene homolog 1 (AKT1) in about 9%, Smoothened, frizzled family receptor (SMO) in 6%, and Phosphatidylinositol-4,5-Bisphosphonate 3-Kinase Catalytic Subunit Alpha (PIK3CA) in 7%.[30–32] Mutations in AKT, PIK3CA, and Krupple-like factor 4 (KLF4) frequently co-occur with tumor necrosis factor (TNF) receptor-associated factor 7 (TRAF7).[32] Interestingly, there appears to be a genotypic relationship with intracranial location of skull base meningiomas, with SMO-mutant tumors arising frequently from the olfactory groove, NF2-mutant tumors clustering posteriorly and laterally, KLF4-mutant tumors cluster anteriorly and laterally, and AKT-mutant tumors clustering anteriorly in the midline.[31]

In higher grade tumors, inactivating germline mutations in SMARCE1 are described in clear cell meningiomas, and may be especially common in familial cases of clear cell meningioma.[26] Similarly, BAP1 mutations have been shown in both germline and somatic forms in patients with rhabdoid meningiomas, though there is no familial risk reported to date with this gene.[27] Somatic deletions involving the Cyclin-Dependent Kinase Inhibitor 2A (CDKN2A) gene are commonly seen in anaplastic tumors and are associated with shorter survival,[33] whereas mutations in the promoter region for Telomerase reverse transcriptase (TERT) are common in higher-grade tumors and significantly worsen prognosis.[34]

Therapy

Surgery

The primary therapeutic modality for meningiomas is surgical resection. Extent of resection has been linked with recurrence risk for intracranial meningiomas and is graded according to the Simpson Scale (**Table 1**).[35] Additional factors influencing the risk of recurrence include higher grade, older age, and female gender.[28] Although gross total resection of a benign meningioma may be considered curative, there remains a small risk of local recurrence even with complete resection. One recent literature review cited a 5-year recurrence risk of 7% to 23%, 10-year recurrence risk of 20% to 39%, and 15-year recurrence risk of 24% to 60% after gross total resection,

Table 1	
Simpson scale describes the extent of resection for intracranial meningiomas	
Simpson Grade	**Extent of Resection**
I	Macroscopically complete removal of the tumor, with excision of dural attachment and of any abnormal bone for tumors arising from the dural venous sinus, including resection of the sinus
II	Macroscopically complete removal of the tumor and of its visible extensions, with coagulation of its dural attachment
III	Macroscopically complete removal of intradural tumor, without resection or coagulation of dural attachment or its extradural extensions
IV	Partial removal, leaving intradural tumor in situ
V	Simple decompression, with or without biopsy

and posited that the higher end of these estimates likely reflects increased use of se-rial, high-quality MRI.[29]

Radiotherapy

For recurrent meningiomas, surgically inaccessible meningiomas, or incompletely resected meningiomas, radiotherapy may be undertaken as an adjuvant treatment. Fractionated radiation therapy provided to incompletely resected or recurrent benign tumors results in greater than 90% local control rate at 5, 10, and 15 years.[36,37] Because of this longer term survival, patients may be at risk of late effects of radiation, such as radiation-induced tumors or cognitive side effects. Stereotactic radiosurgery (SRS), a radiotherapy technique providing a high dose of radiation to a small target in a single dose, may be used as an alternative to fractionated radiotherapy for small tumors, resulting in a smaller treatment field. In tumors small enough to treat with SRS, local control rates with SRS are approximately 80% at 8 years[38,39]; therefore, this may be a viable alternative to fractionated radiotherapy in certain patients. An infrequent consequence of radiotherapy for meningioma is malignant transformation; a single-center report found the risk of malignant transformation of SRS treated meningiomas at 2.2%.[40]

Chemotherapy

Despite surgery and radiation, meningiomas may recur. At such times, although repeat surgery or radiation may be considered, these modalities may not always be possible or preferred. Many systemic therapies have been studied to treat recurrent or progressive meningiomas[41] but none have demonstrated survival benefit to date. Based on the female predominance of meningiomas, as well as the high prevalence of progesterone and estrogen receptors on meningiomas,[9] hormonal therapies were once a prominent focus of therapeutic trials. However, treatment with the oral progesterone agonist megestrol acetate (Megace),[42] the progesterone antagonist mifepristone (RU-486),[43] and the estrogen receptor antagonist tamoxifen[44] did not improve clinical outcomes. Other attempts using more traditional chemotherapies such as temozolomide,[45] irinotecan,[46] and hydroxyurea[47–49] similarly did not definitively extend patient survival.

Trials using biologically targeted approaches with imatinib (inhibitor of platelet-derived growth factor receptor [PDGFR] and c-KIT),[50] erlotinib (inhibitor of epithelial growth factor receptor [EGFR]),[51] and gefitinib (inhibitor of EGFR)[51] also failed to show clinical benefit. A small phase II study of sunitinib (inhibitor of vascular endothelial growth factor receptor-2 [VEGFR2], EGFR, and PDGFR) for recurrent grade II and III meningioma demonstrated a 6-month progression-free survival of 42%.[52]

More recent study of everolimus (inhibitor of mTORC1) demonstrated a cytostatic effect on meningiomas.[53] There is an ongoing multicenter trial of vistusertib (inhibitor of mTORC1/mTORC2) for recurrent grade II and III tumors (NCT03071874). Another ongoing trial uses somatic mutational status to allocate subjects to treatment with vismodegib (Hedgehog pathway inhibitor) for SMO-mutant or PTCH-mutant meningiomas, whereas NF2-mutant tumors are allocated to treatment with GSK2256098 (FAK inhibitor) (NCT02523014).

SCHWANNOMA
Key Points

- Schwannoma is a benign tumor arising from Schwann cells within the nerve sheath.
- Most occur sporadically and singly, though certain genetic diseases and exposures may increase the risk of multiple tumors.

- Surgery and radiation are treatment options, though hearing loss and facial nerve dysfunction are a major concern when used for vestibular nerve tumors.
- Bevacizumab (anti-vascular endothelial growth factor [VEGF] antibody) may shrink tumors or improve hearing for vestibular schwannomas.

Epidemiology

Schwannomas are a common, benign tumor arising from the Schwann cells of nerve sheaths, accounting for 8% of all intracranial tumors, 85% of all cerebellopontine angle tumors, and 29% of all spinal nerve root tumors.[54] Other common intracranial locations include the trigeminal nerve or, less commonly, other lower cranial nerves, although there are also a large proportion of schwannomas diagnosed in peripheral nerves and skin. The annual incidence of schwannomas is 1.82 per 100,000, and the risk of schwannoma increases with age, with a peak annual incidence rate of 4.75 per 100,000 for individuals 65 to 74 years of age.[1] Autopsy studies of sporadic schwannomas suggest a lifetime risk of 4.8% with greater than 85% representing vestibular schwannomas.[55] Although there is no clear predilection by patient sex, the incidence of schwannoma diagnosis is nearly 2 times greater in white patients than black patients.[1]

Approximately 90% of schwannomas are solitary and sporadic,[54] though there are various exogenous and genetic factors that may increase the risk of schwannoma development significantly. The only known exogenous risk factor for schwannoma, to date, is exposure to ionizing radiation. One retrospective cohort study determined the average latency between radiotherapy and schwannoma diagnosis was 24.5 years, and survival was 65.2% at 10 years from schwannoma development.[56]

Similar to meningiomas, the risk of schwannoma development is also greatly increased by various genetic diseases, including NF2 and schwannomatosis. Although the background of these diseases is previously outlined, the risk of schwannoma development differs between them. Bilateral vestibular schwannomas are the hallmark of NF2, are pathognomonic for the disease, and are present in at least 90% of patients diagnosed with NF2.[14,57] Unilateral vestibular schwannomas are present in a much smaller proportion of patents with NF2, whereas peripheral schwannomas are found in about 70% of patients with NF2, and such individuals must have additional disease specific findings to meet clinical diagnostic criteria for NF2 (**Table 2**).[14,57]

Schwannomas are the defining feature of schwannomatosis, a distinct neurogenetic disease, which is described previously.[20,58] Schwannomatosis is associated with chronic pain in most patients,[59] which is a distinguishing feature from the more commonly painless NF2. Also distinguishing from NF2, vestibular schwannomas are rare in schwannomatosis, and schwannomatosis-associated schwannomas are never present on bilateral vestibular nerves. For those infrequent cases of schwannomatosis with unilateral vestibular schwannomas, there is increasing evidence for a genotype-phenotype correlation with *LZTR1* mutations.[23,60] Spinal schwannoma location is common for patients with schwannomatosis and there is a predilection for lumbar spine.[61] Notably, reports are mixed for the utility of tumor excision for targeted pain relief, with a suggestion of better pain-related outcomes for spinal schwannomas than peripheral schwannomas.[59,61] Studies are ongoing to better understand determinants of schwannomatosis-associated schwannoma growth, associated pain, and opportunities for therapy.

Finally, Carney complex is an autosomal dominant disorder characterized by multiple schwannomas, including the rare histologic subtype of melanotic schwannomas, as well as lentiginous facial pigmentation, cardiac myxoma, and endocrine hyperactivity, including Cushing syndrome.[62] Most cases of Carney complex are due to

Table 2 Diagnostic criteria for NF2	
NIH Diagnostic Criteria	**Expanded (Manchester) Criteria**
Bilateral vestibular schwannomas (VS) *or* Family history of NF2 *plus either* • Unilateral VS; *or* • ANY TWO OF[a]: meningioma, glioma, neurofibroma, schwannoma, posterior subcapsular cataract	Bilateral vestibular schwannomas (VS) *or* Family history of NF2 *plus either* • Unilateral VS, *or* • ANY TWO OF[a]: meningioma, glioma, neurofibroma, schwannoma, posterior subcapsular cataract *or* Unilateral VS *plus* ANY TWO OF[a]: meningioma, glioma, neurofibroma, schwannoma, posterior subcapsular cataract or cortical wedge cataract *or* Multiple meningiomas *plus either* • Unilateral VS, *or* • ANY TWO OF: glioma, neurofibroma, schwannoma, posterior subcapsular cataract or cortical wedge cataract

[a] ANY TWO OF includes two of any tumor type such as two schwannomas.

mutations in the Protein Kinase CAMP-Dependent Type 1 Regulatory Subunit Alpha (*PRKAR1A*) gene, with a smaller contribution from mutations in Protein Kinase CAMP-Activated Catalytic Subunit Alpha (*PRKACA*) or Protein Kinase CAMP-Activated Catalytic Subunit Beta (*PRKACB*), and still a smaller proportion of cases whose cause remain uncertain.[63]

Imaging

Visualization of schwannomas may be challenging on CT scan because tumors tend to be isodense to normal surrounding structures, and may be quite small and not necessarily placing mass effect on adjacent structures. Bony remodeling may occasionally be seen, and the internal auditory canal may be widened in the case of large vestibular schwannomas.

On MRI, schwannomas appear as isointense to parenchyma on T1-weighted and T2-weighted images but have bright, homogeneous enhancement on postcontrast images. In this way, schwannomas are similar to meningiomas and the precise cause of some lesions may be unsure if otherwise distinguishing features (eg, dural tail, intracanalicular location) are not present. Occasionally, large schwannomas may have internal cysts, which is also helpful in distinguishing from meningiomas. Large intracranial schwannomas, including vestibular or other cranial nerve schwannomas, may cause mass effect on adjacent structures, whereas very small tumors may require 1 mm T2-weighted slices through affected cranial nerves to visualize the lesion. MRIs are best ordered with fine T2-weighted cuts through the internal auditory canals in the case of a suspected vestibular schwannoma, whereas short tau inversion recovery (STIR) imaging is useful for suspected peripheral nerve (extracranial) schwannomas. **Fig. 3** shows an exemplary case of bilateral vestibular schwannomas on MRI. Although PET imaging is not routinely used in practice for schwannoma care, it is important to note that schwannomas avidly uptake fluorodeoxyglucose. Thus, a positive PET scan does not necessarily indicate malignancy in the case of schwannomas.

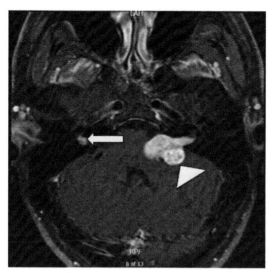

Fig. 3. Postgadolinium T1-weighted MRI showing bilateral vestibular schwannomas, with a small intracanalicular homogeneously enhancing lesion in the right internal auditory canal (*arrow*) and a right homogeneously enhancing tumor causing mass effect on the cerebello-pontine angle (*arrowhead*).

In fact, the rate of malignancy for nerve sheath tumors is less than 1% overall.[1] A recent publication showed 0% malignancy in greater than 2000 unirradiated schwannomas in patients with NF2.[64]

Pathology

Schwannomas are generally solitary, well-circumscribed tumors, with a smooth border and surrounding capsule. Histologically, schwannomas have areas of fascicles of Schwann cells with a spindle morphology and occasional nuclear palisading (ie, Antoni A pattern), with interspersed areas of looser and sometimes microcystic areas (ie, Antoni B pattern).[54] Additionally, schwannomas often contain marked parallel, palisading nuclear arrangements (ie, Verocay bodies), though these are less common in vestibular schwannomas than from other origins.[54] By contrast, neurofibromas (another type of nerve sheath tumor that primarily occurs extracranially) can be distinguished by a lack of capsule, lack of Antoni A or B patterns, and presence of axons within the tumor.[65] Hybrid tumors, containing both neurofibroma and schwannomas features, are also described.[66] Schwannomas may have extensive degenerative changes and nuclear atypia, and are referred to as ancient schwannomas in such a setting. Notably, these changes may occasionally be misinterpreted as malignant changes.

Cellular schwannomas, a separate histologic category, have increased mitoses, no Verocay bodies, and are primarily Antoni A patterned.[54] These tumors are more commonly sporadic, and occur along the spine. Clinically, their distinction is important due to a reported increased risk of local recurrence, in up to 40% depending on extent of resection.[67,68]

Genetics

The genetic landscape of schwannomas is overall quite bland, without evidence of a high mutation burden to date. Vestibular schwannomas universally have loss of Moesin-Ezrin-Radixin–Like Protein (MERLIN), the protein product of the *NF2* gene, regardless of whether they arise sporadically or in a patient with NF2.[69] Related to this, most sporadic vestibular schwannomas have identifiable somatic mutations in the *NF2* gene.[70] Interestingly, among patients with NF2, vestibular schwannomas have been noted to have multiple somatic *NF2* mutations within the same tumor, suggesting polyclonality.[71] The loss of MERLIN function is so important to schwannoma development that schwannomas arising in the setting of schwannomatosis must still functionally lose both alleles of *NF2* in addition to losing both copies of the underlying mutated schwannomatosis gene (*SMARCB1* or *LZTR1*). A process of 4 genetic hits in 3 steps (the final step representing a large deletion event) has been hypothesized.[20,72]

A recent study in sporadic schwannomas showed recurrent mutations in AT-Rich Interaction Domain 1A (*ARID1A*), AT-Rich Interaction Domain 1B (*ARID1B*), and Discoidin Domain Receptor Tyrosine Kinase 1 (*DDR1*), as well as a newly described SH3 and PX domains S1 (*SH3PXD2A*) and high temperature requirement A serine peptidase 1 (*HTRA1*) fusion protein present in 10% of tumors.[73] Notably, this fusion was much more common in men and may provide a targeted therapeutic opportunity.[73] Another recent a genomic study of schwannomas described a propensity for mutations in axonal guidance pathways, as well as in the Cell Division Cycle 27 (*CDC27*) and Ubiquitin Specific Peptidase 8 (*USP8*) genes.[70] Finally, methylation analysis recently showed distinct epigenetic characteristics between vestibular and spinal meningiomas.[73]

Therapy

Surgery

Whereas the risk of spontaneous malignant transformation of schwannomas is less than 1%,[1] intervention is not necessarily required for tumors that are asymptomatic, radiographically stable, and are not adversely effecting adjacent structures. In such a setting, the risk of intervention may outweigh the benefit thereof. However, a subgroup of tumors does grow and therefore requires treatment. A natural history study of 162 vestibular schwannomas from Denmark showed 55% of tumors grew less than or equal to 1 mm per year, yet 23% grew greater than 1 mm per year.[74] A more recent study following only intracanalicular vestibular schwannomas reported that about 37% of tumors grow within 10 years.[75] As such, for growing tumors, or tumors that cause neurologic symptoms that affect quality of life, intervention may be indicated.

Similar to meningioma, the first choice of therapy for safely accessible schwannomas is surgical resection, which may be curative. For vestibular schwannoma, the risk of surgical resection leading to ipsilateral deafness is nearly 43% to 73%, and the risk of facial nerve dysfunction is 15% to 72%, both depending on the size and location of the tumor along the facial nerve.[76,77] For progressive lower cranial nerve schwannomas, resection is sometimes possible but may result in intolerable dysfunction of lower cranial nerves, including dysphonia, dysphagia, and risk of aspiration. Surgery for painful spinal schwannomas may improve pain and neurologic dysfunction, whereas pain from peripheral schwannoma resection is less likely to improve.[59,61]

Radiation therapy and radiosurgery are effective means of obtaining local control for sporadic schwannomas, with roughly 90% progression-free survival for both therapies at 5 years.[78] Similar to surgery, both hearing and facial nerve function are at risk with radiation therapy but on more of a long-term basis. The risk of losing ipsilateral serviceable hearing after radiotherapy is 45% at 3 years, 63% at 5 years, and 71% at 7 years. The risk of facial nerve dysfunction is 15% at 10 years.[78] Malignant transformation has been reported in 0.3% of radiation-treated schwannomas at a median of 4.9 years and so is of greatest concern in treating younger patients.[40]

Finally, chemotherapy is an increasingly noteworthy consideration for the treatment of NF2-associated schwannomas. For NF2-related vestibular schwannomas specifically, bevacizumab (an anti-VEGF antibody) has been described to improve hearing in approximately 50% of patients, and to reduce tumor size in about 50% of patients, though tumor size does not correlate with hearing and so hearing and size response may not be seen in the same individual.[79,80] Everolimus, an mTORC1 inhibitor, shows cytostatic effects for NF2-associated vestibular schwannomas, similar to its use in meningiomas.[81] Erlotinib, an EGFR tyrosine kinase inhibitor, showed no objective radiographic responses in a retrospective series.[82] However, lapatinib, also an EGFR tyrosine kinase inhibitor, showed objective activity in a small number of progressive NF2-associated vestibular schwannomas in a phase 2 trial.[83] There are ongoing clinical trials of axitinib (VEGF, c-KIT, and PDGFR tyrosine kinase inhibitor, NCT02129647), AR-42 (histone deacetylase inhibitor, NCT02282917), and selumetinib (MEK inhibitor, NCT03095248). Finally, there is recent retrospective evidence of routine aspirin use slowing the growth of vestibular schwannomas,[84] and so a prospective clinical trial is planned (NCT03079999).

SUMMARY

Meningiomas and schwannomas are the most common benign intracranial tumors in adults and are associated with several genetic driver events, including both germline mutations (especially in the disorders of NF2 and schwannomatosis) and somatic tumor initiating events. Although not all tumors require treatment, surgery remains the primary therapeutic modality for many of these tumors. However, surgery may not always be feasible or sufficient for every tumor; therefore, radiation is a commonly used adjuvant or even alternative option. Finally, for multiple recurrent meningiomas or for individuals with many benign tumors, such as with a genetic disorder, chemotherapy is an enticing option but has historically been ineffective. Novel findings in genetic drivers and cellular growth pathway activation have identified promising new systemic therapeutic options.

REFERENCES

1. Ostrom QT, Gittleman H, Xu J, et al. CBTRUS statistical report: primary brain and other central nervous system tumors diagnosed in the United States in 2009-2013. Neuro Oncol 2016;18(suppl_5):v1–75.
2. Kuratsu J, Ushio Y. Epidemiological study of primary intracranial tumours in elderly people. J Neurol Neurosurg Psychiatry 1997;63(1):116–8.
3. Neglia JP, Robison LL, Stovall M, et al. New primary neoplasms of the central nervous system in survivors of childhood cancer: a report from the Childhood Cancer Survivor Study. J Natl Cancer Inst 2006;98(21):1528–37.
4. Phillips LE, Frankenfeld CL, Drangsholt M, et al. Intracranial meningioma and ionizing radiation in medical and occupational settings. Neurology 2005;64(2):350–2.
5. Yamanaka R, Hayano A, Kanayama T. Radiation-induced meningiomas: an exhaustive review of the literature. World Neurosurg 2017;97:635–44.e8.
6. Sioka C, Kyritsis AP. Chemotherapy, hormonal therapy, and immunotherapy for recurrent meningiomas. J Neurooncol 2009;92(1):1–6.
7. Phillips LE, Koepsell TD, van Belle G, et al. History of head trauma and risk of intracranial meningioma: population-based case-control study. Neurology 2002;58(12):1849–52.
8. Huisman TW, Tanghe HL, Koper JW, et al. Progesterone, oestradiol, somatostatin and epidermal growth factor receptors on human meningiomas and their CT characteristics. Eur J Cancer 1991;27(11):1453–7.

9. Chamberlain M. Chemotherapy for intracranial meningiomas. In: DeMonte F, McDermott MW, Al-Mefty O, editors. Al-Mefty's meningiomas. 2nd edition. New York: Thieme; 2011. p. 399–406.

10. Beauchamp RL, James MF, DeSouza PA, et al. A high-throughput kinome screen reveals serum/glucocorticoid-regulated kinase 1 as a therapeutic target for NF2-deficient meningiomas. Oncotarget 2015;6(19):16981–97.

11. James MF, Stivison E, Beauchamp R, et al. Regulation of mTOR complex 2 signaling in neurofibromatosis 2-deficient target cell types. Mol Cancer Res 2012;10(5):649–59.

12. Goutagny S, Kalamarides M. Meningiomas and neurofibromatosis. J Neurooncol 2010;99(3):341–7.

13. Smith MJ, Higgs JE, Bowers NL, et al. Cranial meningiomas in 411 neurofibromatosis type 2 (NF2) patients with proven gene mutations: clear positional effect of mutations, but absence of female severity effect on age at onset. J Med Genet 2011;48(4):261–5.

14. Mautner VF, Lindenau M, Baser ME, et al. The neuroimaging and clinical spectrum of neurofibromatosis 2. Neurosurgery 1996;38(5):880–5 [discussion: 885–6].

15. Ruggieri M, Iannetti P, Polizzi A, et al. Earliest clinical manifestations and natural history of neurofibromatosis type 2 (NF2) in childhood: a study of 24 patients. Neuropediatrics 2005;36(1):21–34.

16. Smith MJ, Kulkarni A, Rustad C, et al. Vestibular schwannomas occur in schwannomatosis and should not be considered an exclusion criterion for clinical diagnosis. Am J Med Genet A 2012;158A(1):215–9.

17. Gripp KW, Baker L, Kandula V, et al. Constitutional LZTR1 mutation presenting with a unilateral vestibular schwannoma in a teenager. Clin Genet 2017;92(5):540–3.

18. Mehta GU, Feldman MJ, Wang H, et al. Unilateral vestibular schwannoma in a patient with schwannomatosis in the absence of LZTR1 mutation. J Neurosurg 2016;125(6):1469–71.

19. Wu J, Kong M, Bi Q. Identification of a novel germline SMARCB1 nonsense mutation in a family manifesting both schwannomatosis and unilateral vestibular schwannoma. J Neurooncol 2015;125(2):439–41.

20. Plotkin SR, Blakeley JO, Evans DG, et al. Update from the 2011 International Schwannomatosis Workshop: from genetics to diagnostic criteria. Am J Med Genet Part A 2013;161A(3):405–16.

21. Rousseau G, Noguchi T, Bourdon V, et al. SMARCB1/INI1 germline mutations contribute to 10% of sporadic schwannomatosis. BMC Neurol 2011;11:9.

22. Smith MJ, Wallace AJ, Bowers NL, et al. SMARCB1 mutations in schwannomatosis and genotype correlations with rhabdoid tumors. Cancer Genet 2014;207(9):373–8.

23. Smith MJ, Isidor B, Beetz C, et al. Mutations in LZTR1 add to the complex heterogeneity of schwannomatosis. Neurology 2015;84(2):141–7.

24. Piotrowski A, Xie J, Liu YF, et al. Germline loss-of-function mutations in LZTR1 predispose to an inherited disorder of multiple schwannomas. Nat Genet 2014;46(2):182–7.

25. Gerkes EH, Fock JM, den Dunnen WF, et al. A heritable form of SMARCE1-related meningiomas with important implications for follow-up and family screening. Neurogenetics 2016;17(2):83–9.

26. Smith MJ, Wallace AJ, Bennett C, et al. Germline SMARCE1 mutations predispose to both spinal and cranial clear cell meningiomas. J Pathol 2014;234(4):436–40.

27. Shankar GM, Abedalthagafi M, Vaubel RA, et al. Germline and somatic BAP1 mutations in high-grade rhabdoid meningiomas. Neuro Oncol 2017;19(4):535–45.

28. Perry A, Louis DN, Budka H, et al. Meningiomas. In: Louis DN, Ohgaki H, Wiestler OD, et al, editors. WHO classification of tumours of the central nervous system. 4th edition. Lyon (France): International Agency for Research on Cancer; 2016. p. 231–46.

29. Rogers L, Barani I, Chamberlain M, et al. Meningiomas: knowledge base, treatment outcomes, and uncertainties. A RANO review. J Neurosurg 2015;122(1): 4–23.

30. Brastianos PK, Horowitz PM, Santagata S, et al. Genomic sequencing of meningiomas identifies oncogenic SMO and AKT1 mutations. Nat Genet 2013;45(3): 285–9.

31. Clark VE, Erson-Omay EZ, Serin A, et al. Genomic analysis of non-NF2 meningiomas reveals mutations in TRAF7, KLF4, AKT1, and SMO. Science 2013; 339(6123):1077–80.

32. Abedalthagafi M, Bi WL, Aizer AA, et al. Oncogenic PI3K mutations are as common as AKT1 and SMO mutations in meningioma. Neuro Oncol 2016;18(5): 649–55.

33. Bostrom J, Meyer-Puttlitz B, Wolter M, et al. Alterations of the tumor suppressor genes CDKN2A (p16(INK4a)), p14(ARF), CDKN2B (p15(INK4b)), and CDKN2C (p18(INK4c)) in atypical and anaplastic meningiomas. Am J Pathol 2001; 159(2):661–9.

34. Sahm F, Schrimpf D, Olar A, et al. TERT promoter mutations and risk of recurrence in meningioma. J Natl Cancer Inst 2016;108(5).

35. Simpson D. The recurrence of intracranial meningiomas after surgical treatment. J Neurol Neurosurg Psychiatry 1957;20(1):22–39.

36. Sanford NN, Yeap BY, Larvie M, et al. Prospective, randomized study of radiation dose escalation with combined proton-photon therapy for benign meningiomas. Int J Radiat Oncol Biol Phys 2017;99(4):787–96.

37. Mendenhall WM, Morris CG, Amdur RJ, et al. Radiotherapy alone or after subtotal resection for benign skull base meningiomas. Cancer 2003;98(7):1473–82.

38. Miralbell R, Linggood RM, de la Monte S, et al. The role of radiotherapy in the treatment of subtotally resected benign meningiomas. J Neurooncol 1992; 13(2):157–64.

39. Hakim R, Alexander E 3rd, Loeffler JS, et al. Results of linear accelerator-based radiosurgery for intracranial meningiomas. Neurosurgery 1998;42(3):446–53 [discussion: 453–4].

40. Pollock BE, Link MJ, Stafford SL, et al. The risk of radiation-induced tumors or malignant transformation after single-fraction intracranial radiosurgery: results based on a 25-year experience. Int J Radiat Oncol Biol Phys 2017;97(5):919–23.

41. Kaley T, Barani I, Chamberlain M, et al. Historical benchmarks for medical therapy trials in surgery- and radiation-refractory meningioma: a RANO review. Neuro Oncol 2014;16(6):829–40.

42. Grunberg SM, Weiss MH. Lack of efficacy of megestrol acetate in the treatment of unresectable meningioma. J Neurooncol 1990;8(1):61–5.

43. Ji Y, Rankin C, Grunberg S, et al. Double-Blind Phase III Randomized Trial of the Antiprogestin Agent Mifepristone in the Treatment of Unresectable Meningioma: SWOG S9005. J Clin Oncol 2015;33(34):4093–8.

44. Goodwin JW, Crowley J, Eyre HJ, et al. A phase II evaluation of tamoxifen in unresectable or refractory meningiomas: a Southwest Oncology Group study. J Neurooncol 1993;15(1):75–7.

45. Chamberlain MC, Tsao-Wei DD, Groshen S. Temozolomide for treatment-resistant recurrent meningioma. Neurology 2004;62(7):1210–2.
46. Chamberlain MC, Tsao-Wei DD, Groshen S. Salvage chemotherapy with CPT-11 for recurrent meningioma. J Neurooncol 2006;78(3):271–6.
47. Newton HB, Scott SR, Volpi C. Hydroxyurea chemotherapy for meningiomas: enlarged cohort with extended follow-up. Br J Neurosurg 2004;18(5):495–9.
48. Loven D, Hardoff R, Sever ZB, et al. Non-resectable slow-growing meningiomas treated by hydroxyurea. J Neurooncol 2004;67(1–2):221–6.
49. Rosenthal MA, Ashley DL, Cher L. Treatment of high risk or recurrent meningiomas with hydroxyurea. J Clin Neurosci 2002;9(2):156–8.
50. Wen PY, Yung WK, Lamborn KR, et al. Phase II study of imatinib mesylate for recurrent meningiomas (North American Brain Tumor Consortium study 01-08). Neuro Oncol 2009;11(6):853–60.
51. Norden AD, Raizer JJ, Abrey LE, et al. Phase II trials of erlotinib or gefitinib in patients with recurrent meningioma. J Neurooncol 2010;96(2):211–7.
52. Kaley TJ, Wen P, Schiff D, et al. Phase II trial of sunitinib for recurrent and progressive atypical and anaplastic meningioma. Neuro Oncol 2015;17(1):116–21.
53. Karajannis M, Osorio D, Filatov A, et al. Effects of everolimus on meningioma growth in patients with neurofibromatosis type 2. Neuro Oncol 2014;16(suppl 5) [abstract: AT-30].
54. Antonescu CR, Louis DN, Hunter S, et al. Schwannoma. In: Louis DN, Ohgaki H, Wiestler OD, et al, editors. WHO classification of tumours of the central nervous system. 4th edition. Lyon (France): International Agency for Research on Cancer; 2016. p. 214–6.
55. Schneider J, Warzok R, Schreiber D, et al. Tumors of the central nervous system in biopsy and autopsy material. 7th communication: neurinomas and neurofibromatoses with CNS involvement. Zentralbl Allg Pathol 1983;127(5–6):305–14 [in German].
56. Yamanaka R, Hayano A. Radiation-induced schwannomas and neurofibromas: a systematic review. World Neurosurg 2017;104:713–22.
57. Evans DG, Huson SM, Donnai D, et al. A clinical study of type 2 neurofibromatosis. Q J Med 1992;84(304):603–18.
58. MacCollin M, Chiocca EA, Evans DG, et al. Diagnostic criteria for schwannomatosis. Neurology 2005;64(11):1838–45.
59. Merker VL, Esparza S, Smith MJ, et al. Clinical features of schwannomatosis: a retrospective analysis of 87 patients. Oncologist 2012;17(10):1317–22.
60. Smith MJ, Bowers NL, Bulman M, et al. Revisiting neurofibromatosis type 2 diagnostic criteria to exclude LZTR1-related schwannomatosis. Neurology 2017; 88(1):87–92.
61. Li P, Zhao F, Zhang J, et al. Clinical features of spinal schwannomas in 65 patients with schwannomatosis compared with 831 with solitary schwannomas and 102 with neurofibromatosis type 2: a retrospective study at a single institution. J Neurosurg Spine 2016;24(1):145–54.
62. Carney JA. Psammomatous melanotic schwannoma. A distinctive, heritable tumor with special associations, including cardiac myxoma and the Cushing syndrome. Am J Surg Pathol 1990;14(3):206–22.
63. Bosco Schamun MB, Correa R, Graffigna P, et al. Carney complex review: genetic features. Endocrinol Diabetes Nutr 2018;65(1):52–9.
64. King AT, Rutherford SA, Hammerbeck-Ward C, et al. Malignant peripheral nerve sheath tumors are not a feature of neurofibromatosis type 2 in the unirradiated patient. Neurosurgery 2018;83(1):38–42.

65. Perry A, von Deimling A, Louis DN, et al. Neurofibroma. In: Louis DN, Ohgaki H, Wiestler OD, et al, editors. WHO classification of tumours of the central nervous system. 4th edition. Lyon (France): International Agency for Research on Cancer; 2016. p. 219–21.

66. Hornick JL, Bundock EA, Fletcher CD. Hybrid schwannoma/perineurioma: clinicopathologic analysis of 42 distinctive benign nerve sheath tumors. Am J Surg Pathol 2009;33(10):1554–61.

67. Casadei GP, Scheithauer BW, Hirose T, et al. Cellular schwannoma. A clinicopathologic, DNA flow cytometric, and proliferation marker study of 70 patients. Cancer 1995;75(5):1109–19.

68. White W, Shiu MH, Rosenblum MK, et al. Cellular schwannoma. A clinicopathologic study of 57 patients and 58 tumors. Cancer 1990;66(6):1266–75.

69. Stemmer-Rachamimov AO, Xu L, Gonzalez-Agosti C, et al. Universal absence of merlin, but not other ERM family members, in schwannomas. Am J Pathol 1997; 151(6):1649–54.

70. Håvik AL, Bruland O, Myrseth E, et al. Genetic landscape of sporadic vestibular schwannoma. J Neurosurg 2018;128(3):911–22.

71. Dewan R, Pemov A, Kim HJ, et al. Evidence of polyclonality in neurofibromatosis type 2-associated multilobulated vestibular schwannomas. Neuro Oncol 2015; 17(4):566–73.

72. Sestini R, Bacci C, Provenzano A, et al. Evidence of a four-hit mechanism involving SMARCB1 and NF2 in schwannomatosis-associated schwannomas. Hum Mutat 2008;29(2):227–31.

73. Agnihotri S, Jalali S, Wilson MR, et al. The genomic landscape of schwannoma. Nat Genet 2016;48(11):1339–48.

74. Mirz F, Pedersen CB, Fiirgaard B, et al. Incidence and growth pattern of vestibular schwannomas in a Danish county, 1977-98. Acta Otolaryngol Suppl 2000;543: 30–3.

75. Kirchmann M, Karnov K, Hansen S, et al. Ten-year follow-up on tumor growth and hearing in patients observed with an intracanalicular vestibular schwannoma. Neurosurgery 2017;80(1):49–56.

76. Wiet RJ, Mamikoglu B, Odom L, et al. Long-term results of the first 500 cases of acoustic neuroma surgery. Otolaryngol Head Neck Surg 2001;124(6): 645–51.

77. Samii M, Matthies C, Tatagiba M. Management of vestibular schwannomas (acoustic neuromas): auditory and facial nerve function after resection of 120 vestibular schwannomas in patients with neurofibromatosis 2. Neurosurgery 1997;40(4):696–705 [discussion: 705–6].

78. Lo A, Ayre G, Ma R, et al. Population-based study of stereotactic radiosurgery or fractionated stereotactic radiation therapy for vestibular schwannoma: long-term outcomes and toxicities. Int J Radiat Oncol Biol Phys 2018;100(2):443–51.

79. Plotkin SR, Merker VL, Halpin C, et al. Bevacizumab for progressive vestibular schwannoma in neurofibromatosis type 2: a retrospective review of 31 patients. Otol Neurotol 2012;33(6):1046–52.

80. Plotkin SR, Stemmer-Rachamimov AO, Barker FG 2nd, et al. Hearing improvement after bevacizumab in patients with neurofibromatosis type 2. N Engl J Med 2009;361(4):358–67.

81. Goutagny S, Raymond E, Esposito-Farese M, et al. Phase II study of mTORC1 inhibition by everolimus in neurofibromatosis type 2 patients with growing vestibular schwannomas. J Neurooncol 2015;122(2):313–20.

82. Plotkin SR, Halpin C, McKenna MJ, et al. Erlotinib for progressive vestibular schwannoma in neurofibromatosis 2 patients. Otol Neurotol 2010;31(7):1135–43.
83. Karajannis MA, Legault G, Hagiwara M, et al. Phase II trial of lapatinib in adult and pediatric patients with neurofibromatosis type 2 and progressive vestibular schwannomas. Neuro Oncol 2012;14(9):1163–70.
84. Kandathil CK, Cunnane ME, McKenna MJ, et al. Correlation between aspirin intake and reduced growth of human vestibular schwannoma: volumetric analysis. Otol Neurotol 2016;37(9):1428–34.

Primary Central Nervous System Lymphoma

Kaylyn Sinicrope, MD[a], Tracy Batchelor, MD, MPH[a,b,c],*

KEYWORDS

- Primary central nervous system lymphoma • Brain • Non-Hodgkin's lymphoma
- Methotrexate

KEY POINTS

- Primary central nervous system lymphoma (PCNSL) is an aggressive form of Non-Hodgkin's lymphoma restricted to the central nervous system.
- Stereotactic biopsy is the gold-standard for diagnosis of PCNSL.
- Methotrexate-based chemotherapy is the standard induction for PCNSL patient.
- Optimal treatment for relapsed and refractory PCNSL has not been defined.

INTRODUCTION

Primary central nervous system lymphoma (PCNSL) is an aggressive Non-Hodgkin's lymphoma (NHL) confined to the CNS, including the brain, spinal cord, eyes, and leptomeninges. It is a rare disease that makes up approximately 1% to 2% of all NHL cases and about 4% of primary brain tumors.[1–3] Although PCNSL can develop in both the immunocompetent and immunocompromised host, the focus of this article is on the former.

EPIDEMIOLOGY

Data from population-based studies on PCNSL are limited due to its low incidence of 7 cases per 1,000,000 population in the United States per year.[4] Over time, the incidence of PCNSL has fluctuated, with an increase in the 1980s that was thought to be due to the acquired immunodeficiency syndrome (AIDS) pandemic. The incidence

[a] Department of Neurology, Massachusetts General Hospital, Harvard Medical School, 55 Fruit Street, Boston, MA 02114, USA; [b] Radiation Oncology, Massachusetts General Hospital, Harvard Medical School, 55 Fruit Street, Boston, MA 02114, USA; [c] Division of Hematology and Oncology, Massachusetts General Hospital, Harvard Medical School, 55 Fruit Street, Boston, MA 02114, USA
* Corresponding author. Massachusetts General Hospital, Pappas Center for Neuro Oncology, 55 Fruit Street, Boston, MA 02114.
E-mail address: tbatchelor@mgh.harvard.edu

Neurol Clin 36 (2018) 517–532
https://doi.org/10.1016/j.ncl.2018.04.008
0733-8619/18/© 2018 Elsevier Inc. All rights reserved.
neurologic.theclinics.com

increased until the mid-1990s, when it peaked; it has subsequently declined.[4] In the immunocompetent population, PCNSL tends to occur in older individuals with a median age at diagnosis of 65.[5–7] For unclear reasons, this older population is the only subgroup that continues to have an increasing incidence of PCNSL despite the overall decline reported in the United States.[4,8,9]

PATHOPHYSIOLOGY

Most (>90%) PCNSL cases are diffuse large B cell lymphomas (DLBCLs), a lymphoma histologically indistinct from systemic NHL.[10] PCNSLs are highly proliferative, and demonstrate an angiocentric growth pattern.[10]

Genetic profiling has allowed for lymphomas to be subdivided into classes based on the specific differentiation stage during which malignant transformation is assumed to occur. These groups include germinal center B cell-like (GCB), activated B cell-like (ABC), and type 3. PCNSL displays a unique molecular signature (MUM1+, BCL6+, CD10-), consistent with features of both GCB and ABC types. Most PCNSL cases are considered to be of the ABC immunophenotype, which, in systemic DLBCL, is associated with more aggressive disease and poor prognosis.[10]

In PCNSL, additional mutations in the B cell signaling pathway affect the downstream target nuclear factor kappa B (NFkB), particularly mutations in MYD88.[11] Studies have shown elevated but variable percentages of mutations in these genes from 29% to 86% of patients with PCNSL.[12,13] Interestingly, the increase in mutations in the MYD88 genes has been reported to be significantly more frequent in PCNSL compared with systemic ABC-type DLBCL.[12,13] The presence of this mutation suggests that targeted therapies focused on this pathway may be useful in the treatment of PCNSL.

CLINICAL PRESENTATION

PCNSL can be a diagnostic challenge, as presentation is variable and nonspecific. In a retrospective study of 248 immunocompetent individuals with PCNSL, the most common symptoms on presentation were focal neurologic deficits (70%), neuropsychiatric symptoms (43%), seizures (14%), and symptoms attributable to increased intracranial pressure such as headache, nausea, and vomiting (33%).[6]

Isolated leptomeningeal (LM) lymphoma is rare, comprising only 7% of all cases of PCNSL in immunocompetent hosts. However, LM lymphoma occurs simultaneously with intracranial disease in approximately 15% to 20% of all PCNSL patients.[14] LM disease is asymptomatic in the majority of patients, although cranial nerve palsies have been reported variably in the literature (5%–31% of cases).[15]

In some cases, PCNSL patients will have involvement of the eye or spine. Approximately 10% to 20% of PCNSL cases are found to have intraocular involvement at the time of diagnosis, although isolated intraocular lymphoma is much less common.[16] Typically patients with eye involvement report nonspecific symptoms such as floaters and blurred vision.[5,6] Spinal involvement of PCNSL is rare (<5%) and typically presents with symptoms that localize to the spinal cord such as limb paresthesias, weakness (often asymmetric), bowel or bladder dysfunction, impaired gait, and perineal numbness.[17]

DIAGNOSIS
Imaging

PCNSL has a characteristic appearance on both computed tomography (CT) and MRI due to its hypercellularity and disruption of the blood-brain barrier (**Fig. 1**).[17] On MRI,

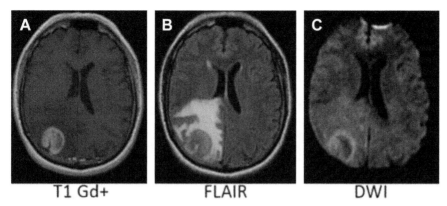

T1 Gd+   FLAIR   DWI

Fig. 1. Characteristic pattern of PCNSL on MRI. (*A*) Axial T1 weighted imaging after contrast demonstrates a single contrast-enhancing lesion. (*B*) Fluid-attenuated inversion recovery (FLAIR) image visualizes an area of edema surrounding the lesion. (*C*) Diffusion-weighted imaging (DWI) with corresponding bright appearance suggesting increased cellularity.

most lesions show decreased signal compared with gray matter on T1 sequences, and demonstrate homogenous enhancement after the administration of contrast. Most PCNSL cases have a moderate amount of vasogenic edema, appearing on MRI as high T2 weighted signal surrounding the lesion.[18] In the immunocompetent host, approximately two-thirds of PCNSL patients present with a single, supratentorial lesion. Lesions are typically located near the gray-white junction in the cerebral hemispheres (49%), with another 15% found in the basal ganglia and thalamus.[19,20] As many as 12% of PCNSL lesions arise in the corpus callosum, a site that is particularly suggestive of the diagnosis.[6] The lesions are often larger than 1 cm, and are well circumscribed. They are rarely associated with hemorrhage, reported in just 2% to 8% of cases.[19]

Cerebrospinal Fluid

Ideally, cerebrospinal fluid (CSF) analysis should be performed on patients in whom the diagnosis of PCNSL is being considered. However, in patients with increased intracranial pressure or mass effect, lumbar puncture may be contraindicated. If there is doubt about the safety of obtaining CSF, neurosurgical consultation should be obtained. Diagnosis of PCNSL from CSF cytology occurs in only 10% to 20% of patients (**Fig. 2**).[17,21] Flow cytometry, a method of immunophenotyping, has a higher sensitivity in the diagnosis of PCNSL than cytology. However, most authorities suggest that cytology and flow cytometry are complementary tests and thus should be performed together.[22,23] PCNSL may have a clonally mutated immunoglobulin heavy chain (IgH) that can be detected via polymerase chain reaction (PCR) of CSF, providing an efficient and sensitive diagnostic test. In an untreated PCNSL patient cohort, 1 study found that 60% of patients had a positive result, showing that PCR integration with cytology enhances the sensitivity of CSF analysis.[24] However, given the importance of early diagnosis and treatment of PCNSL, it is generally not recommended to await results of CSF studies in patients who could otherwise have a stereotactic biopsy of a coexisting brain lesion.

Brain Biopsy

The diagnosis of PCNSL should be confirmed histologically. In most cases this is achieved by performing a stereotactic biopsy. The robust response of lymphoma cells to steroids can alter the diagnostic yield of biopsy and thus should be held until a diagnostic work up is complete.[25]

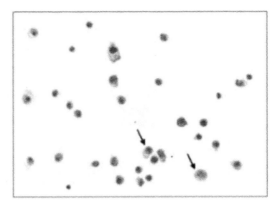

Fig. 2. Photomicrograph demonstrating positive cytopathological results in a sample of CSF from a patient with leptomeningeal involvement in PCNSL. The sample demonstrates multiple lymphocytes (*arrows*) with features of malignancy including pleomorphic nuclei, coarse chromatin, and excess cytoplasm. H&E, magnification unknown. (*From* Fitzsimmons A, Upchurch K, Batchelor T. Clinical features and diagnosis of primary central nervous system lymphoma. Hematol Oncol Clin North Am 2005;19(4):696, vii; with permission.)

Extent of Disease Evaluation

The International PCNSL Lymphoma Collaborative Group (IPCG) has developed consensus guidelines for the diagnostic evaluation of patients with PCNSL.[26] The purpose of the guidelines is to determine the extent of disease within the CNS and to exclude the presence of disease outside of the nervous system. This work up is critical, as up to 12.5% of individuals presenting with presumed primary CNS lymphoma are found to have systemic disease.[27,28] A combined positron emission tomography (PET)/CT scan of the chest, abdomen, and pelvis is indicated to assess for systemic lymphoma. Older males should also have a testicular ultrasound to assess for testicular lymphoma. A bone marrow biopsy is recommended to assess for evidence of systemic disease. Given the tendency of lymphoma to involve the leptomeninges, a lumbar puncture should be performed, when safe, with CSF analysis for glucose, total protein, cell counts, cytology, flow cytometry, and IgH gene rearrangement. An ophthalmologic evaluation that includes a slit lamp examination by an ophthalmologist is needed to screen for intraocular involvement. Testing of the serum for cell counts, creatinine, lactate dehydrogenase (LDH), and HIV should be performed.[26] Given the risk of neurocognitive impairment with treatment and disease, serial cognitive assessment should be performed, and the IPCG has developed a battery for this evaluation.

PROGNOSIS

Evaluating and understanding prognostic factors in PCNSL is useful to patients, clinicians, and investigators, as they can guide expectations and influence therapeutic approaches. Factors that affect prognosis have been evaluated in several studies, and the most consistent factors found to impact prognosis are age and performance status.[21,29,30]

Prior to treatment, it is recommended that patients with PCNSL be evaluated with a prognostic score in an attempt to stratify by risk. The International Extranodal Lymphoma Study Group (IELSG) score, Memorial Sloan Kettering Cancer Center (MSKCC) score, and the Nottingham-Barcelona (NB) model[21,29,30] represent 3 prognostic scoring systems. The NB prognostic score was developed from a study of 77 patients and includes 4 factors: age, Karnofsky Performance status (KPS), multifocal, or meningeal disease.[30] The IELSG model is a prognostic scoring system based on the evaluation of 378 patients that includes 5 variables associated with poor prognosis: age greater than 60, Eastern Cooperative Oncology Group performance score greater than 1, elevated serum lactate dehydrogenase, and involvement of the deep structures of the brain. Patients with 1 to 2 variables were found to have a 5-year overall survival of 80%, while those with 4 to 5 variables had a 5-year overall survival of 15%.[21] The MSKCC prognostic score is simpler model based on age and KPS, separating patients into 3 classes. The MSKCC score was validated with an external cohort of 194 patients; within this cohort, individuals in class 1 (age <50) were found to have a median survival of 5.2 years, while those in class 3 (age >50 and KPS <70) had an median survival of 0.8 years.[29]

PRIMARY CENTRAL NERVOUS SYSTEM LYMPHOMA TREATMENT

Historically, the treatment of PCNSL has focused on regimens similar to those used in the treatment of systemic DLBCL. However, these regimens proved ineffective because of the poor penetration of these agents across the blood-brain barrier. Alternate treatment regimens will be outlined and involve surgery, corticosteroids, radiation, chemotherapy, and high-dose chemotherapy with stem cell transplantation. In typical treatment of PCNSL, the initial phase of treatment is referred to as remission-induction. Once remission is achieved, the second phase of treatment, called remission-consolidation, is typically pursued with the intent to eradicate any residual lymphoma cells and reduce the risk of relapse.

Surgery

In PCNSL, the role of resection has been limited to biopsy because of the infiltrative nature of lymphoma. Although no randomized controlled trials evaluating the efficacy of surgical resection exist, surgery is avoided due to limited observational data, suggesting that it does not offer any survival benefit and has higher associated risks.[31,32]

Recently, the role of surgery in PCNSL has been challenged by retrospective studies. In the German PCNSL study group 1 randomized trial, there was an unexpectedly high number of individuals who underwent subtotal resections (STRs) and gross total resections (GTRs). Outcomes were compared between those with resection and those who underwent biopsy in a post hoc analysis. In the population undergoing resection, 56% of the GTR and 46% of the STR groups achieved complete remission with radiation therapy compared to 34% with biopsy and radiation. Progression-free survival (PFS) and overall survival (OS) were also significantly longer in the patients who underwent resection.[33] The role of selection bias in this retrospective analysis is difficult to determine.

Despite emerging data challenging the role of surgical resection, there remain insufficient data to support its routine use. The role of surgery is limited at this point to diagnostic biopsy, and resection is appropriate only in special cases of mass lesions leading to increased intracranial pressure and impending herniation.

Corticosteroids

Corticosteroids are useful in the treatment of lymphoma. The use of steroids in the initial treatment of PCNSL has been reported to cause partial radiographic regression in up to 40% of patients[25,33] In addition to its cytolytic effects, steroids are effective at restoring the blood-brain barrier. There are conflicting data regarding whether the diagnostic yield of biopsy is negatively impacted by pretreatment with corticosteroids.[34] However, the standard practice is to avoid corticosteroids prior to biopsy in this patient population.

Radiation

Whole-brain radiation therapy (WBRT) is an effective treatment for PCNSL that results in tumor regression and is often part of multimodality treatment regimens used in practice. WBRT is required due to the diffuse, microscopic nature of PCNSL. Focal forms of radiation have not been systematically assessed for PCNSL and are not advised at this point.

Given the low overall survival in patients with PCNSL treated with WBRT alone, investigations have also assessed WBRT plus chemotherapy (**Table 1**). There is 1 randomized phase 3 trial that specifically investigated the efficacy of WBRT as part of a multimodality treatment regimen. In this study, all patients received chemotherapy with high-dose methotrexate (HD-MTX) with or without ifosfamide. Those who achieved complete remission were randomized to WBRT or observation. The WBRT arm had a longer progression-free survival of 18 months versus 12 months in the observation arm. However, there was no difference in overall survival between the 2 arms, and patients in the WBRT arm had higher rates of delayed neurotoxicity. Interpretations of this study vary, but it appears that deferral of WBRT does not negatively impact overall survival.[35]

The primary concern with the use of WBRT in PCNSL is its association with neurotoxicity. WBRT may lead to neurotoxicity, most apparent in cognitive function, particularly in the elderly.[36] In addition to the clinical evidence suggesting neurotoxicity, imaging evaluations have found that WBRT leads to leukoencephalopathy and atrophy of the subcortical and cortical white matter.[37]

Chemotherapy

The foundation of effective chemotherapeutic regimens used in the treatment of PCNSL is methotrexate (**Table 2**). Methotrexate is an antimetabolite of the antifolate type that competitively inhibits dihydrofolate reductase (DHFR) and effectively inhibits the activation of folate. Folate is critical for the synthesis of DNA and RNA, and MTX is thus a cytotoxic agent. There are multiple prospective trials evaluating the use of HD-MTX for PCNSL.[38–41] These studies demonstrated a response to treatment in at least 50% of the patients studied. In a multicenter, prospective phase 2 trial, 25 patients were treated with 8 g/m^2 of intravenous methotrexate. In this group, 52% of the patients achieved complete remission, although progression-free survival was 12.8 months.[38] The benefit of using methotrexate in the treatment of PCNSL is clear; however, the optimal dose of methotrexate has not been defined. It is possible to achieve therapeutic levels of methotrexate in the CSF through intravenous infusion at high doses, but the concentration in the CNS is affected by both the dose and the rate of infusion. A study evaluating the CSF concentrations of intravenous MTX found that a dose of 3 g/m^2 was the minimum dose required to achieve therapeutic CSF levels.[42]

Several prospective studies have subsequently evaluated the efficacy of methotrexate in combination with other chemotherapies. Most have demonstrated good radiographic response rates and improved survival (see **Table 1**). Ferreri and colleagues[43] found that combination chemotherapy was superior to HD-MTX alone in a clinical trial of HD-MTX versus HD-MTX plus cytarabine. Patients who received HD-MTX plus cytarabine had significantly higher complete responses, 46%, versus 18% with MTX alone. Data from the first part of the IELSG32 trial, a multicenter randomized phase 2 trial evaluating 3 immunochemotherapy induction regimens at initial randomization: (A) methotrexate, cytarabine; (B) methotrexate, cytarabine, rituximab;

Table 1
Select prospective trials of multimodality treatment regimens in primary central nervous system lymphoma

Chemotherapy, Reference	Whole-Brain Radiation Treatment	Intrathecal Therapy	Complete Response (%)	Partial Response (%)	Progression-Free Survival (mos)	Overall Survival (mos)	Neurotoxicity (%)	N
MTX (3.5 g/m²), cytarabine, idarubicin (13 mg/m²), thiotepa (20 mg/m²)[80]	Y (30 Gy if CR, 36 Gy if PR, 45 Gy if stable or progressive disease)	N	44	32	NR	15	NR	41
MTX (2.5 g/m²), vincristine, procarbizine[81]	Y (45 Gy, if ocular involvement included eyes in the RT field to a total dose of 36 Gy)	Intraventicular MTX	58	36	24	36.9	15	98
MTX (3.5 g/m²), rituximab, procarbazine, vincristine, ara-C[82,83]	Y (23.4 Gy if CR, 45 Gy if not CR)	N	77	NR	3.3 y	6.6 y	NR	30
MTX (3.5 g/m²), Belomycin, Cyclophosphamide, vincristine, dexamethasone[84]	Delayed at recurrence, 45 Gy	N	69.4	19.4	NR	48	NR	36
MTX (8 g/m²)[85]	Y (30 Gy)	N	56	32	32	33	8	25
MTX (3 g/m²), teniposide, carmustine, methylprednisolone[86]	Y (40 Gy)	MTX, ara-C, hydrocortisone	69.2	11.5	NR	46	11.5	52

Abbreviations: CR, complete response; gy, gray; MTX, methotrexate; N, number of patients; NR, not recorded; y, year.

Table 2
Select published prospective trials of chemotherapy for newly diagnosed primary central nervous system lymphoma patients

Treatment, Reference	Intrathecal Treatment	Complete Response (%)	Partial Response (%)	Overall Survival (mos)	Progression-Free Survival (mos)	Toxicity	N
MTX (8 g/m²)[38,39]	None	52	22	55	12.8	6%	25
MTX (8 g/m²)[41]	None	65	35	30.4	25.9	NR	31
MTX (8 g/m²)[40]	None	30	NR	25	10	20	37
MTX (3.5 g/m²), cytarabine[43]	None	46	23	3y OS 46%	3 y FFS 21%	3%	39
MTX 8 g/m², temozolmide, rituximab[79]	None	66	11	Not reached	2.4 YRS	0	47
MTX (5 g/m²) cytarabine, vincristine, ifosfamide, dexamethasine, cysclophasphamide[45]	MTX, prednisolone, ara-C	61	40	50	21	3%	65
MTX (1 g/m²), lomustine, procarbazine, methylprednisolone[66]	MTX, ara-C	42	6	14	11	8%	50
MTX (3.5 g/m²) (a), cytarabine or MTX/cytarabine/rituximab (b), or MTX/cytarabine/rituximab/thiotepa (c)[44]	None	a. 23 b. 30 c. 49	a. 31 b. 43 c. 37%	a. 12 b. 30 c. NR	a. 6 b. 20 c. NR	1%	a. 75 b. 69 c. 75

Abbreviations: FFS, failure-free survival; MTX, methotrexate; N, number of patients; NR, not recorded.

or (C) methotrexate, cytarabine, rituximab, thiotepa, reported that arm C (methotrexate, cytarabine, rituximab, thiotepa) had a higher proportion of complete response (49%) compared with the other 2 arms.[44]

Intrathecal chemotherapy

Intrathecal chemotherapy (IT) is the infusion of chemotherapeutic agents into the CSF either through lumbar puncture or into the ventricular space through an Ommaya reservoir. IT chemotherapy has been incorporated into several combination regimens (see **Table 1**), but has not been evaluated in the setting of a randomized trial. Consequently, its efficacy remains unclear. There have been prospective trials that have shown benefit with regimens containing IT chemotherapy when added to HD-MTX regimens; however, it is unknown whether the benefit was from the IT chemotherapy or another agent in the systemic regimen.[45,46] Furthermore, several retrospective trials have evaluated the addition of IT chemotherapy to HD-MTX with conflicting results.[45,47–49]

There are limitations to the use of IT chemotherapy in the PCNSL patient population. Patients may have elevated intracranial pressure that might make lumbar puncture dangerous. There is also an increased risk of neurotoxicity, particularly in patients who have undergone prior HD-MTX or WBRT. Given the lack of data demonstrating clear efficacy of IT chemotherapy, and the associated toxicities, the use of IT chemotherapy in the treatment of PCNSL has largely been deferred as part of induction therapy.

Rituximab

Rituximab is a chimeric monoclonal antibody against the B cell-specific CD20 antigen that has had a substantially positive impact in the treatment of several systemic B cell malignancies, including DLBCL. The effect of rituximab in the treatment of PCNSL was first evaluated as a monotherapy in a small study of 12 individuals with recurrent or refractory PCNSL following MTX-based chemotherapy regimens. Patients were treated with a 375 mg/m^2 intravenous infusion weekly for up to 8 weeks. Of the 12 patients, one-third had a radiographic response (partial or complete).[50] The promising results of this study prompted incorporation of rituximab into methotrexate-based chemotherapy induction regimens (see **Table 2**). Other studies have evaluated the use of rituximab as a salvage therapy.[51,52] Additional evidence supporting the efficacy of rituximab in the treatment of PCNSL has come from retrospective studies evaluating rituximab plus MTX versus MTX monotherapy. Both studies demonstrated a substantial improvement in complete response and overall response with the addition of rituximab, although interpretation of these results should be cautious due to the limited generalizability of small retrospective studies.[53,54]

HIGH-DOSE CHEMOTHERAPY AND AUTOLOGOUS STEM CELL TRANSPLANTATION

The use of high-dose chemotherapy followed by autologous stem cell transplant (HDC/SCT) is based on its efficacy in the treatment of recurrent systemic lymphoma. PCNSL patients typically undergo an initial step (termed conditioning) where they receive myeloablative chemotherapy or radiation to rid the body of lymphoma cells. Following conditioning therapy, the patient undergoes a hematopoietic stem cell transplant with his or her own stem cells (autologous transplant). A unique problem to CNS lymphoma is the existence of the blood-brain barrier (BBB). Its presence may create a sanctuary for lymphoma, allowing PCNSL to evade the host immune response and protecting it from a number of chemotherapy agents. Even when chemotherapy drugs can penetrate the BBB, they often require very high doses to achieve cytotoxic levels within the brain, which is the rationale behind HDC/SCT.[55]

Studies have evaluated the efficacy of HDC/SCT in the treatment of PCNSL with promising results. Initial studies investigating HDC/SCT focused on its use following WBRT, but as evidence began to suggest neurotoxicity associated with WBRT, studies shifted to evaluate HDC/SCT after induction chemotherapy without radiation.[56,57] Several studies evaluated HDC/SCT in both the upfront and salvage settings with promising results.[58–61]

To date, the largest prospective phase 2 study of HDC/SCT in PCNSL evaluated the response of newly diagnosed patients to induction with HD MTX 8 g/m^2 (days 1,11,21,31), rituximab 375 mg/m^2 (days −7, 0, 10, 20, 30), cytarabine 3 g/m^2 (days 2 and 3), and thiotepa 40 mg/m^2 (day 3). Three weeks following the last dose of chemotherapy, participants began a conditioning regimen with rituximab 375 mg/m^2 (day 1), carmustine 400 mg/m^2 (day 2), and thiotepa 40 mg/m^2 (day 3), with autologous stem cell transplant 7 days following conditioning. The investigators evaluated response rates at 30 days and found an overall response rate of 91%, with 77% of participants achieving complete response. Median progression-free survival was 74 months. Data from this study suggest that the this regimen with HDT/SCT has a high rate of remission, with manageable toxicity in patients with newly diagnosed PCNSL.[62]

Although current data are promising, it must be highlighted that these studies are enrolling younger patients with better performance status given the minimum organ function requirements to be eligible for HDC/SCT.

Treatment of Elderly Patients

PCNSL disproportionately effects elderly individuals (>65 years old), making treatment of this group, with frequent medical comorbidities and enhanced sensitivity to the toxicity of chemoradiation therapies, a unique challenge. Despite the need for optimal treatment strategies in this group, it remains an understudied population.

Because of the high rate of neurotoxicity in the elderly population treated with WBRT, recent studies have focused on chemotherapy-based regimens, avoiding the use of radiation.[63,64] Several studies have been performed evaluating older patients and have found that MTX-based chemotherapy regimens are effective and well-tolerated.[65–68] A meta-analysis of a cohort of 741 PCNSL patients over the age of 60 showed no outcome differences between HD-MTX and oral chemotherapy compared with more aggressive chemotherapeutic regimens.[63] At present, there appears to be benefit from treating elderly individuals with MTX-based chemotherapy regimens, although the optimal combination remains unclear.

Salvage Therapy

Relapse is common in PCNSL, with 30% to 60% of individuals treated with methotrexate- based chemotherapy experiencing disease recurrence at 1 to 2 years.[69] Relapse almost always occurs in the CNS, and is associated with a poor prognosis. There is no standard of care for the treatment of PCNSL at recurrence. Studies have evaluated a variety of chemotherapeutic agents including temozolomide, pemetrexed, topotecan, bendamustine, and temsirolimus, with modest benefit.[50,70–72] Repeat challenge of patients with methotrexate has also shown efficacy, with an overall response rate ranging from 85% to 91%.[73–76] Additionally, HDC/SCT has been evaluated in a prospective multicenter trial and found to have an overall survival of 58.6 months.[77] More recently, studies have shown promising preliminary results with the use of ibrutinib, an inhibitor of Bruton's tyrosine kinase that leads to apoptosis and/or disrupted cellular migration, with a clinical response in 77% in relapsed or refractory PCNSL patients.[11] Another strategy with promising initial results is immunotherapy in recurrent or refractory PCNSL patients.[78] Nivolumab, a checkpoint inhibitor, may be effective in relapsed/refractory PCNSL via inhibition of programmed cell death protein 1.[78] Additional research into these targeted therapies and immunotherapies is underway.

SUMMARY

PCNSL is a rare type of NHL that is associated with a poor prognosis. The diagnosis of PCNSL relies on brain biopsy. The optimal treatment for newly diagnosed PCNSL patients is not well defined; at present the foundation of treatment is methotrexate-based induction chemotherapy in combination with additional, consolidative chemotherapy, radiation, or stem cell transplant. New treatments such as targeted agents and immunotherapy are being investigated with promising preliminary results.

REFERENCES

1. Krogh-Jensen M, D'Amore F, Jensen MK, et al. Clinicopathological features, survival and prognostic factors of primary central nervous system lymphomas: trends in incidence of primary central nervous system lymphomas and primary malignant brain tumors in a well-defined geographical area. population-based data from the Danish lymphoma registry, LYFO, and the Danish cancer registry. Leuk Lymphoma 1995;19(3–4):223–33.
2. Villano JL, Koshy M, Shaikh H, et al. Age, gender, and racial differences in incidence and survival in primary CNS lymphoma. Br J Cancer 2011;105(9):1414–8.
3. Panageas KS, Elkin EB, DeAngelis LM, et al. Trends in survival from primary central nervous system lymphoma, 1975-1999: a population-based analysis. Cancer 2005;104(11):2466–72.
4. O'Neill BP, Decker PA, Tieu C, et al. The changing incidence of primary central nervous system lymphoma is driven primarily by the changing incidence in young and middle-aged men and differs from time trends in systemic diffuse large B-cell non-Hodgkin's lymphoma. Am J Hematol 2013;88(12):997–1000.
5. Feuerhake F, Baumer C, Cyron D, et al. Primary CNS lymphoma in immunocompetent patients from 1989 to 2001: a retrospective analysis of 164 cases uniformly diagnosed by stereotactic biopsy. Acta Neurochir (Wien) 2006;148(8):831–8 [discussion: 838].
6. Bataille B, Delwail V, Menet E, et al. Primary intracerebral malignant lymphoma: report of 248 cases. J Neurosurg 2000;92(2):261–6.
7. Ostrom QT, Gittleman H, Xu J, et al. CBTRUS statistical report: primary brain and other central nervous system tumors diagnosed in the united states in 2009-2013. Neuro Oncol 2016;18(suppl_5):v1–75.
8. Enblad G, Martinsson G, Baecklund E, et al. Population-based experience on primary central nervous system lymphoma 2000-2012: the incidence is increasing. Acta Oncol 2017;56(4):599–607.
9. Shiels MS, Pfeiffer RM, Besson C, et al. Trends in primary central nervous system lymphoma incidence and survival in the U.S. Br J Haematol 2016;174(3):417–24.
10. Camilleri-Broet S, Criniere E, Broet P, et al. A uniform activated B-cell-like immunophenotype might explain the poor prognosis of primary central nervous system lymphomas: analysis of 83 cases. Blood 2006;107(1):190–6.
11. Grommes C, Pastore A, Palaskas N, et al. Ibrutinib unmasks critical role of Bruton tyrosine kinase in primary CNS lymphoma. Cancer Discov 2017;7(9):1018–29.
12. Ngo VN, Young RM, Schmitz R, et al. Oncogenically active MYD88 mutations in human lymphoma. Nature 2011;470(7332):115–9.

13. Chapuy B, Roemer MG, Stewart C, et al. Targetable genetic features of primary testicular and primary central nervous system lymphomas. Blood 2016;127(7): 869–81.
14. Kiewe P, Fischer L, Martus P, et al. Meningeal dissemination in primary CNS lymphoma: diagnosis, treatment, and survival in a large monocenter cohort. Neuro Oncol 2010;12(4):409–17.
15. Herrlinger U, Schabet M, Bitzer M, et al. Primary central nervous system lymphoma: from clinical presentation to diagnosis. J Neurooncol 1999;43(3):219–26.
16. Peterson K, Gordon KB, Heinemann M, et al. The clinical spectrum of ocular lymphoma. Cancer 1993;72(3):843–9.
17. Fitzsimmons A, Upchurch K, Batchelor T. Clinical features and diagnosis of primary central nervous system lymphoma. Hematol Oncol Clin North Am 2005; 19(4):689–703, vii.
18. Bühring U, Herrlinger U, Krings T, et al. MRI features of primary central nervous system lymphomas at presentation. Neurology 2001;57(3):393–6.
19. Kuker W, Nagele T, Korfel A, et al. Primary central nervous system lymphomas (PCNSL): MRI features at presentation in 100 patients. J Neurooncol 2005; 72(2):169–77.
20. Haldorsen IS, Krakenes J, Krossnes BK, et al. CT and MR imaging features of primary central nervous system lymphoma in norway, 1989-2003. AJNR Am J Neuroradiol 2009;30(4):744–51.
21. Ferreri AJ, Blay JY, Reni M, et al. Prognostic scoring system for primary CNS lymphomas: the international extranodal lymphoma study group experience. J Clin Oncol 2003;21(2):266–72.
22. Bromberg JE, Breems DA, Kraan J, et al. CSF flow cytometry greatly improves diagnostic accuracy in CNS hematologic malignancies. Neurology 2007;68(20): 1674–9.
23. Schroers R, Baraniskin A, Heute C, et al. Diagnosis of leptomeningeal disease in diffuse large B-cell lymphomas of the central nervous system by flow cytometry and cytopathology. Eur J Haematol 2010;85(6):520–8.
24. Ekstein D, Ben-Yehuda D, Slyusarevsky E, et al. CSF analysis of IgH gene rearrangement in CNS lymphoma: relationship to the disease course. J Neurol Sci 2006;247(1):39–46.
25. Pirotte B, Levivier M, Goldman S, et al. Glucocorticoid-induced long-term remission in primary cerebral lymphoma: case report and review of the literature. J Neurooncol 1997;32(1):63–9.
26. Abrey LE, Batchelor TT, Ferreri AJ, et al. Report of an international workshop to standardize baseline evaluation and response criteria for primary CNS lymphoma. J Clin Oncol 2005;23(22):5034–43.
27. Loeffler JS, Ervin TJ, Mauch P, et al. Primary lymphomas of the central nervous system: patterns of failure and factors that influence survival. J Clin Oncol 1985;3(4):490–4.
28. Ferreri AJM, Reni M, Zoldan MC, et al. Importance of complete staging in non-Hodgkin's lymphoma presenting as a cerebral mass lesion. Cancer 1996;77(5):827.
29. Abrey LE, Ben-Porat L, Panageas KS, et al. Primary central nervous system lymphoma: the Memorial Sloan-Kettering Cancer Center prognostic model. J Clin Oncol 2006;24(36):5711–5.
30. Bessell EM, Graus F, Lopez-Guillermo A, et al. Primary non-Hodgkin's lymphoma of the CNS treated with CHOD/BVAM or BVAM chemotherapy before radiotherapy: long-term survival and prognostic factors. Int J Radiat Oncol Biol Phys 2004;59(2):501–8.

31. DeAngelis LM, Yahalom J, Heinemann MH, et al. Primary CNS lymphoma: combined treatment with chemotherapy and radiotherapy. Neurology 1990;40(1):80–6.

32. Bellinzona M, Roser F, Ostertag H, et al. Surgical removal of primary central nervous system lymphomas (PCNSL) presenting as space occupying lesions: a series of 33 cases. Eur J Surg Oncol 2005;31(1):100–5.

33. Weller M, Martus P, Roth P, et al, German PCNSL Study Group. Surgery for primary CNS lymphoma? challenging a paradigm. Neuro Oncol 2012;14(12):1481–4.

34. Binnahil M, Au K, Lu JQ, et al. The influence of corticosteroids on diagnostic accuracy of biopsy for primary central nervous system lymphoma. Can J Neurol Sci 2016;43(5):721–5.

35. Thiel E, Korfel A, Martus P, et al. High-dose methotrexate with or without whole brain radiotherapy for primary CNS lymphoma (G-PCNSL-SG-1): a phase 3, randomised, non-inferiority trial. Lancet Oncol 2010;11(11):1036–47.

36. Dropcho EJ. Neurotoxicity of radiation therapy. Neurol Clin 2010;28(1):217–34.

37. Armstrong CL, Hunter JV, Ledakis GE, et al. Late cognitive and radiographic changes related to radiotherapy: initial prospective findings. Neurology 2002; 59(1):40–8.

38. Batchelor T, Carson K, O'Neill A, et al. Treatment of primary CNS lymphoma with methotrexate and deferred radiotherapy: a report of NABTT 96-07. J Clin Oncol 2003;21(6):1044–9.

39. Gerstner ER, Carson KA, Grossman SA, et al. Long-term outcome in PCNSL patients treated with high-dose methotrexate and deferred radiation. Neurology 2008;70(5):401–2.

40. Herrlinger U, Kuker W, Uhl M, et al. NOA-03 trial of high-dose methotrexate in primary central nervous system lymphoma: final report. Ann Neurol 2005;57(6): 843–7.

41. Guha-Thakurta N, Damek D, Pollack C, et al. Intravenous methotrexate as initial treatment for primary central nervous system lymphoma: response to therapy and quality of life of patients. J Neurooncol 1999;43(3):259–68.

42. Lippens RJ, Winograd B. Methotrexate concentration levels in the cerebrospinal fluid during high-dose methotrexate infusions: an unreliable prediction. Pediatr Hematol Oncol 1988;5(2):115–24.

43. Ferreri AJ, Reni M, Foppoli M, et al. High-dose cytarabine plus high-dose methotrexate versus high-dose methotrexate alone in patients with primary CNS lymphoma: a randomised phase 2 trial. Lancet 2009;374(9700):1512–20.

44. Ferreri AJ, Cwynarski K, Pulczynski E, et al. Chemoimmunotherapy with methotrexate, cytarabine, thiotepa, and rituximab (MATRix regimen) in patients with primary CNS lymphoma: results of the first randomisation of the international extranodal lymphoma study group-32 (IELSG32) phase 2 trial. Lancet Haematol 2016;3(5):e217–27.

45. Pels H, Schmidt-Wolf IG, Glasmacher A, et al. Primary central nervous system lymphoma: results of a pilot and phase II study of systemic and intraventricular chemotherapy with deferred radiotherapy. J Clin Oncol 2003;21(24):4489–95.

46. Peyrl A, Chocholous M, Azizi AA, et al. Safety of ommaya reservoirs in children with brain tumors: a 20-year experience with 5472 intraventricular drug administrations in 98 patients. J Neurooncol 2014;120(1):139–45.

47. Khan RB, Shi W, Thaler HT, et al. Is intrathecal methotrexate necessary in the treatment of primary CNS lymphoma? J Neurooncol 2002;58(2):175–8.

48. Ferreri AJ, Blay JY, Reni M, et al. Relevance of intraocular involvement in the management of primary central nervous system lymphomas. Ann Oncol 2002;13(4): 531–8.

49. Sierra del Rio M, Ricard D, Houillier C, et al. Prophylactic intrathecal chemotherapy in primary CNS lymphoma. J Neurooncol 2012;106(1):143–6.
50. Batchelor TT, Grossman SA, Mikkelsen T, et al. Rituximab monotherapy for patients with recurrent primary CNS lymphoma. Neurology 2011;76(10):929–30.
51. Mappa S, Marturano E, Licata G, et al. Salvage chemoimmunotherapy with rituximab, ifosfamide and etoposide (R-IE regimen) in patients with primary CNS lymphoma relapsed or refractory to high-dose methotrexate-based chemotherapy. Hematol Oncol 2013;31(3):143–50.
52. Nayak L, Abrey LE, Drappatz J, et al. Multicenter phase II study of rituximab and temozolomide in recurrent primary central nervous system lymphoma. Leuk Lymphoma 2013;54(1):58–61.
53. Holdhoff M, Ambady P, Abdelaziz A, et al. High-dose methotrexate with or without rituximab in newly diagnosed primary CNS lymphoma. Neurology 2014;83(3):235–9.
54. Birnbaum T, Stadler EA, von Baumgarten L, et al. Rituximab significantly improves complete response rate in patients with primary CNS lymphoma. J Neurooncol 2012;109(2):285–91.
55. Muldoon LL, Soussain C, Jahnke K, et al. Chemotherapy delivery issues in central nervous system malignancy: a reality check. J Clin Oncol 2007;25(16):2295–305.
56. Illerhaus G, Marks R, Ihorst G, et al. High-dose chemotherapy with autologous stem-cell transplantation and hyperfractionated radiotherapy as first-line treatment of primary CNS lymphoma. J Clin Oncol 2006;24(24):3865–70.
57. Colombat P, Lemevel A, Bertrand P, et al. High-dose chemotherapy with autologous stem cell transplantation as first-line therapy for primary CNS lymphoma in patients younger than 60 years: a multicenter phase II study of the GOELAMS group. Bone Marrow Transplant 2006;38(6):417–20.
58. Illerhaus G, Muller F, Feuerhake F, et al. High-dose chemotherapy and autologous stem-cell transplantation without consolidating radiotherapy as first-line treatment for primary lymphoma of the central nervous system. Haematologica 2008;93(1):147–8.
59. Alimohamed N, Daly A, Owen C, et al. Upfront thiotepa, busulfan, cyclophosphamide, and autologous stem cell transplantation for primary CNS lymphoma: a single centre experience. Leuk Lymphoma 2012;53(5):862–7.
60. Cote GM, Hochberg EP, Muzikansky A, et al. Autologous stem cell transplantation with thiotepa, busulfan, and cyclophosphamide (TBC) conditioning in patients with CNS involvement by non-hodgkin lymphoma. Biol Blood Marrow Transplant 2012;18(1):76–83.
61. Schorb E, Kasenda B, Atta J, et al. Prognosis of patients with primary central nervous system lymphoma after high-dose chemotherapy followed by autologous stem cell transplantation. Haematologica 2013;98(5):765–70.
62. Illerhaus G, Kasenda B, Ihorst G, et al. High-dose chemotherapy with autologous haemopoietic stem cell transplantation for newly diagnosed primary CNS lymphoma: a prospective, single-arm, phase 2 trial. Lancet Haematol 2016;3(8):e388–97.
63. Kasenda B, Ferreri AJM, Marturano E, et al. First-line treatment and outcome of elderly patients with primary central nervous system lymphoma (PCNSL)-a systematic review and individual patient data meta-analysis. Ann Oncol 2015;26(7):1305–13.
64. Abrey LE, DeAngelis LM, Yahalom J. Long-term survival in primary CNS lymphoma. J Clin Oncol 1998;16(3):859–63.

65. Gavrilovic IT, Hormigo A, Yahalom J, et al. Long-term follow-up of high-dose methotrexate-based therapy with and without whole brain irradiation for newly diagnosed primary CNS lymphoma. J Clin Oncol 2006;24(28):4570–4.

66. Hoang-Xuan K, Taillandier L, Chinot O, et al. Chemotherapy alone as initial treatment for primary CNS lymphoma in patients older than 60 years: a multicenter phase II study (26952) of the european organization for research and treatment of cancer brain tumor group. J Clin Oncol 2003;21(14):2726–31.

67. Zhu JJ, Gerstner ER, Engler DA, et al. High-dose methotrexate for elderly patients with primary CNS lymphoma. Neuro Oncol 2008;11(2):211–5.

68. Omuro A, Chinot O, Taillandier L, et al. Methotrexate and temozolomide versus methotrexate, procarbazine, vincristine, and cytarabine for primary CNS lymphoma in an elderly population: an intergroup ANOCEF-GOELAMS randomised phase 2 trial. Lancet Haematol 2015;2(6):e251–9.

69. Jahnke K, Thiel E, Martus P, et al. Relapse of primary central nervous system lymphoma: clinical features, outcome and prognostic factors. J Neurooncol 2006; 80(2):159–65.

70. Makino K, Nakamura H, Hide T, et al. Salvage treatment with temozolomide in refractory or relapsed primary central nervous system lymphoma and assessment of the MGMT status. J Neurooncol 2012;106(1):155–60.

71. Wong SF, Gan HK, Cher L. A single centre study of the treatment of relapsed primary central nervous system lymphoma (PCNSL) with single agent temozolomide. J Clin Neurosci 2012;19(11):1501–5.

72. Fischer L, Thiel E, Klasen HA, et al. Prospective trial on topotecan salvage therapy in primary CNS lymphoma. Ann Oncol 2006;17(7):1141–5.

73. Plotkin SR, Betensky RA, Hochberg FH, et al. Treatment of relapsed central nervous system lymphoma with high-dose methotrexate. Clin Cancer Res 2004; 10(17):5643–6.

74. Pentsova E, Deangelis LM, Omuro A. Methotrexate re-challenge for recurrent primary central nervous system lymphoma. J Neurooncol 2014;117(1):161–5.

75. Nguyen PL, Chakravarti A, Finkelstein DM, et al. Results of whole-brain radiation as salvage of methotrexate failure for immunocompetent patients with primary CNS lymphoma. J Clin Oncol 2005;23(7):1507–13.

76. Hottinger AF, DeAngelis LM, Yahalom J, et al. Salvage whole brain radiotherapy for recurrent or refractory primary CNS lymphoma. Neurology 2007;69(11):1178–82.

77. Soussain C, Hoang-Xuan K, Taillandier L, et al. Intensive chemotherapy followed by hematopoietic stem-cell rescue for refractory and recurrent primary CNS and intraocular lymphoma: Societe Francaise de Greffe de Moelle Osseuse-Therapie Cellulaire. J Clin Oncol 2008;26(15):2512–8.

78. Nayak L, Iwamoto FM, LaCasce A, et al. PD-1 blockade with nivolumab in relapsed/refractory primary central nervous system and testicular lymphoma. Blood 2017;129(23):3071–3.

79. Rubenstein JL, Hsi ED, Johnson JL, et al. Intensive chemotherapy and immunotherapy in patients with newly diagnosed primary CNS lymphoma: CALGB 50202 (alliance 50202). J Clin Oncol 2013;31(25):3061–8.

80. Ferreri AJ, Dell'Oro S, Foppoli M, et al. MATILDE regimen followed by radiotherapy is an active strategy against primary CNS lymphomas. Neurology 2006;66(9):1435–8.

81. DeAngelis LM, Seiferheld W, Schold SC, et al, Radiation Therapy Oncology Group Study 93-10. Combination chemotherapy and radiotherapy for primary central nervous system lymphoma: radiation therapy oncology group study 93-10. J Clin Oncol 2002;20(24):4643–8.

82. Shah GD, Yahalom J, Correa DD, et al. Combined immunochemotherapy with reduced whole-brain radiotherapy for newly diagnosed primary CNS lymphoma. J Clin Oncol 2007;25(30):4730–5.
83. Morris PG, Correa DD, Yahalom J, et al. Rituximab, methotrexate, procarbazine, and vincristine followed by consolidation reduced-dose whole-brain radiotherapy and cytarabine in newly diagnosed primary CNS lymphoma: final results and long-term outcome. J Clin Oncol 2013;31(31):3971–9.
84. Silvani A, Salmaggi A, Eoli M, et al. Methotrexate based chemotherapy and deferred radiotherapy for primary central nervous system lymphoma (PCNSL): single institution experience. J Neurooncol 2007;82(3):273–9.
85. Glass J, Gruber ML, Cher L, et al. Preirradiation methotrexate chemotherapy of primary central nervous system lymphoma: long-term outcome. J Neurosurg 1994;81(2):188–95.
86. Poortmans PM, Kluin-Nelemans HC, Haaxma-Reiche H, et al. High-dose methotrexate-based chemotherapy followed by consolidating radiotherapy in non-AIDS-related primary central nervous system lymphoma: European Organization for Research and Treatment of Cancer Lymphoma Group phase II trial 20962. J Clin Oncol 2003;21(24):4483–8.

Pediatric Brain Tumors

Yoko T. Udaka, MD[a,b], Roger J. Packer, MD[a,c],*

KEYWORDS

- Brain tumors • Pediatric brain tumors • Medulloblastoma • Gliomas
- Embryonal tumors

KEY POINTS

- Pediatric central nervous system tumors are the most common solid tumors in children and the leading cause of cancer-related morbidity and mortality.
- The World Health Organization brain tumor classification is in flux and now includes some molecular parameters.
- Recent understandings of tumor biology and genomic aberrations have led to better prediction of outcome and alteration of treatment approaches for children with brain tumors.

INTRODUCTION

Pediatric central nervous system (CNS) tumors are the second most common childhood malignancy and the most common solid tumor in children. The incidence rate of childhood and adolescent primary malignant and nonmalignant brain and other CNS tumors in the United States is approximately 5.67 per 100,000 person-years.[1] Brain tumors are the most common cause of death among all childhood cancers according to the Surveillance, Epidemiology, and End Results Program. Signs and symptoms depend on a variety of factors, including location of the tumor, age of child, and rate of tumor growth. Supratentorial tumors are more common in infants and children up to 3 years of age and again after age 10, whereas between ages 4 and 10 infratentorial tumors are more common. The most common tumor types by age are shown in **Figs. 1** and **2**. Younger children have a higher incidence of tumors of embryonal origin, such as medulloblastoma or atypical teratoid/rhabdoid tumor (ATRT), whereas older patients tend to have tumors of glial origin.

Disclosures: None.
a The Brain Tumor Institute, Center for Neuroscience and Behavioral Medicine, Children's National Health System, 111 Michigan Avenue Northwest, Washington, DC 20010, USA; b Division of Oncology, Center for Cancer and Blood Disorders, 111 Michigan Avenue Northwest, Washington, DC 20010, USA; c The Brain Tumor Institute, Gilbert Family Neurofibromatosis Institute, Children's National Medical Center, 111 Michigan Avenue Northwest, Washington, DC 20010, USA
* Corresponding author. The Brain Tumor Institute, Center for Neuroscience and Behavioral Medicine, Children's National Health System, 111 Michigan Avenue Northwest, Washington, DC 20010.
E-mail address: RPacker@childrensnational.org

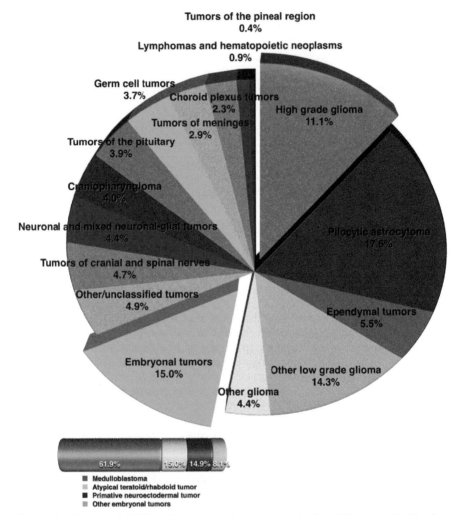

Fig. 1. Distribution of childhood primary brain tumors and other CNS tumors by histology from the Central Brain Tumor Registry of the United States (CBTRUS) for children between ages 0 and 14 years.

Little is known regarding the pathogenesis of most brain tumors in children. There are genetic syndromes that can predispose patients to getting brain tumors, such as neurofibromatosis type 1 (NF-1), tuberous sclerosis, Li-Fraumeni syndrome, and other less common inherited conditions, such as Gorlin syndrome or Turcot syndrome. Recent data demonstrate that more than 8% of childhood and adolescent cancers arise in the setting of germline predisposition syndromes and it is likely this number will rise as investigations increase.[2] Aside from inherited syndromes, the only other uniformly agreed on environmental risk factor that has consistently been shown to increase the risk of developing brain tumors is radiation exposure.[3]

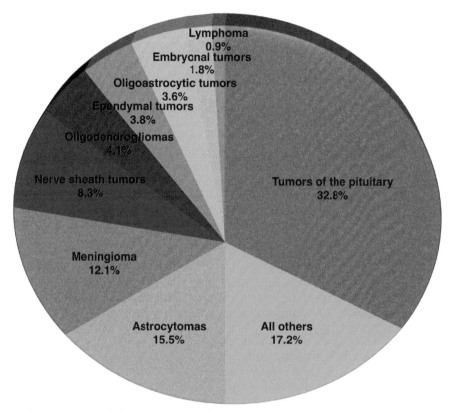

Fig. 2. Distribution of childhood primary brain tumors and other CNS tumors by histology from the CBTRUS for adolescents between ages 15 and 19 years.

PRESENTATION

The clinical presentation primarily depends on location of tumor and age of the patient. Infants tend to exhibit relatively nonspecific symptoms, such as macrocephaly, irritability, failure to thrive, loss of developmental milestones, and vomiting.[4] Older children most commonly present with localizing neurologic deficits and symptoms related to increased intracranial pressure secondary to obstruction of the normal flow of cerebral spinal fluid (CSF) leading to hydrocephalus. Nonlocalizing symptoms due to increased pressure may include headaches, nausea, vomiting, and cranial nerve deficits and most often are seen in posterior fossa tumors that represent approximately half of all pediatric brain tumors.[1]

CLASSIFICATION

Brain tumor classification is difficult given that many pediatric CNS tumors may have multiple cell types. Previous classifications tried to identify morphologic appearance on histology and stages of development within the nervous system. As a result, the

2007 World Health Organization (WHO) classification of CNS tumors was based primarily on histologic appearance. However, with recent advancements in tumor biology, in 2016, this classification was changed to incorporate some molecular parameters, as well as histologic similarities[5] (discussed further as follows). This tiered approach will hopefully allow for easier identification of tumor types and their respective treatments. Further molecular understanding will, no doubt, result in further changes in classifications in the near future.

MEDULLOBLASTOMA

Medulloblastoma is, by definition, an embryonal tumor of the posterior fossa and is thought to be the most common malignant brain tumor in children. It comprises up to 20% of all pediatric brain tumors.[1] Primarily a tumor of childhood, medulloblastoma is most commonly diagnosed before 15 years of age and has a male predominance.[6] There is a biphasic incidence with peaks at 3 to 4 years of age and again at 8 to 9 years of age.[7] Previously, in the 2007 WHO classification, medulloblastoma was divided into 4 histologic variants, including classic histology, anaplastic/large-cell variant, desmoplastic/nodular, and medulloblastoma with extensive nodularity.[8] In 2016, the WHO classification system changed, and medulloblastoma was also subdivided by molecular subgroups: wingless (WNT), Sonic hedgehog (SHH), group 3, and group 4 in a 2-tiered system incorporating both histology and molecular findings.[5,9] These subgroups have distinct tumor biology in addition to having a diverse and wide range of phenotypes, including demographics, dissemination, and patient outcome (**Fig. 3**).[9–11] The molecular subgroups have been further broken into in as many as eleven subtypes which are thought to even better predict outcome and allow more exact treatment stratification.

Traditional therapies for medulloblastoma in children older than 3 years include a combination of surgical resection, radiation therapy, and chemotherapy, regardless of molecular subtype. Surgical resection is the initial step in management and it has consistently been reported that total or near-total resection of the primary tumor correlates with improved outcomes, especially in patients with nondisseminated disease.[12] Posterior fossa syndrome, or cerebellar mutism, is seen in up to 25% of patients following resection of midline cerebellar tumors.[13] The mechanism underlying this syndrome is unclear, but is thought to be related to unilateral or bilateral dentate

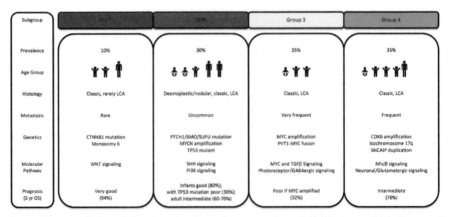

Fig. 3. Characteristics of the 4 molecular subgroups of medulloblastoma. LCA, large cell anaplastic; NF, nuclear factor; OS, overall survival; WNT, wingless.

nuclear damage with resultant denta-thalamo-rubral pathway damage. Patients have late-onset mutism associated with other neurologic symptoms that may persist for weeks to months with residual sequelae even 1 year after surgery.

Following maximal resection, patients are conventionally risk stratified into average or high risk based on extent of surgical resection and dissemination status at the time of diagnosis (**Table 1**).[14] Children older than 3 years receive between 2400 and 3600 cGy of craniospinal radiation (CSI) depending on risk status with 5580 cGy local boost radiotherapy followed by cisplatin-based chemotherapy.[15–17] Recent trials have attempted to decrease the dose of craniospinal radiation in average-risk patients (to 1800 cGy) so as to reduce the extent of neurocognitive deficits while maintaining efficacy of treatment.[18] Five-year disease-free survival is more than 80% in those with "average-risk" disease and 60% to 65% for those with "high-risk" disease after such treatment. Treatment of infants has been more challenging because of the impact that high-dose radiation can have on the developing brain. Infants also have a higher incidence of dissemination with up to 40% having disseminated disease at diagnosis, making treatment options more complicated.[6] In younger children, primarily those younger than 3 or 4 years at diagnosis, postsurgical treatment is usually undertaken with chemotherapy alone; the later use of focal or craniospinal radiation is unsettled. With improving survival, children often have significant morbidity from treatment, which includes neurocognitive deficits, neuroendocrine sequelae, and permanent neurologic dysfunction.[19] Late treatment-related complications may also include sequelae of cerebrovascular damage and secondary malignancies, especially in those with an underlying genetic predisposition.[20]

WNT medulloblastoma is approximately 10% of medulloblastomas and occurs most frequently among children older than 3 years and has a >95% 5-year survival and likely cure.[21] WNT subgroup affects boys and girls equally and has the most favorable prognosis. WNT medulloblastoma is almost always located near the brainstem and fourth ventricle and is thought to originate from progenitor cells from the lower rhombic lip and may be hemorrhagic at diagnosis.[22] The WNT family of receptors plays an important role in cell cycle control and embryogenesis and was first identified in Turcot syndrome, as patients with this syndrome had a higher incidence of medulloblastoma.[23] Turcot syndrome is characterized with mutations in the adenomatous polyposis coli (*APC*) gene, a negative regulator of WNT signaling. However, the most common WNT signaling mutation seen in this subgroup is the *CTNNB1* gene, which encodes for β-catenin and results in nuclear accumulation of β-catenin (**Fig. 4**).[24,25] The loss of chromosome 6 has also been associated with this subgroup.[24] The most recent clinical trials for WNT tumors are designed to minimize potential long-term side effects of current treatments by reducing the dose of radiation and chemotherapy because current therapies have such favorable outcomes.[18]

SHH medulloblastoma comprise approximately 30% of medulloblastomas and occurs most frequently in infants and adults. Sequencing of SHH tumors has shown that SHH medulloblastomas are now considered at least 3 variations, infants, children, and

Table 1
Risk stratification of medulloblastoma in children

Tumor Characteristic	Average Risk	High Risk
Dissemination	Localized	Disseminated
Tumor resection	Gross total/near total resection Residual tumor <1.5 cm^2	Subtotal resection/biopsy Residual tumor >1.5 cm^2
Histology	Classic, desmoplastic/nodular	Anaplastic/large cell

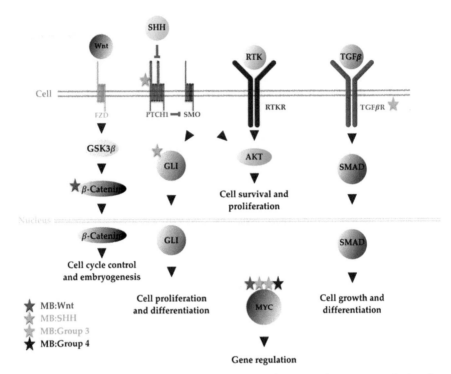

Fig. 4. Key signaling molecules involved in medulloblastoma formation and signaling. MB.WNT has been associated with mutations in β-Catenin, whereas MB.SHH has been associated with mutations along the PTCH1-SMO-GLI pathway. Group 3 has been associated with mutations in the TGFα receptor and all 4 subgroups have been associated with mutations in Myc. AKT, serine/threonine protein kinases; FZD, Frizzled; GLI, glioma associated oncogene homolog; GSK, glycogen synthase kinase; MB, medulloblastoma; RTK, receptor tyrosine kinase PTCH1, Patched1; SMAD, main signal transducer protein for TGF-B superfamily receptors; SMO, Smoothened.

adults, and are a very heterogeneous group of tumors with a diverse set of genetic aberrations that differ from each other.[26] Hereditary predisposition syndromes involving germline mutations of suppressor of fused gene (SUFU) are seen in some infants. Germline TP53 mutations (Li-Fraumeni syndrome) can occur in older children, especially between the ages of 8 and 17. Almost all adults harbor somatic mutations in the TERT promoter, a less common finding in pediatric patients with SHH medulloblastoma.[26] SHH medulloblastoma is thought to originate from granule neuron precursor cells of the external granule layer, neural stem cells in the subventricular zone, or from brainstem progenitors,[27] although recent data suggest that infant SHH medulloblastomas may have a different cellular origin compared with childhood or adult SHH medulloblastomas.[26,28] SHH signaling is essential in cell proliferation and differentiation and was first recognized in Gorlin syndrome, characterized by craniofacial abnormalities, basal cell carcinomas of the skin, and medulloblastoma.[29] Further studies have identified many key genes involved in SHH signaling and medulloblastoma formation, such as SUFU, smoothened (SMO), SHH, GLI2, and MYCN.[30] Patients with SHH tumors containing TP53 mutations have a peak incidence in late childhood and adolescence and have a particularly poor prognosis.[31] Similarly, an overlapping subset of patients with MYCN amplification in SHH medulloblastomas are also associated with poor outcomes.[26,32] Current therapies have targeted all aspects of SHH signaling, including upstream targets (see **Fig. 4**), with small-molecule inhibitors like erismodegib/sonidegib[33] and vismodegib, with better results in adults than children.[34] Downstream target inhibition also has shown activity in preclinical models with antifungal agents, such as itraconazole, saridegib, arsenic trioxide, bromodomain inhibitors, aurora kinase A inhibitors, and Polo-like kinase inhibitors.[30] The diverse heterogeneity of SHH tumors with multiple mutations and resistance mechanisms makes appropriate therapy selection difficult.

Group 3 medulloblastoma accounts for approximately 25% of medulloblastomas and overall has a poor prognosis. Male individuals are more likely to be affected than female individuals and more infants and children are affected than adults. Five-year survival is poor, with approximately 50% overall survival.[35] At diagnosis, nearly one-half of the group 3 patients have metastatic disease. Group 3 tumors are normally located in the midline of the brainstem near the fourth ventricle, possibly facilitating access to the CSF, resulting in metastasis.[30] Although no specific gene has been identified in group 3, somatic copy number aberrations are commonly found (~17%) in the *MYC* gene, leading to tumor promotion or formation (see **Fig. 4**).[36] Other possible pathways include transforming growth factor-β (TGF-β), which has been found in approximately 20% of group 3 medulloblastomas.[36] Current therapies include use of craniospinal radiation therapy with focal boost with intensified chemotherapy following surgical resection. Studies using mouse models have suggested that histone deacetylase (HDAC) inhibitors, such as panobinostat, as well as bromodomain inhibitors, such as JQ1, may be potential therapeutic agents for group 3 medulloblastomas with *MYC* amplification.[37,38]

Group 4 medulloblastoma is the most prevalent subgroup, making up more than 30% of all medulloblastomas; however, it is the least well biologically characterized. Group 4 medulloblastoma has many similarities to group 3, including chromosomal instability, especially in the formation of isochromosome 17q, which is more often found in patients with group 4 tumors than group 3. Furthermore, somatic copy number aberrations are also observed, resulting from chromosomal instability. The most common unique somatic copy number aberration is found in a gain of function of the *SNCAIP* gene. *SNCAIP* encodes synphilin 1, a crucial protein involved in Parkinson disease.[39] Somatic copy number aberrations affecting nuclear factor κB signaling have also been observed in group 4 (see **Fig. 4**).[36] Given similarities with group 3 medulloblastoma, potential therapies are also similar, including bromodomain inhibitors and HDAC inhibitors.

SUPRATENTORIAL EMBRYONAL TUMORS

Non–posterior fossa embryonal tumors, formally known as CNS-primitive neuroectodermal tumors (PNETs), are a group of rare pediatric brain tumors comprising fewer than 3% of pediatric brain tumors and carry a poor prognosis.[40,41] The 2016 WHO classification system incorporates the presence or absence of amplification of the C19MC region on chromosome 19 in defining several subgroups.[5] All CNS embryonal tumors are highly malignant and are considered WHO grade IV tumors. Molecular studies have shown that many tumors histologically classified as supratentorial embryonal tumors molecularly cluster with other tumor types, such as high-grade gliomas and ependymomas; this has major therapeutic implications with regard to the volume of radiotherapy needed for tumor control and the choice of adjuvant chemotherapy or biologic therapy. They are poorly differentiated, rapidly growing neuroepithelial tumors that histologically resemble and share features with that of medulloblastoma but with very different biology.[42] Older children will typically present with signs of increased intracranial pressure, whereas younger children and infants can present with nonspecific symptoms, such as irritability, fatigue, or progressive macrocephaly. Depending on tumor location, patients may also present with more focal neurologic deficits or seizures.

Current management includes aggressive (if possible) surgical resection, craniospinal and local boost radiation, and intensive chemotherapy, similar to therapy directed at high-risk patients with medulloblastoma. It is thought that adjuvant chemotherapy enhances survival but the optimal regimen has not been established. Prolonged and intensive multiagent chemotherapy regimens have been used in younger patients to avoid or delay radiation with limited success in improving survival rates in this group of patients.[43–45] There is clearly biological complexity that is not being addressed with the current treatment strategies. It is hoped that molecular subclassifications within this group of heterogeneous tumors will lead to more exact diagnosis and molecularly directed tumor treatment.[46]

ATYPICAL TERATOID/RHABDOID TUMORS

ATRTs are rare malignant intracranial neoplasms most commonly occurring in infants and young children. They account for only 1% to 2% of all pediatric brain tumors but approximately 10% to 20% of CNS tumors in patients younger than 3 years.[47,48] ATRTs were previously misclassified until being described as a discrete clinical entity in the 1980s. The genetic hallmark of ATRTs are mutations in *SMARCB1*.[49] In addition to the somatic mutation detected in tumor tissue, approximately a third of the patients harbor a germline mutation in SMARCB1, or less commonly SMARCA4.[50]

Histologically they are characterized by atypical cells with eccentric nuclei, small nucleoli, and abundant amounts of eosinophilic cytoplasm with frequent mitotic figures. Immunohistochemistry plays a large role in confirming the diagnosis, with a loss of INI1 nuclear staining indicating biallelic mutations of *SMARCB1* on chromosome 22 in the tumors.[51] Although overall ATRTs have a very poor prognosis, there are some with better clinical outcomes, suggesting molecular intertumor heterogeneity. DNA methylation profiling has identified 3 distinct molecular subgroups: ATRT-TYR, ATRT-SHHS, and ATRT-MYC. Similar to other brain tumors, each ATRT subgroup has a predilection for specific locations within the brain.[52]

The treatment of ATRT is controversial, with no consensus on optimal treatment given the lack of randomized control studies. Various strategies with multiagent chemotherapy and radiation therapy are being used; however, the young age of presentation often precludes the use of radiation.[53–55] Survival has improved with intensive multimodality regimens and outcome has been more favorable in older patients with up to 50% survival in those with localized disease. Targeted therapies are under investigation with a large number of potentially promising agents, such as the aurora kinase A inhibitor, alisertib, that has shown antitumor activity in some patients with recurrent or progressive ATRT.[56]

GLIOMAS
High-Grade Gliomas

In children, high-grade gliomas (HGGs) occur at an incidence of 0.8 per 100,000 children per year.[30] Approximately 20% of all childhood gliomas are HGGs, and include anaplastic astrocytoma (AA), diffuse intrinsic pontine glioma (DIPG), and glioblastoma multiforme (GBM).[57] Children with HGGs have an overall poor prognosis despite intensive therapy. Patients may present with headaches, weakness, behavioral changes, or seizures.[58] The extent of surgical resection remains one of the most important prognostic factors in predicting outcome in children with HGGs, with improved 5-year progression-free survival in those who have a >90% resection.[59–61] Local site radiation to 5000 to 6000 cGy remains the mainstay of therapy for children with HGG. The benefits of chemotherapy remain controversial. Adjuvant therapy with CCNU (lomustine), vincristine and prednisone was initially thought to improve survival based on a study performed in the 1970s; on retrospective central histologic review, the significance of this report was put in question as a portion of the patients were found to have low-grade gliomas (LGGs).[62] Temozolomide, both during and after radiation, was found not to improve survival compared with CCNU and vincristine.[63] The combination of CCNU and temozolomide concurrent and after radiotherapy may be more effective.[64] High-dose chemotherapy has shown a possible small survival benefit but with significantly more toxicities.[65]

DNA methylation studies have identified 6 molecular subgroups for pediatric GBM. These include IDH, K27, G34, Receptor Tyrosine Kinase I and II, and mesenchymal.[66] K27 (Lys27Met) and G34 (Gly34Arg) are mostly found in pediatric HGGs, the other groups have a wider range of ages (**Table 2**). Pediatric HGGs are histologically the same as adult HGGs, but molecularly very different entities, making translation of adult clinical data to pediatrics essentially impossible. Although nearly half of all adult GBMs are O^6-methylguanine-DNA methyltransferase (MGMT) methylated, resulting in impaired DNA repair, the significance of MGMT methylation in pediatric patients is less conclusive. Most recent clinical trials have attempted to target specific biological markers relevant to the formation of HGGs. Targeted therapies, such as erlotinib (epidermal growth factor receptor inhibitor), imatinib (platelet-derived growth factor receptor [PDGFR] inhibitor), and bevacizumab (vascular endothelial growth factor inhibitor) have demonstrated only minimal effects in pediatric AA or GBM.[67] Some recent studies are also using oncolytic viruses, such as the herpes simplex virus 1716,[35] cytomegalovirus,[68] and parvovirus H-1[69] as potential immunotherapeutic agents in pediatric GBM. Inhibitors against essential targets within survival pathways, such as Akt and Notch, also are under investigation[70] (**Fig. 5**).

Brain Stem Gliomas

Brain stem gliomas (BSGs), now classified as diffuse midline gliomas, H3 K27M-mutant, account for 10% to 15% of all pediatric CNS tumors.[5] Approximately 80% arise in the pons and have a characteristic appearance on MRI and are one of the few brain tumors that can be diagnosed without histologic confirmation.[71] On MRI DIPGs characteristically expand the pons, are usually hypointense, and typically do

Table 2
Clinical features of pediatric high-grade gliomas

Methylation Subgroup	IDH Wt	IDH Mut	K27 Mut	G34 Mut
Subdivisions	PDGFRA, EGFR, MYCN, and so forth	NA	H3.1 K27M	H3.3 K27M or H3.3 G34R/V
Location	Hemispheric	Mostly frontal lobe and hemispheric	DIPG – Pons	DIPG – midline structures Hemispheric
Mean age	8–10 y old	Teen to young adult	4.5 y old	7 y old – young adult
Prognosis (overall survival)	14–44 mo	>5 y	~15 mo	10–24 mo

Abbreviations: DIPG, diffuse intrinsic pontine glioma; EGFR, epidermal growth factor receptor; Mut, mutant; NA, not applicable; PDGFR, platelet-derived growth factor receptor; Wt, Wildtype.

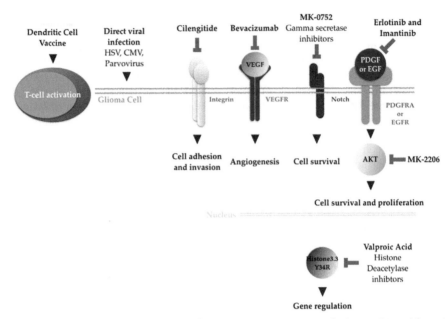

Fig. 5. Potential therapeutic targets for HGGs. CMV, cytomegalovirus; EGF, epidermal growth factor; EGFR, EGF receptor; HSV, herpes simplex virus; VEGF, vascular endothelial growth factor; VEGFR, VEGF receptor.

not enhance (**Fig. 6**). Histologically, they are high grade and resemble GBMs. Historically, these tumors were not biopsied because of safety concerns, but recent studies show that stereotactic biopsy of the tumor is safe with minimal morbidity and high diagnostic, including molecular, utility.[72,73] Patients with BSGs often present with multiple cranial neuropathies, most commonly sixth and/or seventh nerve palsies.

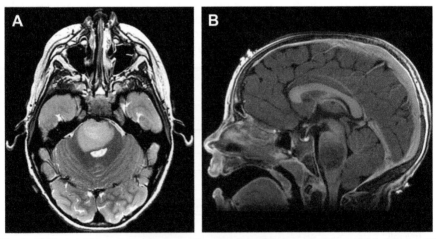

Fig. 6. DIPG. Axial T2-weighted image (*A*) and postcontrast sagittal T1-weighted image (*B*) reveal a T2-hyperintense tumor that occupies most of the pons, causing expansion of the pons and mass effect on the fourth ventricle. The tumor has low T1 signal and shows no appreciable enhancement on the postcontrast image (*B*).

Prognosis remains dismal with more than 90% of patients succumbing to the disease within 18 months with a median survival of 9 months. On the other hand, tumors of the medulla and midbrain tend to be lower-grade lesions and have better prognosis with a more indolent course.

Standard treatment involves radiation therapy and has been the only treatment that has altered the course of the disease. Despite multiple trials, including radiosensitization, increasing radiation doses, and single or multiagent postradiation and preradiation chemotherapeutic regimens, overall survival has not changed.[74–79] More recently, an understanding of the molecular biology of DIPGs has led to trials targeting specific mutations. Approximately 80% of DIPGs harbor the H3K27M mutation.[5] Other commonly found mutations include amplification or overexpression of the PDGFRA, activating mutations in PI3K, and somatic mutations in *ACVR1*.[80–83] *IDH1* or *IDH2* mutations often seen in adult diffuse gliomas are generally absent in pediatric DIPGs.

Low-Grade Gliomas

LGGs are the most common form of brain tumor in children and represent approximately 40% of all CNS tumors in children younger than 18.[1] Pilocytic astrocytomas are the most common form, but pediatric LGGs include a wide range of histologic subtypes, including pilomyxoid astrocytoma, oligoastrocytoma, oligodendroglioma, and ganglioglioma. Although the WHO classification for many tumors now includes genetic features, as of the 2016 update, LGGs are not classified by molecular features. Clinical presentation depends on tumor location. They are most commonly found in the cerebellum, but midline diencephalon tumors also are common. There is a distinct clinical entity called diencephalic syndrome, which occurs as a result of a tumor, often an LGG or astrocytoma, in the hypothalamus. These children present with failure to thrive and profound emaciation despite normal caloric intake.

Surgical resection is curative for LGGs, especially pilocytic astrocytomas, when tumors can be totally resected. In some cases, a partial resection also results in long-term control. Treatment can become challenging when the tumors arise in close proximity to vital structures, making resection difficult without causing significant morbidity or functional compromise. Traditionally, radiation was first-line therapy for unresectable or incompletely resected LGGs; however, the potential for radiation-induced injury in the developing brain of young children has led clinicians to move away from radiation as first-line treatment. Various chemotherapy regimens have been developed with varying response rates and most commonly the combination of carboplatin and vincristine has been used in pediatrics. Vinblastine has also been recently extensively used.[84,85] Despite initial response, as measured by radiographic shrinkage or disease stabilization in 90% to 95% of newly diagnosed LGGs, approximately half of the patients will show tumor progression/growth within 3 years of initiation of chemotherapy.

More recent understanding of the genomic alterations in many of the LGGs has led to use of small-molecule inhibitors to treat unresectable, progressive, or refractory tumors. Alterations involving the BRAF gene are common, with the most common being a gene fusion between KIAA1549 and BRAF, resulting in a fusion protein that lacks the BRAF regulatory domain. This fusion is seen in most cerebellar pilocytic astrocytomas and 40% of chiasmatic/hypothalamic tumors. MEK-inhibitors have been successfully used in children with recurrent disease. Outside of the cerebellum, the BRAF V600E point mutation has been frequently seen.[86] For these tumors, BRAF point mutation inhibitors also have been successfully used. Unlike adult LGGs, pediatric grade II astrocytomas rarely harbor IDH/IDH2 abnormalities,[66] partially explaining the lack of pediatric astrocytomas mutating into higher-grade lesions.

Visual Pathway Gliomas

Visual pathway gliomas are low-grade astrocytic tumors and can involve the optic nerve, chiasm, tract, and optic radiations. They account for 4% to 8% of all brain tumors in children.[87] They are slow-growing neoplasms that occur mostly in younger children.[88] These tumors are frequently associated with NF-1. It is imperative to assess for other signs of NF-1 when patients present with visual pathway tumors, as the diagnosis can then be made without a biopsy. The rationale for biopsy of non-NF children at diagnosis is driven by the understanding that BRAF aberrations are frequent. Recent data suggest that 40% of visual pathway gliomas harbor BRAF fusions, 40% BRAF point mutations, and 20% harbor less frequent molecular aberrations or have no discernible abnormality with current testing. The clinical presentation depends on the tumor location and can include isolated findings of or a combination of visual loss, strabismus, nystagmus, or proptosis. In some cases, patients can be asymptomatic and the tumor identified on routine screening for NF-1.[89] Tumors can extend into the hypothalamus and present with hypothalamic-pituitary dysfunctions.[90]

The location of the tumor precludes extensive surgical excision in most cases. In asymptomatic patients, treatment is often deferred until there is clear-cut radiographic or clinical progression. In general, visual pathway gliomas in patients with NF-1 often behave less aggressively.[89] Younger age at presentation can be a risk factor for more aggressive growth requiring treatment.[91] There can be infrequent to rare spontaneous regression of optic gliomas reported in patients with NF-1 and non–NF-1.[92] First-line treatment is often chemotherapy, whereas radiotherapy is usually reserved for older non–NF-1 children. Chemotherapy with carboplatin and vincristine has shown tumor response with shrinkage in 40% and disease stability in an additional 50% of children younger than 5 years.[93] The incorporation of bevacizumab with irinotecan has shown dramatic recovery of vision in some patients. Recent understanding of the molecular pathways of LGGs has allowed targeting of the BRAF pathway in ongoing clinical trials.

EPENDYMOMAS

Ependymomas are the third most common brain tumor in children and account for approximately 8% to 10% of all childhood CNS tumors.[94] They are neuroepithelial malignancies that occur in the supratentorial brain, posterior fossa, and spinal cord and can affect both children and adults. In children, most occur intracranially with two-thirds located in the posterior fossa.[8,95] There is an increased risk for intramedullary spinal cord ependymomas in patients with NF-2.[96] The clinical presentation depends on the tumor location. Most children with posterior fossa tumors present with signs of increased intracranial pressure with headache, vomiting, papilledema, ataxia, and multiple cranial nerve palsies, whereas those with supratentorial lesions can present with focal neurologic deficits or seizures.[97] Dissemination at diagnosis is seen in fewer than 10% of cases.[98]

Currently, WHO classifies ependymomas based on histopathology into 4 major subtypes (subependymoma, myxopapillary ependymoma, classic ependymoma, and anaplastic ependymoma) with the RELA fusion-positive ependymomas added as a subcategory to the classification in 2016.[5] More recently, DNA methylation profiling has been used to identify molecular subgroups within each anatomic compartment to better predict prognosis[99] (**Fig. 7**). Patients with infratentorial posterior fossa ependymoma group A (PF-EPN-A) or supratentorial RELA-positive ependymoma comprise the largest molecular subgroups and have the worst prognosis.[100] PF-EPN-A occurs primarily in infants and young children and are often lateral and difficult to resect with a high recurrence rate, whereas PF-EPN-B occurs more in adolescents and young

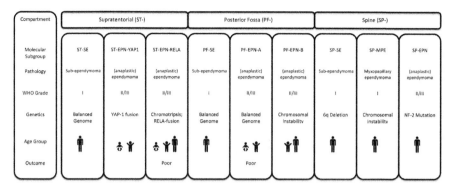

Fig. 7. Summary of molecular and clinical characteristics of ependymal tumor subgroups.

adults and has a more favorable prognosis.[101,102] The molecular subgroup of supratentorial ependymomas with the YAP1 fusion are primarily seen in children and have an excellent prognosis.

The standard of care for ependymomas remains maximal safe surgical resection followed by adjuvant postoperative radiation therapy directed at the primary site. The use of irradiation in children younger than 3 years remains controversial, but chemotherapy is typically used to delay or avoid irradiation to avoid the long-term consequences, including neurocognitive deficits, increased risk of stroke, and secondary malignancies.

CRANIOPHARYNGIOMA

Craniopharyngiomas are slow-growing benign epithelial tumors that arise from embryonic remnants of the Rathke pouch in the suprasellar region adjacent to the optic chiasm. They account for approximately 5% to 10% of pediatric brain tumors.[103,104] Symptoms occur as a result of compression of nearby neural structures and can include visual deficits, endocrinopathies, panhypopituitarism from compression of the pituitary gland or stalk, and symptoms of increased intracranial pressure from obstruction of the CSF pathways.[105–107] Visual symptoms are frequent and can vary, including decreased visual acuity or visual field deficits in 1 or both eyes, depending on direct or indirect damage to the optic chiasm by the solid or cystic portion of the tumor. Patients are often diagnosed months after they present with endocrine abnormalities, such as growth failure, sexual dysfunction, amenorrhea, and, less commonly, diabetes insipidus if the pituitary stalk is involved.[108] Tumors are frequently large at the time of diagnosis, classically with calcifications in the suprasellar region, and the presence of one or more cysts present (**Fig. 8**). They are divided into adamantinomatous and papillary types, with those with adamantinomatous features associated with higher recurrence rates.[109]

Although considered histologically benign tumors, pediatric craniopharyngiomas remain a challenge with respect to treatment options due to the close proximity to many vital structures[110] and in the long-term management of the treatment-related late-effects. Despite controversy over optimal management, surgery remains the mainstay of treatment, with a >85% progression-free survival rate after total resection, but often at the cost of neurocognitive difficulties and permanent hormonal deficiencies. Malignant transformation is extremely rare, especially in children.[111] When gross total resection is not achieved or is considered inadvisable, radiation provides

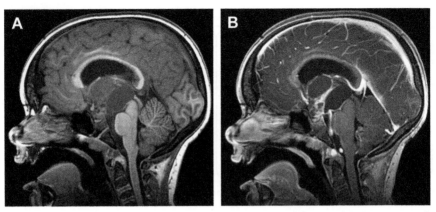

Fig. 8. Craniopharyngioma. Precontrast (*A*) and postcontrast (*B*) sagittal T1 images reveal a sellar and suprasellar mass that extends superiorly into the third ventricle and posteriorly to the interpeduncular cistern. Two dominant superior and posterior cysts show rim enhancement, whereas the more inferior component is mostly solid and shows heterogeneous enhancement.

excellent long-term control.[112] Alternative less-invasive treatment options may involve endoscopic cyst fenestration or placement of an Ommaya reservoir into the tumor cyst for antineoplastic or radiolabeled agent delivery.[113,114]

CHOROID PLEXUS TUMORS

Choroid plexus tumors are very rare and account for fewer than 1% of all brain tumors and 3% to 4% of pediatric intracranial tumors.[115] Patients often present with symptoms of hydrocephalus due to overproduction of CSF by the tumor and less commonly obstruction.[116,117] They are intraventricular papillary neoplasms derived from the choroid plexus epithelium. Histologically they can range from benign well-differentiated choroid plexus papillomas (CPPs) (WHO grade I), atypical CPPs (WHO grade II) to highly aggressive choroid plexus carcinomas (CPCa) (WHO grade III). Approximately 50% of choroid plexus tumors are found in the lateral ventricles, 40% in the fourth ventricle and 5% in the third ventricle and multiple ventricles in the remaining 5%.[118,119] Although extraventricular choroid plexus tumors are rare, they have been reported to occur in various other locations throughout the brain, including brainstem and posterior fossa.[115,120] CPCa occurs at a higher frequency in patients with Li-Fraumeni syndrome, although most patients with CPCa do not have a germline TP53 mutation.[121] Aicardi syndrome has been associated with CPPs.

Gross total resection is typically curative for CPP, whereas the invasive nature of CPCa makes it difficult to achieve complete resection, necessitating the use of adjuvant therapy. Radiation therapy has been shown to be beneficial, but is often avoided in younger children. In this group of patients, multiagent chemotherapy can be used to delay or obviate irradiation.[115,122,123] Prognosis remains poor, with 5-year survival less than 50% in patients with CPCa.[121,124,125]

GERM CELL TUMORS

Intracranial germ cell tumors (GCTs) represent approximately 3% of pediatric brain tumors and most commonly arise in midline locations, such as the pineal or suprasellar region of the brain.[126] The incidence can vary according to geography, with CNS

GCTs accounting for up to 11% of all pediatric brain tumors in Asian countries such as Japan.[126–128] The WHO classification system divides intracranial GCTs into germinomas and non-germinomatous GCTs (NGGCTs). NGGCTs comprise a heterogeneous group of various histologies, including embryonal carcinoma, endodermal sinus tumor (yolk sac tumor), choriocarcinoma, teratoma (mature and immature), and mixed GCTs. The histologic subtype varies with age, with mature and immature teratomas predominating in the neonatal period; an increasing proportion of malignant tumors arise in adolescence. Germinomas are the most common, accounting for 50% to 60% of all intracranial GCTs.

Although histologic examination is often needed for a definitive diagnosis, the tumor markers alpha-fetal protein (AFP) or beta human chorionic gonadotropin (beta-hCG) in the CSF or blood can be diagnostic and can distinguish a germinoma from an NGGCT. Highly elevated levels of beta-hCG (>1000 IU/L) or AFP (>500 IU/L) can be diagnostic of a choriocarcinoma or yolk sac tumor, respectively, and may obviate the need for surgical intervention. A mild elevation in beta-hCG can be seen in some beta-hCG secreting germinomas, but tend to be <50 IU/L.[129] AFP is not elevated in germinomas, so a high AFP is sufficient to classify a tumor as an NGGCT.

Presenting symptoms depend on tumor location. Delay in diagnosis of up to 12 months is not uncommon, especially when symptoms involve endocrinopathies, school difficulties, or behavioral problems.[130] Pineal tumors often cause obstructive hydrocephalus, and patients may present with signs of increased intracranial pressure or signs related to direct tectal damage with neuroophthalmologic abnormalities. Parinaud syndrome (characterized by several neuro-ophthalmologic findings including pupillary abnormalities and vertical gaze limitation) can be present in up to 50% of cases. Patients with tumors in the suprasellar region more commonly present with hypothalamic or pituitary dysfunction, but also may have visual deficits due to chiasmatic or optic nerve compression, classically a bitemporal hemianopsia.

Germinomas have a more favorable prognosis and require less-intensive therapy compared with NGGCTs. Germinomas are exquisitely sensitive to radiation and can be effectively treated with a cure rate of greater than 90% with craniospinal and local boost.[131–133] Germinomas are also chemosensitive, and treatment with preradiation chemotherapy followed by reduced dose radiotherapy in the form of whole ventricular therapy supplemented with radiotherapy to the local tumor site has been shown to be as effective as craniospinal radiotherapy, with excellent 5-year overall survival rates.[131,134,135] NGGCTs, on the other hand, are less radiosensitive and radiotherapy alone resulted in much lower rates of disease control, ranging anywhere from 20% to 60%.[136,137] In this group of patients, administering multiagent chemotherapy regimens in addition to craniospinal plus local boost radiation therapy has improved survival significantly.[138–140]

SPINAL CORD TUMORS

Primary spinal cord tumors are rare CNS tumors in childhood with an annual incidence of less than 1 per 100,000 children per year[141] and account for fewer than 6% of all childhood CNS tumors.[142] They are difficult to diagnose due to the vague nature of symptoms that can be difficult to characterize. Spinal cord tumors are unique in that they can cause both local and distal symptoms due to tumors interrupting ascending and descending spinal cord pathways. Symptoms typically have a gradual onset and can be especially hard to detect in infants. Although duration of symptoms have not been correlated with survival and patients typically report symptom duration of longer than 6 months before diagnosis,[143] severity of neurologic deficits at presentation is directly associated with worse outcomes following surgery, emphasizing the need for early intervention.[144,145] Spinal cord tumors can be classified based on location: intramedullary, intradural-extramedullary, and extradural.

The most common subtype of pediatric spinal cord tumors are gliomas followed by ependymomas.[146–148] Surgical resection remains the mainstay of treatment for spinal cord LGGs. When complete resection cannot be obtained, radiotherapy and chemotherapy have been somewhat effective in treating the tumors,[149] but they usually are reserved for tumors that progress after extensive surgery.[150] Treatment of HGGs includes radiation and usually chemotherapy following surgical resection.

REFERENCES

1. Ostrom QT, Gittleman H, Xu J, et al. CBTRUS statistical report: primary brain and other central nervous system tumors diagnosed in the United States in 2009-2013. Neuro Oncol 2016;18(suppl_5):v1–75.
2. Zhang J, Walsh MF, Wu G, et al. Germline mutations in predisposition genes in pediatric cancer. N Engl J Med 2015;373(24):2336–46.
3. Ron E, Modan B, Boice JD Jr, et al. Tumors of the brain and nervous system after radiotherapy in childhood. N Engl J Med 1988;319(16):1033–9.
4. Wilne S, Collier J, Kennedy C, et al. Presentation of childhood CNS tumours: a systematic review and meta-analysis. Lancet Oncol 2007;8(8):685–95.
5. Louis DN, Ohgaki H, Wiestler OD, et al. WHO classification of tumours of the central nervous system, revised. 4th edition. World Health Organization; 2016.
6. Packer RJ, Cogen P, Vezina G, et al. Medulloblastoma: clinical and biologic aspects. Neuro Oncol 1999;1(3):232–50.
7. Crawford JR, MacDonald TJ, Packer RJ. Medulloblastoma in childhood: new biological advances. Lancet Neurol 2007;6(12):1073–85.
8. Louis DN, Ohgaki H, Wiestler OD, et al. The 2007 WHO classification of tumours of the central nervous system. Acta Neuropathol 2007;114(2):97–109.
9. Taylor MD, Northcott PA, Korshunov A, et al. Molecular subgroups of medulloblastoma: the current consensus. Acta Neuropathol 2012;123(4):465–72.
10. Kool M, Koster J, Bunt J, et al. Integrated genomics identifies five medulloblastoma subtypes with distinct genetic profiles, pathway signatures and clinicopathological features. PLoS One 2008;3(8):e3088.
11. Northcott PA, Buchhalter I, Morrissy AS, et al. The whole-genome landscape of medulloblastoma subtypes. Nature 2017;547(7663):331–7.
12. Albright AL, Sposto R, Holmes E, et al. Correlation of neurosurgical subspecialization with outcomes in children with malignant brain tumors. Neurosurgery 2000;47(4):879–85 [discussion: 885–7].
13. Robertson PL, Muraszko KM, Holmes EJ, et al. Incidence and severity of postoperative cerebellar mutism syndrome in children with medulloblastoma: a prospective study by the Children's Oncology Group. J Neurosurg 2006;105(6 Suppl):444–51.
14. Packer RJ, Macdonald T, Vezina G. Central nervous system tumors. Hematol Oncol Clin North Am 2010;24(1):87–108.
15. Packer RJ, Gajjar A, Vezina G, et al. Phase III study of craniospinal radiation therapy followed by adjuvant chemotherapy for newly diagnosed average-risk medulloblastoma. J Clin Oncol 2006;24(25):4202–8.
16. Gajjar A, Chintagumpala M, Ashley D, et al. Risk-adapted craniospinal radiotherapy followed by high-dose chemotherapy and stem-cell rescue in children

with newly diagnosed medulloblastoma (St Jude Medulloblastoma-96): long-term results from a prospective, multicentre trial. Lancet Oncol 2006;7(10): 813–20.

17. Packer RJ, Sutton LN, Elterman R, et al. Outcome for children with medulloblastoma treated with radiation and cisplatin, CCNU, and vincristine chemotherapy. J Neurosurg 1994;81(5):690–8.

18. Ramaswamy V, Northcott PA, Taylor MD. FISH and chips: the recipe for improved prognostication and outcomes for children with medulloblastoma. Cancer Genet 2011;204(11):577–88.

19. Packer RJ, Gurney JG, Punyko JA, et al. Long-term neurologic and neurosensory sequelae in adult survivors of a childhood brain tumor: childhood cancer survivor study. J Clin Oncol 2003;21(17):3255–61.

20. Neglia JP, Robison LL, Stovall M, et al. New primary neoplasms of the central nervous system in survivors of childhood cancer: a report from the Childhood Cancer Survivor Study. J Natl Cancer Inst 2006;98(21):1528–37.

21. Kool M, Korshunov A, Remke M, et al. Molecular subgroups of medulloblastoma: an international meta-analysis of transcriptome, genetic aberrations, and clinical data of WNT, SHH, Group 3, and Group 4 medulloblastomas. Acta Neuropathol 2012;123(4):473–84.

22. Gibson P, Tong Y, Robinson G, et al. Subtypes of medulloblastoma have distinct developmental origins. Nature 2010;468(7327):1095–9.

23. Hamilton SR, Liu B, Parsons RE, et al. The molecular basis of Turcot's syndrome. N Engl J Med 1995;332(13):839–47.

24. Clifford SC, Lusher ME, Lindsey JC, et al. Wnt/Wingless pathway activation and chromosome 6 loss characterize a distinct molecular sub-group of medulloblastomas associated with a favorable prognosis. Cell Cycle 2006;5(22):2666–70.

25. Fattet S, Haberler C, Legoix P, et al. Beta-catenin status in paediatric medulloblastomas: correlation of immunohistochemical expression with mutational status, genetic profiles, and clinical characteristics. J Pathol 2009;218(1):86–94.

26. Kool M, Jones DT, Jager N, et al. Genome sequencing of SHH medulloblastoma predicts genotype-related response to smoothened inhibition. Cancer Cell 2014;25(3):393–405.

27. Oliver TG, Read TA, Kessler JD, et al. Loss of patched and disruption of granule cell development in a pre-neoplastic stage of medulloblastoma. Development 2005;132(10):2425–39.

28. Grammel D, Warmuth-Metz M, von Bueren AO, et al. Sonic hedgehog-associated medulloblastoma arising from the cochlear nuclei of the brainstem. Acta Neuropathol 2012;123(4):601–14.

29. Smith MJ, Beetz C, Williams SG, et al. Germline mutations in SUFU cause Gorlin syndrome-associated childhood medulloblastoma and redefine the risk associated with PTCH1 mutations. J Clin Oncol 2014;32(36):4155–61.

30. Liu KW, Pajtler KW, Worst BC, et al. Molecular mechanisms and therapeutic targets in pediatric brain tumors. Sci Signal 2017;10(470) [pii:eaaf7593].

31. Zhukova N, Ramaswamy V, Remke M, et al. Subgroup-specific prognostic implications of TP53 mutation in medulloblastoma. J Clin Oncol 2013;31(23): 2927–35.

32. Ryan SL, Schwalbe EC, Cole M, et al. MYC family amplification and clinical risk-factors interact to predict an extremely poor prognosis in childhood medulloblastoma. Acta Neuropathol 2012;123(4):501–13.

33. Rudin CM, Hann CL, Laterra J, et al. Treatment of medulloblastoma with hedgehog pathway inhibitor GDC-0449. N Engl J Med 2009;361(12):1173–8.

34. Gajjar A, Stewart CF, Ellison DW, et al. Phase I study of vismodegib in children with recurrent or refractory medulloblastoma: a pediatric brain tumor consortium study. Clin Cancer Res 2013;19(22):6305–12.

35. Glod J, Rahme GJ, Kaur H, et al. Pediatric brain tumors: current knowledge and therapeutic opportunities. J Pediatr Hematol Oncol 2016;38(4):249–60.

36. Northcott PA, Shih DJ, Peacock J, et al. Subgroup-specific structural variation across 1,000 medulloblastoma genomes. Nature 2012;488(7409):49–56.

37. Delmore JE, Issa GC, Lemieux ME, et al. BET bromodomain inhibition as a therapeutic strategy to target c-Myc. Cell 2011;146(6):904–17.

38. Pei Y, Liu KW, Wang J, et al. HDAC and PI3K antagonists cooperate to inhibit growth of MYC-driven medulloblastoma. Cancer Cell 2016;29(3):311–23.

39. Engelender S, Kaminsky Z, Guo X, et al. Synphilin-1 associates with alpha-synuclein and promotes the formation of cytosolic inclusions. Nat Genet 1999; 22(1):110–4.

40. Reddy AT, Janss AJ, Phillips PC, et al. Outcome for children with supratentorial primitive neuroectodermal tumors treated with surgery, radiation, and chemotherapy. Cancer 2000;88(9):2189–93.

41. Cohen BH, Zeltzer PM, Boyett JM, et al. Prognostic factors and treatment results for supratentorial primitive neuroectodermal tumors in children using radiation and chemotherapy: a Children's Cancer Group randomized trial. J Clin Oncol 1995;13(7):1687–96.

42. Pomeroy SL, Tamayo P, Gaasenbeek M, et al. Prediction of central nervous system embryonal tumour outcome based on gene expression. Nature 2002; 415(6870):436–42.

43. Perez-Martinez A, Lassaletta A, Gonzalez-Vicent M, et al. High-dose chemotherapy with autologous stem cell rescue for children with high risk and recurrent medulloblastoma and supratentorial primitive neuroectodermal tumors. J Neurooncol 2005;71(1):33–8.

44. Friedrich C, von Bueren AO, von Hoff K, et al. Treatment of young children with CNS-primitive neuroectodermal tumors/pineoblastomas in the prospective multicenter trial HIT 2000 using different chemotherapy regimens and radiotherapy. Neuro Oncol 2013;15(2):224–34.

45. Geyer JR, Sposto R, Jennings M, et al. Multiagent chemotherapy and deferred radiotherapy in infants with malignant brain tumors: a report from the Children's Cancer Group. J Clin Oncol 2005;23(30):7621–31.

46. Schwalbe EC, Hayden JT, Rogers HA, et al. Histologically defined central nervous system primitive neuro-ectodermal tumours (CNS-PNETs) display heterogeneous DNA methylation profiles and show relationships to other paediatric brain tumour types. Acta Neuropathol 2013;126(6):943–6.

47. Biegel JA. Molecular genetics of atypical teratoid/rhabdoid tumor. Neurosurg Focus 2006;20(1):E11.

48. Ginn KF, Gajjar A. Atypical teratoid rhabdoid tumor: current therapy and future directions. Front Oncol 2012;2:114.

49. Biegel JA, Zhou JY, Rorke LB, et al. Germ-line and acquired mutations of INI1 in atypical teratoid and rhabdoid tumors. Cancer Res 1999;59(1):74–9.

50. Hasselblatt M, Nagel I, Oyen F, et al. SMARCA4-mutated atypical teratoid/rhabdoid tumors are associated with inherited germline alterations and poor prognosis. Acta Neuropathol 2014;128(3):453–6.

51. Eaton KW, Tooke LS, Wainwright LM, et al. Spectrum of SMARCB1/INI1 mutations in familial and sporadic rhabdoid tumors. Pediatr Blood Cancer 2011; 56(1):7–15.

52. Johann PD, Erkek S, Zapatka M, et al. Atypical teratoid/rhabdoid tumors are comprised of three epigenetic subgroups with distinct enhancer landscapes. Cancer Cell 2016;29(3):379–93.

53. Chi SN, Zimmerman MA, Yao X, et al. Intensive multimodality treatment for children with newly diagnosed CNS atypical teratoid rhabdoid tumor. J Clin Oncol 2009;27(3):385–9.

54. Fischer-Valuck BW, Chen I, Srivastava AJ, et al. Assessment of the treatment approach and survival outcomes in a modern cohort of patients with atypical teratoid rhabdoid tumors using the National Cancer Database. Cancer 2017; 123(4):682–7.

55. Schrey D, Carceller Lechon F, Malietzis G, et al. Multimodal therapy in children and adolescents with newly diagnosed atypical teratoid rhabdoid tumor: individual pooled data analysis and review of the literature. J Neurooncol 2016; 126(1):81–90.

56. Wetmore C, Boyett J, Li S, et al. Alisertib is active as single agent in recurrent atypical teratoid rhabdoid tumors in 4 children. Neuro Oncol 2015;17(6):882–8.

57. Braunstein S, Raleigh D, Bindra R, et al. Pediatric high-grade glioma: current molecular landscape and therapeutic approaches. J Neurooncol 2017;134(3): 541–9.

58. Marchese MJ, Chang CH. Malignant astrocytic gliomas in children. Cancer 1990;65(12):2771–8.

59. Pollack IF. The role of surgery in pediatric gliomas. J Neurooncol 1999;42(3): 271–88.

60. Wisoff JH, Boyett JM, Berger MS, et al. Current neurosurgical management and the impact of the extent of resection in the treatment of malignant gliomas of childhood: a report of the Children's Cancer Group trial no. CCG-945. J Neurosurg 1998;89(1):52–9.

61. Finlay JL, Boyett JM, Yates AJ, et al. Randomized phase III trial in childhood high-grade astrocytoma comparing vincristine, lomustine, and prednisone with the eight-drugs-in-1-day regimen. Children's Cancer Group. J Clin Oncol 1995;13(1):112–23.

62. Sposto R, Ertel IJ, Jenkin RD, et al. The effectiveness of chemotherapy for treatment of high grade astrocytoma in children: results of a randomized trial. A report from the Children's Cancer Study Group. J Neurooncol 1989;7(2):165–77.

63. Yazici G, Zorlu F, Cengiz M, et al. High-grade glioma in children and adolescents: a single-center experience. Childs Nerv Syst 2016;32(2):291–7.

64. Jakacki RI, Cohen KJ, Buxton A, et al. Phase 2 study of concurrent radiotherapy and temozolomide followed by temozolomide and lomustine in the treatment of children with high-grade glioma: a report of the Children's Oncology Group ACNS0423 study. Neuro Oncol 2016;18(10):1442–50.

65. MacDonald TJ, Arenson EB, Ater J, et al. Phase II study of high-dose chemotherapy before radiation in children with newly diagnosed high-grade astrocytoma: final analysis of Children's Cancer Group Study 9933. Cancer 2005; 104(12):2862–71.

66. Sturm D, Witt H, Hovestadt V, et al. Hotspot mutations in H3F3A and IDH1 define distinct epigenetic and biological subgroups of glioblastoma. Cancer Cell 2012; 22(4):425–37.

67. Qaddoumi I, Kocak M, Pai Panandiker AS, et al. Phase II trial of Erlotinib during and after radiotherapy in children with newly diagnosed high-grade gliomas. Front Oncol 2014;4:67.

68. Wakefield A, Pignata A, Ghazi A, et al. Is CMV a target in pediatric glioblastoma? Expression of CMV proteins, pp65 and IE1-72 and CMV nucleic acids in a cohort of pediatric glioblastoma patients. J Neurooncol 2015;125(2):307–15.

69. Josupeit R, Bender S, Kern S, et al. Pediatric and adult high-grade glioma stem cell culture models are permissive to lytic infection with parvovirus H-1. Viruses 2016;8(5) [pii:E138].

70. MacDonald TJ, Aguilera D, Kramm CM. Treatment of high-grade glioma in children and adolescents. Neuro Oncol 2011;13(10):1049–58.

71. Freeman CR, Farmer JP. Pediatric brain stem gliomas: a review. Int J Radiat Oncol Biol Phys 1998;40(2):265–71.

72. Roujeau T, Machado G, Garnett MR, et al. Stereotactic biopsy of diffuse pontine lesions in children. J Neurosurg 2007;107(1 Suppl):1–4.

73. Puget S, Beccaria K, Blauwblomme T, et al. Biopsy in a series of 130 pediatric diffuse intrinsic Pontine gliomas. Childs Nerv Syst 2015;31(10):1773–80.

74. Freeman CR, Kepner J, Kun LE, et al. A detrimental effect of a combined chemotherapy-radiotherapy approach in children with diffuse intrinsic brain stem gliomas? Int J Radiat Oncol Biol Phys 2000;47(3):561–4.

75. Hargrave D, Bartels U, Bouffet E. Diffuse brainstem glioma in children: critical review of clinical trials. Lancet Oncol 2006;7(3):241–8.

76. Korones DN, Fisher PG, Kretschmar C, et al. Treatment of children with diffuse intrinsic brain stem glioma with radiotherapy, vincristine and oral VP-16: a Children's Oncology Group phase II study. Pediatr Blood Cancer 2008;50(2):227–30.

77. Mandell LR, Kadota R, Freeman C, et al. There is no role for hyperfractionated radiotherapy in the management of children with newly diagnosed diffuse intrinsic brainstem tumors: results of a Pediatric Oncology Group phase III trial comparing conventional vs. hyperfractionated radiotherapy. Int J Radiat Oncol Biol Phys 1999;43(5):959–64.

78. Jennings MT, Sposto R, Boyett JM, et al. Preradiation chemotherapy in primary high-risk brainstem tumors: phase II study CCG-9941 of the Children's Cancer Group. J Clin Oncol 2002;20(16):3431–7.

79. Broniscer A, Iacono L, Chintagumpala M, et al. Role of temozolomide after radiotherapy for newly diagnosed diffuse brainstem glioma in children: results of a multiinstitutional study (SJHG-98). Cancer 2005;103(1):133–9.

80. Puget S, Philippe C, Bax DA, et al. Mesenchymal transition and PDGFRA amplification/mutation are key distinct oncogenic events in pediatric diffuse intrinsic pontine gliomas. PLoS One 2012;7(2):e30313.

81. Grill J, Puget S, Andreiuolo F, et al. Critical oncogenic mutations in newly diagnosed pediatric diffuse intrinsic pontine glioma. Pediatr Blood Cancer 2012; 58(4):489–91.

82. Wu G, Diaz AK, Paugh BS, et al. The genomic landscape of diffuse intrinsic pontine glioma and pediatric non-brainstem high-grade glioma. Nat Genet 2014;46(5):444–50.

83. Taylor KR, Mackay A, Truffaux N, et al. Recurrent activating ACVR1 mutations in diffuse intrinsic pontine glioma. Nat Genet 2014;46(5):457–61.

84. Lassaletta A, Scheinemann K, Zelcer SM, et al. Phase II weekly vinblastine for chemotherapy-naïve children with progressive low-grade glioma: a Canadian Pediatric Brain Tumor Consortium Study. J Clin Oncol 2016;34(29):3537–43.

85. Bouffet E, Jakacki R, Goldman S, et al. Phase II study of weekly vinblastine in recurrent or refractory pediatric low-grade glioma. J Clin Oncol 2012;30(12):1358–63.

86. Ramkissoon LA, Horowitz PM, Craig JM, et al. Genomic analysis of diffuse pediatric low-grade gliomas identifies recurrent oncogenic truncating rearrangements in the transcription factor MYBL1. Proc Natl Acad Sci U S A 2013; 110(20):8188–93.

87. Pollack IF. Brain tumors in children. N Engl J Med 1994;331(22):1500–7.

88. Alvord EC Jr, Lofton S. Gliomas of the optic nerve or chiasm. Outcome by patients' age, tumor site, and treatment. J Neurosurg 1988;68(1):85–98.

89. Listernick R, Charrow J, Greenwald M, et al. Natural history of optic pathway tumors in children with neurofibromatosis type 1: a longitudinal study. J Pediatr 1994;125(1):63–6.

90. Sani I, Albanese A. Endocrine long-term follow-up of children with neurofibromatosis type 1 and optic pathway glioma. Horm Res Paediatr 2017;87(3):179–88.

91. Silva MM, Goldman S, Keating G, et al. Optic pathway hypothalamic gliomas in children under three years of age: the role of chemotherapy. Pediatr Neurosurg 2000;33(3):151–8.

92. Parsa CF, Hoyt CS, Lesser RL, et al. Spontaneous regression of optic gliomas: thirteen cases documented by serial neuroimaging. Arch Ophthalmol 2001; 119(4):516–29.

93. Packer RJ. Chemotherapy: low-grade gliomas of the hypothalamus and thalamus. Pediatr Neurosurg 2000;32(5):259–63.

94. Allen JC, Siffert J, Hukin J. Clinical manifestations of childhood ependymoma: a multitude of syndromes. Pediatr Neurosurg 1998;28(1):49–55.

95. Kilday JP, Rahman R, Dyer S, et al. Pediatric ependymoma: biological perspectives. Mol Cancer Res 2009;7(6):765–86.

96. Ebert C, von Haken M, Meyer-Puttlitz B, et al. Molecular genetic analysis of ependymal tumors. NF2 mutations and chromosome 22q loss occur preferentially in intramedullary spinal ependymomas. Am J Pathol 1999;155(2):627–32.

97. Prayson RA. Clinicopathologic study of 61 patients with ependymoma including MIB-1 immunohistochemistry. Ann Diagn Pathol 1999;3(1):11–8.

98. Vanuytsel L, Brada M. The role of prophylactic spinal irradiation in localized intracranial ependymoma. Int J Radiat Oncol Biol Phys 1991;21(3):825–30.

99. Pajtler KW, Witt H, Sill M, et al. Molecular classification of ependymal tumors across all CNS compartments, histopathological grades, and age groups. Cancer Cell 2015;27(5):728–43.

100. Archer TC, Pomeroy SL. Defining the molecular landscape of ependymomas. Cancer Cell 2015;27(5):613–5.

101. Pajtler KW, Mack SC, Ramaswamy V, et al. The current consensus on the clinical management of intracranial ependymoma and its distinct molecular variants. Acta Neuropathol 2017;133(1):5–12.

102. Witt H, Mack SC, Ryzhova M, et al. Delineation of two clinically and molecularly distinct subgroups of posterior fossa ependymoma. Cancer Cell 2011;20(2): 143–57.

103. Garre ML, Cama A. Craniopharyngioma: modern concepts in pathogenesis and treatment. Curr Opin Pediatr 2007;19(4):471–9.

104. Jane JA Jr, Laws ER. Craniopharyngioma. Pituitary 2006;9(4):323–6.

105. Hoffmann A, Boekhoff S, Gebhardt U, et al. History before diagnosis in childhood craniopharyngioma: associations with initial presentation and long-term prognosis. Eur J Endocrinol 2015;173(6):853–62.

106. Rucka E, Wedrychowicz A, Zygmunt-Gorska A, et al. Clinical symptoms at the diagnosis of the craniopharyngioma. Pediatr Endocrinol Diabetes Metab 2012;18(2):58–62 [in Polish].

107. Flitsch J, Muller HL, Burkhardt T. Surgical strategies in childhood craniopharyngioma. Front Endocrinol 2011;2:96.
108. Garnett MR, Puget S, Grill J, et al. Craniopharyngioma. Orphanet J Rare Dis 2007;2:18.
109. Sartoretti-Schefer S, Wichmann W, Aguzzi A, et al. MR differentiation of adamantinous and squamous-papillary craniopharyngiomas. AJNR Am J Neuroradiol 1997;18(1):77–87.
110. Muller HL, Albanese A, Calaminus G, et al. Consensus and perspectives on treatment strategies in childhood craniopharyngioma: results of a meeting of the Craniopharyngioma Study Group (SIOP), Genova, 2004. J Pediatr Endocrinol Metab 2006;19(Suppl 1):453–4.
111. Aquilina K, Merchant TE, Rodriguez-Galindo C, et al. Malignant transformation of irradiated craniopharyngioma in children: report of 2 cases. J Neurosurg Pediatr 2010;5(2):155–61.
112. Minniti G, Esposito V, Amichetti M, et al. The role of fractionated radiotherapy and radiosurgery in the management of patients with craniopharyngioma. Neurosurg Rev 2009;32(2):125–32 [discussion: 132].
113. Caceres A. Intracavitary therapeutic options in the management of cystic craniopharyngioma. Childs Nerv Syst 2005;21(8–9):705–18.
114. Samii M, Tatagiba M. Surgical management of craniopharyngiomas: a review. Neurol Med Chir (Tokyo) 1997;37(2):141–9.
115. Gozali AE, Britt B, Shane L, et al. Choroid plexus tumors; management, outcome, and association with the Li-Fraumeni syndrome: the Children's Hospital Los Angeles (CHLA) experience, 1991-2010. Pediatr Blood Cancer 2012; 58(6):905–9.
116. Koeller KK, Sandberg GD. From the archives of the AFIP. Cerebral intraventricular neoplasms: radiologic-pathologic correlation. Radiographics 2002;22(6): 1473–505.
117. Rostasy KM, Sponholz S, Bahn E, et al. Unusual localization of a choroid plexus papilloma in a 4-year-old female. Pediatr Neurol 2003;28(1):66–8.
118. Bettegowda C, Adogwa O, Mehta V, et al. Treatment of choroid plexus tumors: a 20-year single institutional experience. J Neurosurg Pediatr 2012;10(5): 398–405.
119. Jaiswal AK, Jaiswal S, Sahu RN, et al. Choroid plexus papilloma in children: diagnostic and surgical considerations. J Pediatr Neurosci 2009;4(1):10–6.
120. Ogiwara H, Dipatri AJ Jr, Alden TD, et al. Choroid plexus tumors in pediatric patients. Br J Neurosurg 2012;26(1):32–7.
121. Tabori U, Shlien A, Baskin B, et al. TP53 alterations determine clinical subgroups and survival of patients with choroid plexus tumors. J Clin Oncol 2010;28(12): 1995–2001.
122. Wrede B, Liu P, Wolff JE. Chemotherapy improves the survival of patients with choroid plexus carcinoma: a meta-analysis of individual cases with choroid plexus tumors. J Neurooncol 2007;85(3):345–51.
123. Zaky W, Dhall G, Khatua S, et al. Choroid plexus carcinoma in children: the Head Start experience. Pediatr Blood Cancer 2015;62(5):784–9.
124. Lafay-Cousin L, Mabbott DJ, Halliday W, et al. Use of ifosfamide, carboplatin, and etoposide chemotherapy in choroid plexus carcinoma. J Neurosurg Pediatr 2010;5(6):615–21.
125. Rickert CH, Paulus W. Tumors of the choroid plexus. Microsc Res Tech 2001; 52(1):104–11.

126. Echevarria ME, Fangusaro J, Goldman S. Pediatric central nervous system germ cell tumors: a review. Oncologist 2008;13(6):690–9.
127. Hoffman HJ, Otsubo H, Hendrick EB, et al. Intracranial germ-cell tumors in children. J Neurosurg 1991;74(4):545–51.
128. Lin IJ, Shu SG, Chu HY, et al. Primary intracranial germ-cell tumor in children. Zhonghua Yi Xue Za Zhi (Taipei) 1997;60(5):259–64.
129. Ogino H, Shibamoto Y, Takanaka T, et al. CNS germinoma with elevated serum human chorionic gonadotropin level: clinical characteristics and treatment outcome. Int J Radiat Oncol Biol Phys 2005;62(3):803–8.
130. Sethi RV, Marino R, Niemierko A, et al. Delayed diagnosis in children with intracranial germ cell tumors. J Pediatr 2013;163(5):1448–53.
131. Bamberg M, Kortmann RD, Calaminus G, et al. Radiation therapy for intracranial germinoma: results of the German cooperative prospective trials MAKEI 83/86/89. J Clin Oncol 1999;17(8):2585–92.
132. Packer RJ, Cohen BH, Cooney K. Intracranial germ cell tumors. Oncologist 2000;5(4):312–20.
133. Shirato H, Nishio M, Sawamura Y, et al. Analysis of long-term treatment of intracranial germinoma. Int J Radiat Oncol Biol Phys 1997;37(3):511–5.
134. Bouffet E, Baranzelli MC, Patte C, et al. Combined treatment modality for intracranial germinomas: results of a multicentre SFOP experience. Societe Francaise d'Oncologie Pediatrique. Br J Cancer 1999;79(7–8):1199–204.
135. Cheng S, Kilday JP, Laperriere N, et al. Outcomes of children with central nervous system germinoma treated with multi-agent chemotherapy followed by reduced radiation. J Neurooncol 2016;127(1):173–80.
136. Haas-Kogan DA, Missett BT, Wara WM, et al. Radiation therapy for intracranial germ cell tumors. Int J Radiat Oncol Biol Phys 2003;56(2):511–8.
137. Kanamori M, Kumabe T, Saito R, et al. Optimal treatment strategy for intracranial germ cell tumors: a single institution analysis. J Neurosurg Pediatr 2009;4(6):506–14.
138. Matsutani M. Combined chemotherapy and radiation therapy for CNS germ cell tumors–the Japanese experience. J Neurooncol 2001;54(3):311–6.
139. Ogawa K, Toita T, Nakamura K, et al. Treatment and prognosis of patients with intracranial nongerminomatous malignant germ cell tumors: a multiinstitutional retrospective analysis of 41 patients. Cancer 2003;98(2):369–76.
140. Yoshida J, Sugita K, Kobayashi T, et al. Prognosis of intracranial germ cell tumours: effectiveness of chemotherapy with cisplatin and etoposide (CDDP and VP-16). Acta Neurochir (Wein) 1993;120(3–4):111–7.
141. Hayden Gephart MG, Lober RM, Arrigo RT, et al. Trends in the diagnosis and treatment of pediatric primary spinal cord tumors. J Neurosurg Pediatr 2012;10(6):555–9.
142. DeSousa AL, Kalsbeck JE, Mealey J Jr, et al. Intraspinal tumors in children. a review of 81 cases. J Neurosurg 1979;51(4):437–45.
143. Crawford JR, Zaninovic A, Santi M, et al. Primary spinal cord tumors of childhood: effects of clinical presentation, radiographic features, and pathology on survival. J Neurooncol 2009;95(2):259–69.
144. Epstein F, Epstein N. Surgical treatment of spinal cord astrocytomas of childhood. A series of 19 patients. J Neurosurg 1982;57(5):685–9.
145. Luksik AS, Garzon-Muvdi T, Yang W, et al. Pediatric spinal cord astrocytomas: a retrospective study of 348 patients from the SEER database. J Neurosurg Pediatr 2017;19(6):711–9.

146. Jallo GI, Freed D, Epstein F. Intramedullary spinal cord tumors in children. Childs Nerv Syst 2003;19(9):641–9.
147. Merchant TE, Kiehna EN, Thompson SJ, et al. Pediatric low-grade and ependymal spinal cord tumors. Pediatr Neurosurg 2000;32(1):30–6.
148. Wilson PE, Oleszek JL, Clayton GH. Pediatric spinal cord tumors and masses. J Spinal Cord Med 2007;30(Suppl 1):S15–20.
149. Constantini S, Miller DC, Allen JC, et al. Radical excision of intramedullary spinal cord tumors: surgical morbidity and long-term follow-up evaluation in 164 children and young adults. J Neurosurg 2000;93(2 Suppl):183–93.
150. Ahmed R, Menezes AH, Torner JC. Role of resection and adjuvant therapy in long-term disease outcomes for low-grade pediatric intramedullary spinal cord tumors. J Neurosurg Pediatr 2016;18(5):594–601.

Brain Metastases

Ayal A. Aizer, MD, MHS[a,b], Eudocia Q. Lee, MD, MPH[b,c,d],*

KEYWORDS

- Brain metastases • Breast cancer • Lung cancer • Melanoma
- Whole brain radiation • Stereotactic radiosurgery

KEY POINTS

- Which treatment(s) to offer a patient with brain metastases depends on the primary cancer, the number and location of the metastases, the extent of systemic disease, functional status, age, and prognosis.
- The 2 main local therapies available to patients with brain metastases are neurosurgical resection and radiation therapy.
- Stereotactic radiation is an approach frequently used in patients with 1 to 4 brain metastases. Trials exploring the benefit with more than 4 brain metastases are underway.

INTRODUCTION

Brain metastases (BM) from solid tumors are associated with increased morbidity and mortality. Patients can present with focal neurologic deficits, seizures, neurocognitive impairments, or symptoms of increased intracranial pressure depending on the number, size, and location of the BMs. Standard treatment to date is local therapy with surgery and/or radiation therapy, although there is increasing interest in systemic therapies that can control both intracranial and extracranial disease. Unfortunately, few available systemic agents sufficiently control disease inside the central nervous system (CNS).[1]

The decision on which treatment(s) to offer a BM patient depends on several factors, including the primary cancer, the molecular subtype, the number and location of BMs, the extent of systemic disease, functional status, age, and prognosis. Although survival is generally poor, subsets of patients with BM can live longer than expected. The Diagnosis-Specific Graded Prognostic Assessment is a prognostic index for

Disclosure Statement: A.A. Aizer – None. E.Q. Lee – Consulting for Eli Lilly.
[a] Department of Radiation Oncology, Brigham and Women's Hospital, 75 Francis Street, Boston, MA 02115, USA; [b] Harvard Medical School, 25 Shattuck Street, Boston, MA 02115, USA; [c] Center for Neuro-Oncology, Dana-Farber Cancer Institute, 450 Brookline Avenue, Boston, MA 02215, USA; [d] Department of Neurology, Brigham and Women's Hospital, Boston, MA 02115, USA
* Corresponding author. Center for Neuro-Oncology, Dana-Farber Cancer Institute, 450 Brookline Avenue, Boston, MA 02215.
E-mail address: eqlee@partners.org

Neurol Clin 36 (2018) 557–577
https://doi.org/10.1016/j.ncl.2018.04.010
0733-8619/18/© 2018 Elsevier Inc. All rights reserved.

patients with BM refined according to diagnosis, for example, breast carcinoma, small cell lung cancer (SCLC), non-SCLC (NSCLC), gastrointestinal cancers, melanoma, or renal cell carcinoma (**Table 1**).[2] The median overall survival for a patient with a low GPA of 0.0 to 1.0 is approximately 3 to 7 months regardless of primary cancer, whereas the median overall survival for a patient with a high GPA varies according to primary cancer. The Diagnosis-Specific Graded Prognostic Assessment has been further updated in lung adenocarcinoma by incorporating the presence or absence of epidermal growth factor receptor (EGFR) or anaplastic lymphoma kinase (ALK) alterations as a prognostic factor.[3] The median overall survival for a patient with lung adenocarcinoma and high GPA score of 4.0 (age <70, Karnofsky performance status 90–100, absence of extracranial metastases, ≤4 BM, and EGFR positive or ALK

Table 1
Summary of diagnosis-specific GPA indices, which estimates survival from brain metastases

| Diagnosis | Prognostic Factors | Median Survival (mo) | | | |
		GPA 0.0–1.0	GPA 1.5–2.0	GPA 2.5–3.0	GPA 3.5–4.0
Breast cancer	KPS Subtype (triple negative, HR+, HER2+, HR/HER2+) Age (y)	3.4	7.7	15.1	25.3
GI cancers	KPS	3.1	4.4	6.9	13.5
Melanoma	KPS Number of BM	3.4	4.7	8.8	13.2

NSCLC
  (adenocarcinoma)
	Age (y)
	KPS
	Presence/absence of
	  extracranial metastases
	Number of BM
	EGFR or ALK positive
		6.9	13.7	26.5	46.8

NSCLC
  (nonadenocarcinoma)
	Age (y)
	KPS
	Presence/absence of
	  extracranial metastases
	Number of BM
		5.3	9.8	12.8	N/A

Renal cell carcinoma	KPS Number of BM	3.3	7.3	11.3	14.8
SCLC	Age (y) KPS Presence/absence of extracranial metastases Number of BM	3.0	5.5	9.4	14.8

Points are added for each prognostic factor according to primary cancer to calculate a GPA score.

Abbreviations: ALK, anaplastic lymphoma kinase; BM, brain metastases; EGFR, epidermal growth factor receptor; GI, gastrointestinal; GPA, graded prognostic assessment; HER2, human epidermal growth factor receptor 2; HR, hormone receptor; KPS, Karnofsky performance status; NSCLS, non-small cell lung cancer; SCLC, small cell lung cancer.

Adapted from Sperduto PW, Kased N, Roberge D, et al. Summary report on the graded prognostic assessment: an accurate and facile diagnosis-specific tool to estimate survival for patients with brain metastases. J Clin Oncol 2012;30(4):421; and Sperduto PW, Yang TJ, Beal K, et al. Estimating survival in patients with lung cancer and brain metastases: an update of the graded prognostic assessment for lung cancer using molecular markers (lung-molGPA). JAMA Oncol 2017;3(6):829; with permission.

positive) is almost 4 years. An on-line application that helps to calculate the Diagnosis-Specific Graded Prognostic Assessment is available at http://brainmetgpa.com.

EPIDEMIOLOGY

Incidence rates of BM in population-based studies range from 3.0 to 14.3 per 100,000.[4] The incidence may be increasing owing to earlier detection and better systemic therapies (leading to longer survival), although data to support this assertion are limited. The incidence of BMs also varies by primary cancer. The incidence proportion of BMs among patients with cancer is greatest for lung cancer (19.9%), followed by melanoma (6.9%), renal (6.5%), breast (5.1%), and colorectal (1.8%) cancers.[5] Patients with melanoma or lung cancer are most likely to have BM at the initial diagnosis of metastatic cancer.[6]

Studies also suggest that the incidence varies by cancer subtype. In patients with breast cancer with BM at the time of initial cancer diagnosis, incidence proportions for BM was highest for hormone receptor-negative/human epidermal growth factor receptor 2 (HER2)-positive and triple-negative subtypes.[7] Some studies suggest that patients with EGFR-mutant NSCLC are more likely to develop BM compared with patients with an EGFR-wildtype NSCLC[8] and that BRAF or NRAS mutations are associated with the presence of BM at first occurrence of stage IV disease.[9]

PATHOPHYSIOLOGY

The mechanisms underlying BM pathogenesis is an active area of research and may yield potential targets to prevent the metastatic process and/or treat established metastases.[10,11] In theory, any step in the metastatic process could represent a target for treatment.[10] The metastatic process generally begins with seeding—invasion of tumor cells from the primary cancer into surrounding tissues, travel through the bloodstream, and extravasation at distant sites. Although treatments against seeding could prevent the reseeding of metastases from established metastases, such treatments would primarily be useful in patients with early stage, local disease whose disease has not established metastases. A subsequent step in the metastatic process, metastatic colonization, requires cancer cells to infiltrate distant tissue, evade immune defenses, adapt to supportive niches, survive as latent tumor-initiating seeds, and eventually break out to replace host tissue.[12] Many signaling pathways support metastatic colonization, including stem cell support pathways (Wnt, transforming growth factor beta, bone morphogenetic proteins, Notch, and signal transducer and activator of transcription 3), pathways that integrate cell metabolism and survival (phosphatidylinositol-4,5-bisphosphate 3-kinase, AKT, mitogen-activated protein kinases, hypoxia-inducible factor), positional and mechanical pathways (Hedgehog, Hippo), and inflammatory pathways (nuclear factor kappa-light-chain-enhancer of activated B cells, Stat1).[12,13] What separates cancer cells from normal cells using these same pathways is the ability to activate pathways efficiently with low levels of activating signals.[12]

In addition to the general pathways responsible for metastatic colonization, brain-specific pathways exist including important tumor–microenvironment functional interactions.[10] This finding may partly explain the variation of metastases distribution patterns and the kinetics of relapse depending on tumor type. For example, prostate cancer almost never metastasizes to the brain parenchyma, whereas melanoma has a propensity for the brain. Lung cancer frequently metastasizes to the brain and other sites early in the disease course, whereas brain relapse is typically a late event in metastatic breast cancer.[12]

The genomic instability seen in cancer leads to many cellular phenotypes, some of which may have the necessary properties to metastasize to the brain. Indeed, genomic studies of matched sets of patient's primary tumor and BM reveal mutations common to both as well as mutations distinct to the BM.[14] This suggests that sequencing of primary biopsies alone (without sequencing BMs) may miss potential targets for treatment.[14]

LOCAL THERAPY

The 2 main local therapies available to patients with BMs are neurosurgical resection and radiation therapy. Whether to operate on a BM depends on several factors (**Table 2**). Generally, most patients with metastases that produce significant neurologic symptoms refractory to steroids should be managed with surgical resection as an initial step given that radiation therapy generally produces unreliable and nonimmediate improvement of neurologic symptomatology, with possible exceptions being patients with SCLC, germ cell tumors, lymphoma, and myeloma given the typical high radiosensitivity of such tumors. Very large tumors (>4-5 cm) or tumors that produce marked edema or mass effect should also be considered for surgery. Patients with a single tumor that is not managed with stereotactic radiosurgery also benefit from neurosurgical resection given the likely improvement in survival with surgery (discussed further elsewhere in this article).[15] Surgery is also generally indicated in cases of diagnostic uncertainty in which it is not clear if intracranial lesions represent metastases and if further surveillance is not an option given disease bulk or associated symptomatology. Patients with an indication for surgery should be evaluated for the viability of surgery, including an assessment of comorbidities and potential risks associated with surgery. Surgery becomes less preferable as a management strategy in cases with a large systemic disease burden given the delays in resumption of systemic therapy when surgery is used. In addition, surgery becomes more challenging when eloquent areas or deep structures are involved, such as the brainstem, thalamus, motor function, or language.

Neurosurgical Resection

Patchell and colleagues[15] conducted a randomized study of surgical resection followed by whole brain radiation therapy (WBRT) versus a needle biopsy followed by WBRT in patients with a single BM. All patients underwent MRI of the brain before the initiation of intracranial management. The arm assigned to resection displayed improved local control, functional independence, and overall survival. Vecht and

Table 2	
General indications for radiation versus neurosurgical management of brain metastases	
Neurosurgery Considered over Radiation	**Radiation Considered over Neurosurgery**
Solitary brain metastasis that is not managed with SRS	Radiosensitive tumors (SCLC, germ cell tumors, lymphoma, myeloma)
Symptomatic lesion refractory to steroids	Poor surgical candidates
Very large tumors (>4–5 cm)	Tumors in deep structures or eloquent areas (eg, brainstem, language areas)
Tumors with marked edema and mass effect	Large systemic disease burden (where surgery may delay resumption of systemic therapy)
Diagnostic uncertainty	Multiple brain metastases

Abbreviations: SCLC, small cell lung cancer; SRS, stereotactic radiosurgery.

colleagues[16] conducted a similar study in patients with a single BM and found that surgery, as opposed to WBRT alone, improved survival with a single metastasis, but only if systemic disease was controlled given the significant competing risk that systemic progression/death represents. It should be noted that a similar study conducted by Mintz and colleagues[17] did not show a benefit to resection in the case of a single lesion consistent with a BM relative to WBRT alone; however, the study was small and patients in had a poorer performance status than in the Patchell study.[15] In summary, these studies show that surgical resection likely improves oncologic outcome in patients with a single BM, although how surgical resection compares with stereotactic radiation alone and how the results of these studies should be interpreted in patients with a systemic option for intracranial control remains unknown. In addition, the benefits of neurosurgical resection of a dominant lesion in patients with a large number of BMs remain unclear. Laser interstitial thermal therapy is an option for patients with recurrent BMs after prior stereotactic radiation or for radiation necrosis, although further studies are needed to evaluate the risks and benefits of this technique and compare with more conventional treatment options.

Radiation Therapy

Radiation therapy is the mainstay of management for most patients with BMs (**Fig. 1**). Although patients with systemic options for intracranial control may be able to defer radiation therapy, such therapies often fail intracranially before extracranially and salvage brain-directed radiation is often used in such scenarios. As mentioned elsewhere in this article, most patients who undergo resection likely benefit from adjuvant radiation therapy to minimize recurrence in or near the cavity.

Whole brain radiation

For most patients with many BMs, WBRT, in which the entirety of the brain is treated with radiation, remains the standard treatment option. This treatment is generally delivered in 5 to 15 daily treatments given on weekdays over 1 to 3 weeks. Typical

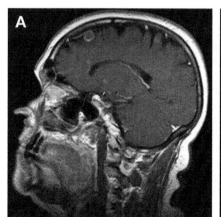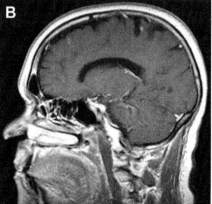

Fig. 1. A 54-year-old woman with metastatic human epidermal growth factor receptor 2+ breast cancer develops slurred speech and difficulty walking. Brain MRI reveals more than 10 brain metastases, some with cystic components (A). She was treated with whole brain radiation to 30 Gy, followed by the human epidermal growth factor receptor 2 inhibitor lapatinib combined with the antimetabolite capecitabine for management of her systemic disease. Repeat brain MRI 6 months later demonstrates partial response to treatment (B).

doses are 20 Gy in 5 fractions, 30 Gy in 10 fractions, 30 Gy in 12 fractions, 35 Gy in 14 fractions, or 37.5 Gy in 15 fractions. There is no consensus as to which regimen is optimal and practice patterns vary widely. Longer courses of WBRT typically used a smaller radiation dose per day. WBRT can be associated with significant fatigue, neurocognitive changes, and other short- and long-term toxicities that can significantly impair quality of life.[18,19] To minimize the long-term side effects of WBRT, a number of approaches have been used. Brown and colleagues[20] published a randomized study of memantine (an N-methyl-D-aspartate receptor antagonist approved for use in moderate to severe Alzheimer's disease) versus placebo in patients receiving WBRT for BMs; memantine generally reduced the likelihood of any cognitive decline in this population. Donepezil (an anticholinergic approved for use in mild to moderate Alzheimer's disease) has also shown promising but not definitive results in patients receiving a multitude of forms of brain-directed radiation for several indications.[21,22] Given the data for memantine and that the study validating its use was conducted in patients receiving WBRT, most providers have used memantine over donepezil for maintenance of cognitive function in patients receiving WBRT.

The hippocampus is integral to learning and memory. Given this fact, excluding the hippocampi from the radiation targets in patients receiving WBRT has theoretic appeal. Gondi and colleagues[23] tested the potential benefits of hippocampal sparing WBRT in patients with BMs by conducting a single arm, phase II trial of hippocampal sparing WBRT therapy in patients with BMs (Radiation Therapy Oncology Group [RTOG] 0933) who did not have metastases near the hippocampi. The authors found lower rates of decline in recall when hippocampal-sparing WBRT was used, relative to historical controls treated with conventional WBRT. The risk of disease progression in the hippocampi was found to be low. Although appealing, there was concern that the historical controls were different than the patients in RTOG 0933 (eg, different median survivals) and, as a result, hippocampal sparing WBRT has not been established as superior to traditional WBRT. In addition, because cognition, including memory, is not solely reliant on the hippocampi, it is unclear how much cognition will be spared by this approach. Ongoing randomized studies are comparing conventional WBRT and hippocampal-sparing WBRT.

Although radiation therapy is commonly used to manage BMs, caution should be exerted not to overuse this approach. The Quality of Life after Treatment for Brain Metastases (QUARTZ) study illustrates the potential detriment of using WBRT in patients with a limited prognosis.[24] This multicenter study randomized 538 patients with NSCLC and BMs to WBRT versus supportive care if they were "unsuitable for either surgery or stereotactic radiotherapy" between 2007 and 2014 in 72 centers in the United Kingdom and Australia. The authors found little benefit to radiation in this setting. However, the fact that the median survival among the entire cohort was only 2 months and that approximately 10% of patients assigned to WBRT either died before receiving WBRT or declined to the point that WBRT could no longer be given suggests that only patients with the poorest of prognoses were enrolled on this study. In addition, most patients had 4 or fewer intracranial lesions; recently published randomized trials[18,19,25,26] indicate that there are few situations where patients with 4 or fewer BMs should be treated with WBRT as opposed to stereotactic radiation. Therefore, if this study enrollment would have started in modern day (2018), it seems that few patients would have met the eligibility criteria. In addition, despite the patient-selection issues noted elsewhere in this article, patients less than 70 years of age and those with a Karnofsky performance status 70 or lower (capable of self-care), as well as those with controlled systemic disease displayed a trend to improved survival with WBRT. Ultimately, the QUARTZ trial shows that, among patients with very limited expected survival, WBRT provides no survival benefit (especially if survival if limited owing to systemic and not intracranial disease), and ultimately the QUARTZ study validates the practice pattern of withholding WBRT in patients that will not live long enough to derive benefit from intracranial control.

Stereotactic radiation

Stereotactic radiation, in which a high dose of radiation is focused on the specific lesion(s) to be treated over 1 to 5 fractions, with minimal dose to the surrounding brain, is an approach frequently used in patients with 1 to 4 BMs. Stereotactic radiation can be delivered in 2 forms: stereotactic radiosurgery (stereotactic radiosurgery, which uses a single highly-targeted dose of radiation) and stereotactic radiotherapy (consisting of multiple smaller doses [fractions] of highly targeted radiation). Doses used for stereotactic radiation have generally been guided by RTOG 9005, a dose escalation study of stereotactic radiation doses administered to patients who had been treated with prior brain-directed radiation for primary or secondary brain tumors.[27] Many modalities for stereotactic radiosurgery/stereotactic radiotherapy exist, including volumetric-modulated arc therapy, Gamma Knife, and CyberKnife, but definitive evidence establishing the superiority of one technique over another is lacking. Stereotactic radiation may carry a more modest acute toxicity profile, but does not treat subclinical disease elsewhere in the brain. In addition, the high doses of radiation used when stereotactic radiation is given place patients at risk for the late effect of radiation necrosis (inflammation/injury to the region of the brain that was targeted by the radiation).[28]

The benefit of stereotactic radiation in patients with a single BM was established by RTOG 9508.[29] In this study, patients with 1 to 3 BMs were randomized to receive WBRT or WBRT followed by a stereotactic radiation boost. The study was powered to examine patients with a single BM. Although stereotactic boost did not confer a survival advantage among the whole cohort, patients with a single BM did display improved overall survival when treated with stereotactic radiation.

Comparisons of whole brain radiation therapy and stereotactic radiation

There has never been a prospective study that has compared WBRT alone versus stereotactic radiation alone as upfront management for BMs. However, several trials have compared the combination of stereotactic radiation plus WBRT versus stereotactic radiation alone.[18,25,30] In all studies, the addition of WBRT to stereotactic radiation decreased the rate of distant intracranial failure, but did not improve overall survival. In addition, the addition of WBRT was associated with a decrease in quality of life and neurocognition in more modern studies using sensitive instruments for these endpoints.[18,19,26,31] As a result, stereotactic radiation is preferred to WBRT in patients with 1 to 4 BMs, including patients who underwent surgical resection for a BM.[19,26,31] Although a small Polish study has suggested that quality of life scores may be improved with adjuvant WBRT versus adjuvant stereotactic radiation after resection of a single BM, the majority of the trials favor omission of WBRT in such a scenario.[31–33] Combinations of WBRT and stereotactic radiation are generally not favored as upfront therapy given the toxicity of this approach, although the trials supporting the use of stereotactic radiation generally incorporated such radiation as a boost to WBRT.

Stereotactic radiation in patients with more than 4 BMs

The use of stereotactic approaches for patients with more than 4 BMs has not been tested in a randomized controlled trial. Among patients with a very limited number of BMs, the risk of distant intracranial failure seems to increase as the number of BMs increases, leading to the need for closer surveillance and more salvage radiotherapeutic treatment when stereotactic treatment is used as initial management. More recent data, however, suggest that the rates of distant intracranial failure do not seem to be closely associated with the number of BMs present in patients with more than one lesion.[34] In addition, a nonrandomized but prospective Japanese study by Yamamoto and colleagues[35] of stereotactic radiation in patients with 5 or more BMs illustrate the potential viability and safety of stereotactic approaches for patients with large numbers of BMs, finding no difference in overall survival, deterioration of neurologic function, local recurrence, new lesions, use of salvage radiation or surgery, or use of systemic anticancer agents between patients with 2 to 4 or 5 to 10 BMs; the Yamamoto and colleagues study is limited, however, by the fact that patients could only be enrolled if the total tumor volume was less than or equal to 15 mL, which disproportionately renders patients with 2 to 4 BMs more eligible for inclusion, even with larger tumors. In addition, the authors anticipated a 1:1 enrollment ratio between patients with 2 to 4 and 5 to 10 brain tumors, respectively. The final cohort had greater than 2:1 enrollment ratio between these respective groups, possibly suggesting that only select (favorable) patients with 5 to 10 brain tumors were enrolled on this study. Randomized studies of stereotactic radiation versus WBRT are desperately needed. One such ongoing study at Brigham and Women's Hospital/Dana-Farber Cancer Institute is actively enrolling patients (NCT03075072).

Cranial irradiation in patients with small cell lung cancer
BMs are common in patients with SCLC. Autopsy series have suggested that approximately 80% of patients with SCLC will develop BMs.[36] Chemotherapy regimens used in SCLC achieve unreliable penetration into the brain and as a result prophylactic cranial irradiation, in which the entire brain is radiated preventatively, improves survival, and remains the standard of care in patients with limited stage SCLC who respond to chemotherapy.[37] In patients with extensive stage SCLC, prophylactic cranial irradiation is also sometimes used, but remains controversial given the greater risk of death owing to extracranial progression.[38,39]

Given the studies supporting the role of prophylactic cranial irradiation, the historic standard approach to patients with SCLC who have BMs, regardless of the number of BMs present, has entailed WBRT. Patients with SCLC were excluded from nearly all studies evaluating the role of stereotactic radiation as monotherapy.[18,25,26,30,40] However, recent studies have questioned whether patients with SCLC and a limited number of BMs can be managed with stereotactic radiation in lieu of WBRT given the improved quality of life and neurocognitive function seen with stereotactic approaches in patients with other primaries.[18,25,26,30,40,41] A recent prospective study involving stereotactic radiation for up to 10 BMs included patients with SCLC for this reason.[35] In addition, multiple retrospective studies have shown that stereotactic radiation in patients with SCLC who have never received prophylactic cranial radiation could be a reasonable option for patients,[42,43] and the role of prophylactic cranial irradiation in patients with extensive stage SCLC has become increasingly questioned.[39] As a result, dedicated prospective studies of stereotactic radiation in the management of patients with SCLC and a limited number of BMs are warranted.

SYSTEMIC THERAPY

Most systemic agents poorly control BMs given their limited penetration across the blood–brain barrier and/or efflux pumps that actively remove these agents from the brain.[1] Indeed, it is not uncommon to see patients with controlled or absent systemic disease who relapse in the CNS on therapy owing to poor penetration of the blood–brain barrier; examples include trastuzumab in HER2-positive breast cancer[44] and crizotinib in ALK-positive NSCLC.[45] Historically, clinical trials of systemic agents excluded patients with BM, partly owing to the misperception that patients with BM make poor clinical trial candidates,[46,47] and thus data on CNS benefit are often generated late in drug development or never at all.[48] However, data from phase I studies suggest that carefully selected patients with BM with good performance status can be safely enrolled in clinical trials without a risk to the patient or damage to the trial.[49] Indeed, perspective papers from the US Food and Drug Administration (FDA) advocate increasing the inclusion of patients with BM in trials of systemic therapy.[50]

Fortunately, interest is increasing in developing systemic therapies with CNS penetration that can treat or prevent intracranial disease as well as treat systemic disease.[51,52] This interest is bolstered by recent trials of systemic therapies with promising CNS as well as systemic benefit (**Fig. 2**, see **Table 2**). More thorough discussions of systemic agents for management of BMs can be found elsewhere.[53–55] The history of ALK inhibitors (targeting ALK rearrangements seen in 2%–7% of NSCLC[56]) exemplifies the importance of developing drugs with intracranial benefit. The brain is the most common site of recurrence in NSCLC patients treated with crizotinib (the first kinase inhibitor approved for the treatment of ALK-positive metastatic NSCLC). Among patients without BM at the time of enrollment on crizotinib trials, 20% developed BMs on study.[45] Alectinib, a next-generation ALK inhibitor, received FDA breakthrough therapy designation in 2013 based on preliminary evidence of clinical activity in patients with metastatic ALK-positive NSCLC previously treated with crizotinib, including activity in CNS metastases.[57] Recently reported results from the randomized, phase III trial comparing alectinib with crizotinib for previously untreated, advanced ALK-positive NSCLC, including those with asymptomatic CNS disease, confirmed alectinib's CNS benefit over crizotinib without compromising extracranial benefit.[58] The time to CNS progression was significantly longer with alectinib than with crizotinib (cause-specific hazard ratio, 0.16; 95% confidence interval, 0.10–0.28; rate of events of CNS progression, 12% with alectinib and 45% with crizotinib).

Other agents with FDA orphan drug or breakthrough therapy designation for BMs include tucatinib[59] (for BM from HER2-positive breast cancer) and ceritinib (for BM

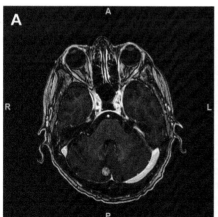
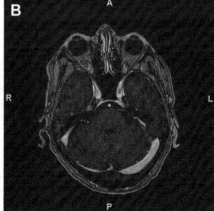

Fig. 2. (*A*) A solitary enhancing brain metastasis in a 63-year-old woman with metastatic non-small cell lung cancer harboring an anaplastic lymphoma kinase (ALK) rearrangement progressed despite treatment with stereotactic radiation. (*B*) Repeat brain MRI 3 months after treatment with the brain-penetrant ALK inhibitor alectinib reveals a partial response to treatment.

from ALK-positive NSCLC).[60] Tucatinib is not currently FDA approved and is only available in clinical trials. From the phase Ib combination study of tucatinib plus capecitabine and/or trastuzumab, CNS responses were reported in patients with BM from HER2+ breast cancer.[61] The ongoing randomized, double-blind, placebo-controlled HER2CLIMB clinical trial comparing capecitabine and trastuzumab with or without tucatinib in patents with locally advanced or metastatic HER2+ breast cancer is enrolling patients with any type of BM (untreated, previously treated but stable, or progressive BM) (NCT02614794).[62]

Choosing Systemic Therapy over Radiation Therapy

No systemic therapy is FDA approved specifically for BMs and only select agents have sufficient data to even support their use in patients with BM. These include the next-generation ALK inhibitors in ALK-positive metastatic NSCLC, BRAF tyrosine kinase inhibitors in BRAF-mutant metastatic melanoma, checkpoint inhibitors in melanoma, and HER2 tyrosine kinase inhibitors in HER2-positive metastatic breast cancer (**Table 3**). In addition, most patients with BMs do not harbor a cancer or mutation that permits the use of one of these select agents. Therefore, local therapy such as surgery and radiation therapy remains the mainstay of management for the majority of patients with BMs. For patients who are candidates for one of these few systemic therapies with demonstrated CNS benefit, whether to pursue upfront brain-directed radiation or systemic therapy remains unclear. Avoiding radiation has the benefit of sparing some patients the adverse effects associated with radiation therapy, whereas using upfront radiation addresses the concern that systemic therapies often fail intracranially before extracranially. Some oncologists consider a trial of systemic therapy first in patients with asymptomatic or minimally symptomatic BMs or in patients whose extracranial disease is significantly more symptomatic than intracranial disease.

Combining Radiation and Systemic Therapy

No clinical trial to date has definitively proven benefit to combining radiation with systemic agents for management of BMs.[51] In addition, some systemic therapies are discontinued during radiation therapy owing to concerns for safety.[63] Nonetheless, interests remains in combining radiation and systemic therapy.

Magnuson and colleagues[64] conducted a multiinstitutional retrospective study of patients with EGFR mutated NSCLC and BMs, and compared overall survival in patients managed with an EGFR-targeting agent alone, stereotactic radiation followed by an EGFR-targeting agent alone, or WBRT followed by an EGFR-targeting agent alone. Overall survival was found to be longest in patients managed with stereotactic radiation and an EGFR-targeting agent alone, suggesting that definitive local therapy may improve outcomes in patients managed with systemic therapy for intracranial metastases. Further evaluation of this association in a randomized trial seems warranted.

The role of brain-directed radiation in patients with BMs who receive immunotherapy also warrants mention. The efficacy of immunotherapy as monotherapy for intracranial control seems limited[65]; in a prospective study from Yale, Goldberg and colleagues[68] found that the intracranial response rate in patients with BMs secondary to NSCLC (PD-L1 positive) and melanoma were 33% and 22%, respectively, although the combination of ipilimumab plus nivolumab in melanoma may be more promising.[64,66] In addition, combining immunotherapy and radiation may improve overall locoregional control and generate abscopal responses (where localized radiation can trigger systemic antitumor effects), potentially yielding better intracranial control rates than immunotherapy alone or stereotactic radiation therapy alone.[69-73]

Table 3
Recently reported clinical trials of systemic therapies enrolling patients with brain metastases from solid tumors

Primary Disease	Subtype (if Applicable)	Agent(s)	Class of Agent	Trial Design	Outcomes
Breast cancer	HER2+	Lapatinib + capecitabine	HER2 TKI + inhibitor of thymidine monophosphate (required for the de novo synthesis of DNA)	Multiple phase II trials in patient with BM from HER2+ metastatic breast cancer.[55]	Greater activity seen with lapatinib + capecitabine than lapatinib alone. CNS response rates for combination therapy range from 18% to 38% in pretreated patients, and a CNS response rate of 66% in the newly diagnosed setting.
		Trastuzumab emtansine (T-DM1)	Antibody-drug conjugate incorporating HER2-targeted antitumor properties of trastuzumab with the cytotoxic activity of the microtubu7le-inhibitor agent DM1	Retrospective, exploratory analysis to characterize the incidence of CNS metastases after treatment with trastuzumab emtansine (T-DM1) vs capecitabine + lapatinib (XL), among patients with preexisting stable CNS metastases in the phase III EMILIA study.[75]	CNS progression occurred in 9 of 450 (2.0%) and 3 of 446 (0.7%) patients without CNS metastases at baseline in the T-DM1 and XL arms, respectively, and in 10 of 45 (22.2%) and 8 of 50 (16.0%) patients with CNS metastases at baseline.
		Tucantinib (ONT-380)	HER2 TKI	Phase Ib study of tucatinib (ONT-380) + T-DM1 in HER2+ metastatic breast cancer. Allowed patients with previously treated CNS lesions (stable or progressive) or untreated asymptomatic CNS lesions.[61]	Preliminary data – 26 patients with CNS metastases enrolled, most with progressive or untreated CNS metastases. In evaluable patients, intracranial response seen in 4 of 12. PFS in patients with BM similar to patients without BM. No patients without BM at baseline developed new clinically apparent BM while on study.
		Pertuzumab + high-dose trastuzumab	Monoclonal antibody against HER2 dimerization + monoclonal antibody against HER2	Phase II study of pertuzumab with high-dose trastuzumab for CNS progression after radiation in patients with HER2+ metastatic breast cancer.[76]	Planned interim analysis of 15 patients – intracranial response seen in 4 of 15 patients (26.7%) and median duration of response was 5.6 mo.

(continued on next page)

Table 3
(continued)

Primary Disease	Subtype (if Applicable)	Agent(s)	Class of Agent	Trial Design	Outcomes
Lung cancer	ALK rearranged NSCLC	Alectinib	Next-generation ALK TKI	Phase I trial of ALK-rearranged NSCLC who progressed/intolerant to crizotinib. Allowed patients with asymptomatic CNS metastases including leptomeningeal metastases, although only 12 of 21 (57%) had progressing CNS metastases at enrollment.[77]	Intracranial responses in 11 of 21 patients (52%). Of the 4 patients who had not had brain radiotherapy, 2 achieved CR, 1 PR, and 1 SD. Measurable concentrations of alectinib noted in CSF samples of the 5 patients in whom paired steady-state and plasma samples were obtained.
				Randomized, phase III trial comparing alectinib vs crizotinib in previously untreated patients with advanced ALK-positive NSCLC. Allowed patients with asymptomatic CNS metastases.[58]	Time to CNS progression was significantly longer with alectinib than with crizotinib (cause-specific hazard ratio, 0.16; 95% CI, 0.10–0.28; rate of events of CNS progression, 12% with alectinib and 45% with crizotinib).
		Brigatinib	Next-generation ALK TKI	Phase II trial of brigatinib in crizotinib-refractory ALK-positive NSCLC. Patients were stratified by BM and randomized to a 90 mg daily dose vs a 180 mg daily dose.[78]	In patients with measurable BMs at baseline, intracranial response seen in 11 of 26 patients (42%) in the 90 mg arm and 12 of 18 patients (67%) in the 180 mg arm. Median intracranial duration of response was not estimable in the 90 mg arm and was 5.6 mo in the 180 mg arm. Among patients who exhibited an intracranial response, 78% of patients in the 90 mg arm and 68% of patients in the 180 mg arm maintained an intracranial response for ≥4 mo.

Category	Drug	Type/Mechanism	Trial	Results
	Ceritinib	Next-generation ALK TKI	Randomized, phase III trial comparing ceritinib vs chemotherapy (pemetrexed or decetaxel by investigator choice) in crizotinib-refractory ALK-positive NSCLC. Patients were stratified by BM.[79]	Among patients with untreated or progressing and measurable BMs selected as active target lesions, intracranial responses seen in 6 of 17 patients (35%) in the certinib arm vs 1 of 20 (5%) in the chemotherapy group.
	Lorlatinib	Next-generation ALK/ROS1 TKI	Phase I/II stud of lorlatinib for ALK-positive or ROS1-positive advanced NSCLC who were treatment naïve or had disease progression after ≥1TKI. Allowed patients with asymptomatic BM, treated or untreated.[80]	Preliminary results – Intracranial response in 18 of 35 patients based on target lesions only ($\geq$5 mm; no prior radiotherapy or progression post prior radiotherapy). Of the 35 patients, 24 had received prior brain radiotherapy and prior ALK TKI therapy.
EGFR-mutant NSCLC	Osimertinib	Irreversible EGFR TKI selective for mutant EGFR and T790M resistance mutations	Randomized, phase III trial comparing osimertinib vs platinum-based doublet chemotherapy in patients with T790M-positive advanced NSCLC who progressed after EGFR-TKI therapy. Patients with asymptomatic, stable BMs allowed to enroll.[81]	In patients with CNS disease who did not have radiotherapy or had radiotherapy $\geq$6 mo before enrollment, CNS ORR was 34% (95% CI, 23–48) for patients assigned to osimertinib (n = 61) vs 16% (95% CI, 5–33) for those assigned to chemotherapy (n = 32).
NSCLC positive for PD-L1 expression	Pembrolizumab	Monoclonal antibody against PD1 (checkpoint inhibitor)	Phase II trial of pembrolizumab in patients with $\geq$1 untreated or progression, asymptomatic BM from NSCLC with tumor tissue positive for PD-L1 expression.[68]	Durable intracranial responses in 6 of 18 patients.
Melanoma	Pembrolizumab	Monoclonal antibody against PD1 (checkpoint inhibitor)	Phase II trial of pembrolizumab in patients with $\geq$1 untreated or progression, asymptomatic BM from melanoma.[68]	Durable intracranial responses in 4 of 18 patients.

(continued on next page)

Table 3
(continued)

Primary Disease	Subtype (if Applicable)	Agent(s)	Class of Agent	Trial Design	Outcomes
		Ipilimumab	Monoclonal antibody against CTLA-4 (a protein receptor that downregulate the immune system)	Phase II trial of ipilimumab in patients with melanoma BM. Cohort A enrolled neurologically asymptomatic patients who were off steroids. Cohort B enrolled neurologically symptomatic on stable dose of steroids.[82]	Stable disease achieved in 12 patients (24%) in cohort A and 2 patients (10%) in cohort B achieved disease control.
		Nivolumab ± ipilimumab	Monoclonal antibodies against PD1 + CTLA-4	Phase II trial of nivolumab with or without ipilimumab in patients with melanoma BM. Cohorts A and B enrolled patients who were asymptomatic and had received no previous local brain therapy. Cohort C enrolled patients with progressive BM after previous local brain therapy or who were symptomatic or with leptomeningeal disease.[67]	Preliminary results – intracranial responses seen in 42% in cohort A with nivolumab + ipilimumab, 20% in cohort B with nivolumab, 6% in cohort C with nivolumab).
	BRAFV600-mutant melanoma	Dabrafenib	BRAF TKI	Phase II trial of dabrafenib in patients with BM from Val600Glu or Val600Lys BRAF-mutant melanoma. Cohort A enrolled patients with no prior local brain therapy. Cohort B enrolled patients with progressive BMs despite prior local brain therapy.[83]	Intracranial responses seen in 29 of 74 patients (39.2%) in cohort A and 20 of 80 patients (22.2%) in cohort B.

Dabrafenib + trametinib	BRAF TKI + MEK TKI	Phase II trial of dabrafenib + trametinib in patients with BM from BRAFV600-mutant melanoma. Cohort A enrolled patients with BRAFV600E, asymptomatic, and previously untreated BM. Cohort B enrolled BRAFV600E, asymptomatic, and progressive BM despite prior local brain therapy. Cohort C enrolled BRAFV600D/K/R, asymptomatic, with or without prior local brain therapy. Cohort D enrolled BRAFV600D/E/D/R, symptomatic, with or without prior local brain therapy.[84]	Intracranial responses seen in 44 of 76 patients (58%) in cohort A, 9 of 16 patients (56%) in cohort B, 7 of 16 (44%; 20–70) in cohort C, and 10 of 17 in cohort D (59%).
Vemurafenib	BRAF TKI	Phase II trial of vemurafenib in patients with BM from BRAFV600-mutant melanoma. Cohort 1 enrolled patients with untreated BM. Cohort 2 enrolled patients with progressive BM despite prior treatment.[85]	Intracranial responses seen in 33% in cohort 1% and 23% in cohort 2.

Abbreviations: ALK, anaplastic lymphoma kinase; BM, brain metastases; CFS, cerebrospinal fluid; CI, confidence interval; CNS, central nervous system; CR, complete response; EGFR, epidermal growth factor receptor; HER2, human epidermal growth factor receptor 2; NSCLC, non-small cell lung cancer; ORR, overall response rate; PFS, progression-free survival; PR, partial response; SD, stable disease; T-DM1, trastuzumab emtansine; TKI, tyrosine kinase inhibitor.

Randomized studies of immunotherapy alone versus immunotherapy plus radiation in the management of patients with BMs seem warranted.

As mentioned, the CNS is a common site of relapse for select targeted agents. In patients whose systemic disease is sufficiently controlled such that the preference is to remain on the targeted agent, patients can be treated with CNS-directed radiotherapy while continuing systemic therapy.[74]

SUMMARY

The brain is a sanctuary site, a common site of relapse, in many patients with cancer owing to the limited ability of most systemic agents to penetrate the blood–brain barrier and remain in the brain. Despite the grim prognosis historically associated with BMs, select patients with BMs are living longer than expected owing to advances in radiation therapy as well as the increasing number of systemic therapies with better CNS penetration. Although overall survival remains an important outcome, studies in radiation oncology are increasingly focused on quality of life and preserving neurocognitive function.

REFERENCES

1. Stewart DJ. A critique of the role of the blood-brain barrier in the chemotherapy of human brain tumors. J Neurooncol 1994;20(2):121–39.
2. Sperduto PW, Kased N, Roberge D, et al. Summary report on the graded prognostic assessment: an accurate and facile diagnosis-specific tool to estimate survival for patients with brain metastases. J Clin Oncol 2012;30(4):419–25.
3. Sperduto PW, Yang TJ, Beal K, et al. Estimating survival in patients with lung cancer and brain metastases: an update of the graded prognostic assessment for lung cancer using molecular markers (lung-molGPA). JAMA Oncol 2017;3(6): 827–31.
4. Nayak L, Lee EQ, Wen PY. Epidemiology of brain metastases. Curr Oncol Rep 2012;14(1):48–54.
5. Barnholtz-Sloan JS, Sloan AE, Davis FG, et al. Incidence proportions of brain metastases in patients diagnosed (1973 to 2001) in the Metropolitan Detroit Cancer Surveillance System. J Clin Oncol 2004;22(14):2865–72.
6. Cagney DN, Martin AM, Catalano PJ, et al. Incidence and prognosis of patients with brain metastases at diagnosis of systemic malignancy: a population-based study. Neuro Oncol 2017;19(11):1511–21.
7. Martin AM, Cagney DN, Catalano PJ, et al. Brain metastases in newly diagnosed breast cancer: a population-based study. JAMA Oncol 2017;3(8):1069–77.
8. Iuchi T, Shingyoji M, Itakura M, et al. Frequency of brain metastases in non-small-cell lung cancer, and their association with epidermal growth factor receptor mutations. Int J Clin Oncol 2015;20(4):674–9.
9. Jakob JA, Bassett RL Jr, Ng CS, et al. NRAS mutation status is an independent prognostic factor in metastatic melanoma. Cancer 2012;118(16):4014–23.
10. Steeg PS. Targeting metastasis. Nat Rev Cancer 2016;16(4):201–18.
11. Fidler IJ. The biology of brain metastasis: challenges for therapy. Cancer J 2015; 21(4):284–93.
12. Massagué J, Obenauf AC. Metastatic colonization. Nature 2016;529(7586): 298–306.
13. Oskarsson T, Batlle E, Massague J. Metastatic stem cells: sources, niches, and vital pathways. Cell Stem Cell 2014;14(3):306–21.

14. Brastianos PK, Carter SL, Santagata S, et al. Genomic characterization of brain metastases reveals branched evolution and potential therapeutic targets. Cancer Discov 2015;5(11):1164–77.

15. Patchell RA, Tibbs PA, Walsh JW, et al. A randomized trial of surgery in the treatment of single metastases to the brain. N Engl J Med 1990;322(8):494–500.

16. Vecht CJ, Haaxma-Reiche H, Noordijk EM, et al. Treatment of single brain metastasis: radiotherapy alone or combined with neurosurgery? Ann Neurol 1993;33: 583–90.

17. Mintz AH, Kestle J, Rathbone MP, et al. A randomized trial to assess the efficacy of surgery in addition to radiotherapy in patients with a single cerebral metastasis. Cancer 1996;78(7):1470–6.

18. Chang EL, Wefel JS, Hess KR, et al. Neurocognition in patients with brain metastases treated with radiosurgery or radiosurgery plus whole-brain irradiation: a randomised controlled trial. Lancet Oncol 2009;10(11):1037–44.

19. Soffietti R, Kocher M, Abacioglu UM, et al. A European Organisation for Research and Treatment of Cancer phase III trial of adjuvant whole-brain radiotherapy versus observation in patients with one to three brain metastases from solid tumors after surgical resection or radiosurgery: quality-of-life results. J Clin Oncol 2013;31(1):65–72.

20. Brown PD, Pugh S, Laack NN, et al. Memantine for the prevention of cognitive dysfunction in patients receiving whole-brain radiotherapy: a randomized, double-blind, placebo-controlled trial. Neuro Oncol 2013;15(10):1429–37.

21. Rapp SR, Case LD, Peiffer A, et al. Donepezil for irradiated brain tumor survivors: a phase iii randomized placebo-controlled clinical trial. J Clin Oncol 2015;33(15): 1653–9.

22. Shaw EG, Rosdhal R, D'Agostino RB Jr, et al. Phase II study of donepezil in irradiated brain tumor patients: effect on cognitive function, mood, and quality of life. J Clin Oncol 2006;24(9):1415–20.

23. Gondi V, Pugh SL, Tome WA, et al. Preservation of memory with conformal avoidance of the hippocampal neural stem-cell compartment during whole-brain radiotherapy for brain metastases (RTOG 0933): a phase II multi-institutional trial. J Clin Oncol 2014;32(34):3810–6.

24. Mulvenna P, Nankivell M, Barton R, et al. Dexamethasone and supportive care with or without whole brain radiotherapy in treating patients with non-small cell lung cancer with brain metastases unsuitable for resection or stereotactic radiotherapy (QUARTZ): results from a phase 3, non-inferiority, randomised trial. Lancet 2016;388(10055):2004–14.

25. Aoyama H, Shirato H, Tago M, et al. Stereotactic radiosurgery plus whole-brain radiation therapy vs stereotactic radiosurgery alone for treatment of brain metastases: a randomized controlled trial. JAMA 2006;295(21):2483–91.

26. Brown PD, Jaeckle K, Ballman KV, et al. Effect of radiosurgery alone vs radiosurgery with whole brain radiation therapy on cognitive function in patients with 1 to 3 brain metastases: a randomized clinical trial. JAMA 2016;316(4):401–9.

27. Shaw E, Scott C, Souhami L, et al. Single dose radiosurgical treatment of recurrent previously irradiated primary brain tumors and brain metastases: final report of RTOG protocol 90-05. Int J Radiat Oncol Biol Phys 2000;47(2):291–8.

28. Blonigen BJ, Steinmetz RD, Levin L, et al. Irradiated volume as a predictor of brain radionecrosis after linear accelerator stereotactic radiosurgery. Int J Radiat Oncol Biol Phys 2010;77(4):996–1001.

29. Andrews DW, Scott CB, Sperduto PW, et al. Whole brain radiation therapy with or without stereotactic radiosurgery boost for patients with one to three brain

metastases: phase III results of the RTOG 9508 randomised trial. Lancet 2004; 363(9422):1665–72.

30. Kocher M, Soffietti R, Abacioglu U, et al. Adjuvant whole-brain radiotherapy versus observation after radiosurgery or surgical resection of one to three cerebral metastases: results of the EORTC 22952-26001 study. J Clin Oncol 2011;29(2):134–41.

31. Brown PD, Ballman KV, Cerhan JH, et al. Postoperative stereotactic radiosurgery compared with whole brain radiotherapy for resected metastatic brain disease (NCCTG N107C/CEC.3): a multicentre, randomised, controlled, phase 3 trial. Lancet Oncol 2017;18(8):1049–60.

32. Mahajan A, Ahmed S, McAleer MF, et al. Post-operative stereotactic radiosurgery versus observation for completely resected brain metastases: a single-centre, randomised, controlled, phase 3 trial. Lancet Oncol 2017;18(8):1040–8.

33. Kepka L, Tyc-Szczepaniak D, Osowiecka K, et al. Quality of life after whole brain radiotherapy compared with radiosurgery of the tumor bed: results from a randomized trial. Clin Transl Oncol 2018;20(2):150–9.

34. Yamamoto M, Kawabe T, Sato Y, et al. Stereotactic radiosurgery for patients with multiple brain metastases: a case-matched study comparing treatment results for patients with 2-9 versus 10 or more tumors. J Neurosurg 2014;121(Suppl):16–25.

35. Yamamoto M, Serizawa T, Shuto T, et al. Stereotactic radiosurgery for patients with multiple brain metastases (JLGK0901): a multi-institutional prospective observational study. Lancet Oncol 2014;15(4):387–95.

36. Nugent JL, Bunn PA Jr, Matthews MJ, et al. CNS metastases in small cell bronchogenic carcinoma: increasing frequency and changing pattern with lengthening survival. Cancer 1979;44(5):1885–93.

37. Auperin A, Arriagada R, Pignon JP, et al. Prophylactic cranial irradiation for patients with small-cell lung cancer in complete remission. Prophylactic Cranial Irradiation Overview Collaborative Group. N Engl J Med 1999;341(7):476–84.

38. Slotman B, Faivre-Finn C, Kramer G, et al. Prophylactic cranial irradiation in extensive small-cell lung cancer. N Engl J Med 2007;357(7):664–72.

39. Takahashi T, Yamanaka T, Seto T, et al. Prophylactic cranial irradiation versus observation in patients with extensive-disease small-cell lung cancer: a multicentre, randomised, open-label, phase 3 trial. Lancet Oncol 2017;18(5):663–71.

40. Kayama T, Sato S, Sakurada K, et al. JCOG0504: a phase III randomized trial of surgery with whole brain radiation therapy versus surgery with salvage stereotactic radiosurgery in patients with 1 to 4 brain metastases. J Clin Oncol 2016; 34(suppl) [abstract: 2003].

41. Patchell RA, Tibbs PA, Regine WF, et al. Postoperative radiotherapy in the treatment of single metastases to the brain: a randomized trial. JAMA 1998;280(17): 1485–9.

42. Wegner RE, Olson AC, Kondziolka D, et al. Stereotactic radiosurgery for patients with brain metastases from small cell lung cancer. Int J Radiat Oncol Biol Phys 2011;81(3):e21–7.

43. Yomo S, Hayashi M. Upfront stereotactic radiosurgery in patients with brain metastases from small cell lung cancer: retrospective analysis of 41 patients. Radiat Oncol 2014;9:152.

44. Bendell JC, Domchek SM, Burstein HJ, et al. Central nervous system metastases in women who receive trastuzumab-based therapy for metastatic breast carcinoma. Cancer 2003;97(12):2972–7.

45. Costa DB, Shaw AT, Ou SH, et al. Clinical experience with crizotinib in patients with advanced ALK-rearranged non-small-cell lung cancer and brain metastases. J Clin Oncol 2015;33(17):1881–8.

46. McCoach CE, Berge EM, Lu X, et al. A brief report of the status of central nervous system metastasis enrollment criteria for advanced non-small cell lung cancer clinical trials: a review of the ClinicalTrials.gov trial registry. J Thorac Oncol 2016;11(3):407–13.
47. Costa R, Gill N, Rademaker AW, et al. Systematic analysis of early phase clinical studies for patients with breast cancer: inclusion of patients with brain metastasis. Cancer Treat Rev 2017;55:10–5.
48. Camidge DR, Lee EQ, Lin NU, et al. Addressing brain metastases from solid tumours within clinical trial designs for systemic agents: a guideline by the Response Assessment in Neuro-Oncology Brain Metastases (RANO-BM) Working Group. Lancet Oncol 2018;19(1):e20–32.
49. Tsimberidou AM, Letourneau K, Wen S, et al. Phase I clinical trial outcomes in 93 patients with brain metastases: the MD Anderson Cancer Center experience. Clin Cancer Res 2011;17(12):4110–8.
50. Beaver JA, Ison G, Pazdur R. Reevaluating eligibility criteria - balancing patient protection and participation in oncology trials. N Engl J Med 2017;376(16): 1504–5.
51. Arvold ND, Lee EQ, Mehta MP, et al. Updates in the management of brain metastases. Neuro Oncol 2016;18(8):1043–65.
52. Chamberlain MC, Baik CS, Gadi VK, et al. Systemic therapy of brain metastases: non-small cell lung cancer, breast cancer, and melanoma. Neuro Oncol 2017; 19(1):i1–24.
53. Shonka N, Venur VA, Ahluwalia MS. Targeted treatment of brain metastases. Curr Neurol Neurosci Rep 2017;17(4):37.
54. Ajithkumar T, Parkinson C, Fife K, et al. Evolving treatment options for melanoma brain metastases. Lancet Oncol 2015;16(13):e486–97.
55. Lin NU, Gaspar LE, Soffietti R. Breast cancer in the central nervous system: multidisciplinary considerations and management. Am Soc Clin Oncol Educ Book 2017;37:45–56.
56. Fan L, Feng Y, Wan H, et al. Clinicopathological and demographical characteristics of non-small cell lung cancer patients with ALK rearrangements: a systematic review and meta-analysis. PLoS One 2014;9(6):e100866.
57. Larkins E, Blumenthal GM, Chen H, et al. FDA approval: alectinib for the treatment of metastatic, ALK-positive non-small cell lung cancer following crizotinib. Clin Cancer Res 2016;22(21):5171–6.
58. Peters S, Camidge DR, Shaw AT, et al. Alectinib versus crizotinib in untreated ALK-positive non-small-cell lung cancer. N Engl J Med 2017;377(9):829–38.
59. Cascadian therapeutics' lead candidate, Tucatinib, receives orphan drug designation from FDA for treatment of breast cancer patients with brain metastases. Seattle (WA): Cascadian Therapeutics, Inc; 2017. Available at: http://ir.cascadianrx.com/releasedetail.cfm?releaseid=1029539.
60. Novartis drug Zykadia receives FDA priority review for first-line use in patients with ALK+ metastatic NSCLC [news release]. Basel (Switzerland): Novartis; 2017. Available at: https://www.novartis.com/news/media-releases/novartis-drug-zykadia-receives-fda-priority-review-first-line-use-patients-alk [press release].
61. Borges VF, Ferrario C, Aucoin N, et al. Efficacy results of a phase 1b study of ONT-380, a CNS-penetrant TKI, in combination with T-DM1 in HER2+ metastatic breast cancer (MBC), including patients (pts) with brain metastases. J Clin Oncol 2016;34(15_suppl):513.
62. Anders CK, Murthy RK, Hamilton EP, et al. A randomized, double-blinded, controlled study of tucatinib (ONT-380) vs. placebo in combination with

capecitabine (C) and trastuzumab (Tz) in patients with pretreated HER2+ unresectable locally advanced or metastatic breast carcinoma (mBC) (HER2CLIMB). J Clin Oncol 2017;35(15_suppl):TPS1107.

63. Verduin M, Zindler JD, Martinussen HM, et al. Use of systemic therapy concurrent with cranial radiotherapy for cerebral metastases of solid tumors. Oncologist 2017;22(2):222–35.

64. Magnuson WJ, Yeung JT, Guillod PD, et al. Impact of Deferring Radiation Therapy in Patients With Epidermal Growth Factor Receptor-Mutant Non-Small Cell Lung Cancer Who Develop Brain Metastases. Int J Radiat Oncol Biol Phys 2016;95: 673–9.

65. Cohen JV, Kluger HM. Systemic immunotherapy for the treatment of brain metastases. Front Oncol 2016;6:49.

66. Tawbi HA-H, Forsyth PAJ, Algazi AP, et al. Efficacy and safety of nivolumab (NIVO) plus ipilimumab (IPI) in patients with melanoma (MEL) metastatic to the brain: results of the phase II study CheckMate 204. J Clin Oncol 2017; 35(15_suppl):9507.

67. Long GV, Atkinson V, Menzies AM, et al. A randomized phase II study of nivolumab or nivolumab combined with ipilimumab in patients (pts) with melanoma brain metastases (mets): the anti-PD1 brain collaboration (ABC). J Clin Oncol 2017;35(15_suppl):9508.

68. Goldberg SB, Gettinger SN, Mahajan A, et al. Pembrolizumab for patients with melanoma or non-small-cell lung cancer and untreated brain metastases: early analysis of a non-randomised, open-label, phase 2 trial. Lancet Oncol 2016;17(7):976–83.

69. Alomari AK, Cohen J, Vortmeyer AO, et al. Possible interaction of anti-PD-1 therapy with the effects of radiosurgery on brain metastases. Cancer Immunol Res 2016;4(6):481–7.

70. Chandra RA, Wilhite TJ, Balboni TA, et al. A systematic evaluation of abscopal responses following radiotherapy in patients with metastatic melanoma treated with ipilimumab. Oncoimmunology 2015;4(11):e1046028.

71. Grimaldi AM, Simeone E, Giannarelli D, et al. Abscopal effects of radiotherapy on advanced melanoma patients who progressed after ipilimumab immunotherapy. Oncoimmunology 2014;3:e28780.

72. Kiess AP, Wolchok JD, Barker CA, et al. Stereotactic radiosurgery for melanoma brain metastases in patients receiving ipilimumab: safety profile and efficacy of combined treatment. Int J Radiat Oncol Biol Phys 2015;92(2):368–75.

73. Qian JM, Yu JB, Kluger HM, et al. Timing and type of immune checkpoint therapy affect the early radiographic response of melanoma brain metastases to stereotactic radiosurgery. Cancer 2016;122(19):3051–8.

74. Rusthoven CG, Doebele RC. Management of brain metastases in ALK-positive non-small-cell lung cancer. J Clin Oncol 2016;34(24):2814–9.

75. Krop IE, Lin NU, Blackwell K, et al. Trastuzumab emtansine (T-DM1) versus lapatinib plus capecitabine in patients with HER2-positive metastatic breast cancer and central nervous system metastases: a retrospective, exploratory analysis in EMILIA. Ann Oncol 2015;26(1):113–9.

76. Lin NU, Stein A, Nicholas A, et al. Planned interim analysis of PATRICIA: an open-label, single-arm, phase II study of pertuzumab (P) with high-dose trastuzumab (H) for the treatment of central nervous system (CNS) progression post radiotherapy (RT) in patients (pts) with HER2-positive metastatic breast cancer (MBC). J Clin Oncol 2017;35(15_suppl):2074.

77. Gadgeel SM, Gandhi L, Riely GJ, et al. Safety and activity of alectinib against systemic disease and brain metastases in patients with crizotinib-resistant ALK-

rearranged non-small-cell lung cancer (AF-002JG): results from the dose-finding portion of a phase 1/2 study. Lancet Oncol 2014;15(10):1119–28.

78. Kim D-W, Tiseo M, Ahn M-J, et al. Brigatinib in patients with crizotinib-refractory anaplastic lymphoma kinase–positive non–small-cell lung cancer: a randomized, multicenter phase II trial. J Clin Oncol 2017;35(22):2490–8.

79. Shaw AT, Kim TM, Crino L, et al. Ceritinib versus chemotherapy in patients with ALK-rearranged non-small-cell lung cancer previously given chemotherapy and crizotinib (ASCEND-5): a randomised, controlled, open-label, phase 3 trial. Lancet Oncol 2017;18(7):874–86.

80. Shaw AT, Ou S-HI, Felip E, et al. Efficacy and safety of lorlatinib in patients (pts) with ALK+ non-small cell lung cancer (NSCLC) with one or more prior ALK tyrosine kinase inhibitor (TKI): a phase I/II study. J Clin Oncol 2017;35(15_suppl): 9006.

81. Mok T, Ahn M-J, Han J-Y, et al. CNS response to osimertinib in patients (pts) with T790M-positive advanced NSCLC: data from a randomized phase III trial (AURA3). J Clin Oncol 2017;35(15_suppl):9005.

82. Margolin K, Ernstoff MS, Hamid O, et al. Ipilimumab in patients with melanoma and brain metastases: an open-label, phase 2 trial. Lancet Oncol 2012;13(5): 459–65.

83. Long GV, Trefzer U, Davies MA, et al. Dabrafenib in patients with Val600Glu or Val600Lys BRAF-mutant melanoma metastatic to the brain (BREAK-MB): a multicentre, open-label, phase 2 trial. Lancet Oncol 2012;13(11):1087–95.

84. Davies MA, Saiag P, Robert C, et al. Dabrafenib plus trametinib in patients with BRAFV600-mutant melanoma brain metastases (COMBI-MB): a multicentre, multicohort, open-label, phase 2 trial. Lancet Oncol 2017;18(7):863–73.

85. McArthur GA, Maio M, Arance A, et al. Vemurafenib in metastatic melanoma patients with brain metastases: an open-label, single-arm, phase 2, multicentre study. Ann Oncol 2017;28(3):634–41.

Metastatic Complications of Cancer Involving the Central and Peripheral Nervous Systems

Joe S. Mendez, MD, Lisa M. DeAngelis, MD*

KEYWORDS

- Neurologic complications • Cancer • CNS • PNS • Epidural cord compression
- Leptomeningeal • Skull base and nerve plexuses

KEY POINTS

- Metastases may involve the central (CNS) and peripheral nervous systems (PNS) with involvement of the brain, leptomeninges, spinal cord, epidural space, plexus, and skull base.
- Excluding the brain parenchyma, metastases to these spaces collectively affect more than 25% of patients with metastatic cancer.
- Metastases to the CNS and PNS can result in significant morbidity and mortality, often causing pain, disability and compromising quality of life.
- Early diagnosis and treatment are essential to optimize quality of life and survival.

INTRODUCTION

Metastatic cancer may involve both the central nervous system (CNS) and peripheral nervous system (PNS). Metastatic complications of the CNS and PNS are relatively rare, but collectively they affect approximately 25% of patients with cancer. The incidence and site of metastatic involvement within the CNS and PNS differ based on the primary histology (**Table 1**). Most patients diagnosed with metastatic complications involving the CNS and PNS have widespread systemic disease, and some have more than one nervous system site involved. These metastatic complications usually occur in the late stages of disease, but rarely are the presenting manifestation of malignancy. The number of patients suffering from metastases to the nervous system is likely to increase with prolonged control of systemic disease. Most importantly,

Funding: This research was supported in part through the NIH/NCI Cancer Center Support Grant P30 CA008748.

The authors have no conflict of interest.

Department of Neurology, Memorial Sloan Kettering Cancer Center, 1275 York Avenue, New York, NY 10065, USA

* Corresponding author.

E-mail address: deangell@mskcc.org

Table 1
Metastatic complications of cancers and common primaries

Metastatic Complication	Common Primary Malignancies	Overall Incidence
Leptomeningeal	Breast, lung (small cell), non-Hodgkin lymphoma, leukemias, stomach, melanoma[1,6]	4%–15%[6]
Intramedullary	Lung (small cell), breast[32]	0.9%–2.1%[32]
Intracranial dural	Breast, lung > head/neck, leukemia, lymphoma, multiple myeloma[36]	9%–10%[36]
Epidural spinal cord compression	Breast, lung, prostate, lymphoma[41]	5%[41]
Nerve plexuses		
Brachial	Lung, breast > lymphoma, sarcoma, melanoma[54]	0.43%[57]
Lumbosacral	Colorectal, sarcoma, breast, lymphoma, genitourinary[56]	0.71%[57]
Skull base	Lung, breast, prostate, lymphoma, and head/neck[59,61]	4%[59]

metastases to the CNS or PNS can result in significant morbidity as well as mortality. This article focuses on leptomeningeal, intramedullary, intradural, epidural, plexus, and skull base metastases. Brain metastases are discussed in Ayal A. Aizer and Eudocia Q. Lee's article, "Brain Metastases," in this issue.

LEPTOMENINGEAL METASTASES
Clinical Presentation

The most common presentation in patients with leptomeningeal metastases (LMs) include symptoms and signs involving several sites along the neuroaxis. The symptoms and signs of LM are considered according to their regional anatomic localization: brain (cerebral), cranial nerves (CN), and spinal cord (**Table 2**).

Pathophysiology

Mechanisms for the invasion of cancer cells to the leptomeninges include arterial and venous hematogenous dissemination, as well as direct extension of metastatic tumor from the brain, spinal cord, or cranial or peripheral nerves.[1] Direct seeding of the cerebrospinal fluid (CSF) can occur in as many as 36% of patients after resection of a posterior fossa brain metastasis.[2]

LM can cause elevated intracranial pressure (ICP) with or without hydrocephalus.[1] Symptoms of elevated ICP can be prominent and are often confused with direct LM involvement. Hydrocephalus develops due to obstruction of CSF outflow by leptomeningeal tumor resulting in impaired CSF absorption.[1] However, elevated ICP also can occur in the absence of hydrocephalus when the ventricular system is unable to dilate

Table 2
Clinical presentation of leptomeningeal metastases

Anatomic Location	Symptoms/Signs
Brain (cerebral)	Headache, lethargy, confusion
Cranial nerves	Vision changes, diplopia, facial numbness/weakness, hearing loss
Spinal cord	Pain (back/neck, but can be radicular), focal weakness, numbness, bladder/bowel symptoms

due to diffuse subarachnoid tumor. As neuro-imaging can be disarmingly normal in this situation, LM is commonly missed, leading to severe headache and intractable nausea and vomiting. Increased baseline ICP prevents the brain from adjusting to transient rises in pressure that occur normally with positional changes in cerebral blood volume and vascular resistance. When these plateau waves occur in the setting of elevated ICP, they lead to decreased cerebral blood flow causing the acute onset of transient neurologic symptoms, including headache, loss of consciousness, and even focal findings, such as weakness or paresthesias that are almost always precipitated by a change in body position.[1] They are often confused with seizures, and a delay in proper diagnosis can be fatal.

Diagnosis

The gold standard for diagnosing LM is the identification of malignant cells in the CSF.[3] However, CSF cytologic examination has a high rate of false negatives, and sensitivity of CSF cytology does not approach 90% until 3 lumbar punctures (LPs) have been performed.[3] Obtaining a large volume of CSF and rapid processing can improve the yield.[3] Cisternal tap has been shown to result in positive cytology in cases in which lumbar tap was negative.[4] In addition to cytology, CSF flow cytometry should be performed in patients with lymphoma or leukemia, as it can be 2 to 3 times more sensitive at detecting LM.[5] The CSF profile often demonstrates elevated protein, pleocytosis in approximately one-half of patients, and hypoglycorrhachia in a minority.[6] An elevated opening pressure is present in at least 50% of patients.[6] Biochemical and molecular markers (**Table 3**) also can be obtained in the CSF and compared with serum concentrations to aid in the diagnosis of LM in specific settings.[1,6] More recently, circulating tumor cells (CTCs) for epithelial primaries have been identified in the CSF and have a 95% sensitivity, which is far superior to CSF cytology.[7] Furthermore, CTCs have been shown to be useful in monitoring response to treatment in breast cancer.[8] The best method for collecting CTCs from CSF is an ongoing area of research, so this approach is not yet routinely used in clinical settings.

MRI of the brain and spine is the imaging study of choice when evaluating for LM with a sensitivity of 34% to 71%.[9] Definitive imaging characteristics of LM include sulcal enhancement, CN deposits, pial enhancement over the spinal cord, and nodular thickening of the cauda equina[9] (**Fig. 1**); these findings can be diagnostic in a patient with known cancer, even if the CSF cytology is negative.[10] LMs from hematologic primaries are less apparent on MRI than solid tumor primaries.[10] Imaging for LM should always include the brain and the complete spine, as the disease can be multifocal. LP should not be delayed for MRI due to concern for inciting pachymeningeal enhancement because this is actually quite rare.[11]

Treatment

Radiation therapy

Current practice for treatment of LM with radiation therapy (RT) is to irradiate symptomatic areas for palliation. It is unclear if treating areas of bulky disease that are asymptomatic prevents the development of symptoms. Craniospinal RT is not used due to its associated toxicities, including bone marrow suppression, which inhibits the ability to deliver subsequent chemotherapy. Whole-brain RT is typically reserved for patients who develop hydrocephalus, hemispheric symptoms, or multiple cranial neuropathies, although RT to the skull base may suffice to treat isolated cranial neuropathies.[1] However, even if RT is symptomatically helpful, it may not prolong survival.[12]

Table 3	
Cerebrospinal fluid evaluation based on suspected malignancy	
Tests/Markers	**Specific Tumor Associations (if Applicable)**
All cancers/unknown	
Standard:	
Cell count with differential	
Glucose	
Protein	
Cytology	
If available:	
Cell-free DNA	
Solid tumors	
Standard:	
CEA	GI/Lung
AFP	Germ cell
βHCG	Germ cell
Melanin	Melanoma
CA 125	Ovarian
CA 15–3	Breast
5-HIAA	Carcinoid
PSA	Prostate
CA 19–9	Adenocarcinoma
If available:	
Circulating tumor cells	Epithelial tumors
FISH (interphase cytogenetics)	
Protein S-100	Melanoma
HMB45	Melanoma
TTF 1	Lung/Thyroid
MAGE, MART-1, tyrosinase	Melanoma
Hematologic cancers	
Standard:	
β-2 microglobulin	Lymphoma
LDH	Lymphoma
Flow cytometry	
IgH gene rearrangement	

Abbreviations: AFP, alphafetoprotein; βHCG, beta human chorionic gonadotropin; CEA, carcinoembryonic antigen; FISH, fluorescence in situ hybridization; GI, gastrointestinal; HMB, human melanoma black; Ig, immunoglobulin; LDH, lactate dehydrogenase; MAGE, melanoma associated antigen; MART-1, melanoma antigen recognized by T cells; PSA, prostate-specific antigen; 5-HIAA, 5-hydroxyindoleacetic acid; TTF 1, thyroid transcription factor 1.

Chemotherapy

Chemotherapy can be delivered systemically or intrathecally for LM. There are no randomized trials comparing these methods of delivery. Depending on the agent, systemic chemotherapy does not always achieve a therapeutic concentration in the CSF. Intrathecal (IT) chemotherapy allows for the direct administration of drug into the CSF via LP or Ommaya reservoir, although IT chemotherapy does not penetrate bulky disease. Compared with LP, intra-Ommaya (IO) chemotherapy achieves better

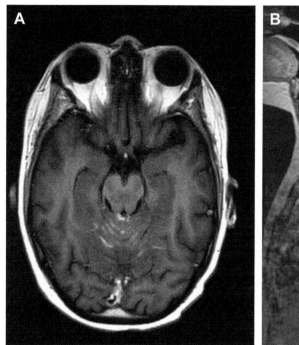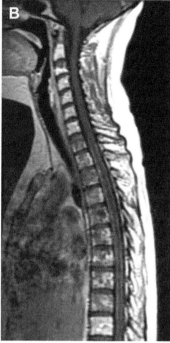

Fig. 1. LMs. (A) Metastatic breast cancer with leptomeningeal disease lining the cerebellar folia on axial, T1 postcontrast imaging. (B) Leptomeningeal disease coating the spinal cord on sagittal, T1 postcontrast imaging.

distribution throughout the CSF, achieves therapeutic concentrations for a longer duration, and guarantees the drug is delivered into the CSF compartment given that approximately 10% of injections via LP actually deliver the drug into the epidural space, despite CSF return.[1,13] For these reasons, along with the ease of administration and patient tolerability, IO delivery is preferred over LP delivery.

Methotrexate (MTX), thiotepa, and cytarabine are the primary agents given intrathecally. Treatment response to MTX has been seen in 36% to 75% of patients with LM from breast cancer and some patients have survived more than 1 year with this approach.[14,15] The primary toxicity associated with IT-MTX is neutropenia,[14] but this can be prevented with oral leucovorin 10 mg twice a day for a few days; leucovorin does not cross the blood-brain barrier and cannot rescue the tumor cells in the CSF. IT combination regimens have failed to show any improvement in response or survival over single-agent use.[15] IT cytarabine is available in a standard formulation and was previously available in a depot formulation (Depocyte),[6] which allowed for every 2-week dosing. MTX and cytarabine are most effective for LM from hematologic malignancies. IT thiotepa has similar response rates and toxicities as MTX.[6] The main side effects for IT chemotherapy are headache and arachnoiditis, which are most severe with Depocyte and require pre-instillation and post-instillation prophylactic glucocorticoids.[6]

IT chemotherapy requires normal CSF flow dynamics to deliver the drug throughout the CSF space. CSF flow can be studied using a radioisotope instilled into the ventricular system via an Ommaya reservoir or by LP.[16] Impaired CSF flow is associated with poor outcome and an increased risk of neurotoxicities.[16] Unfortunately, IT chemotherapy has limited impact on the outcome of patients with LM, except for those with hematologic malignancies in whom it can be curative.[17]

Systemically administered chemotherapies for LM include cytarabine, MTX, and thiotepa. Penetration of the CNS by cytarabine and MTX can be achieved with high-dose regimens, and thiotepa is known to cross the blood-brain barrier. However, these are not usually active agents against the most common solid tumors that cause LM, such as lung and breast cancer. There is also some evidence that administration of drugs or regimens optimal for the primary tumor, regardless of their ability to penetrate the blood-CSF barrier, is the best approach. The presence of tumor in the CSF causes some disruption of the blood-CSF barrier, allowing penetration of drugs that typically do not cross into the CNS.[17]

Targeted and immunotherapies

A significant number of small series have documented response of LM to targeted therapies and immunotherapies. In non–small-cell lung cancer (NSCLC), therapies directed at inhibition of anaplastic lymphoma kinase fusion proteins and epidermal growth factor receptor (EGFR) mutations using alectinib and afatinib, respectively, have produced responses in patients with LM.[18,19] A larger study found that patients with EGFR-mutant NSCLC LM had prolonged survival with treatment of tyrosine kinase inhibitors.[12] Changing the dose and schedule to facilitate access of some agents into the CSF, such as using a pulsatile high-dose schedule for erlotinib, an EGFR inhibitor, can also control CNS disease including LM, even when there is progression on the standard dosing schedule.[20] Choice of agent also can be adjusted on the basis of whether resistance mutations have been acquired within the CNS compartment. These mutations may be identified in the CSF using cell-free DNA technology and can guide treatment decisions.[21]

There are now multiple reports of LM responding to immunotherapy. Patients with NSCLC LM have responded to nivolumab, a monoclonal antibody to programmed cell death-1 (PD-1) that prevents downregulation of the immune system.[22] In a series of 39 patients with melanoma with LM, 21 received targeted therapy with BRAF inhibitors (vemurafenib/dabrafenib) or immunotherapy with antibodies to CTLA-4 (ipilimumab) with or without radiation, and were found to have increased survival with long-term survivors.[23]

Surgery

Surgical intervention for LM is reserved for those patients who develop elevated ICP (with or without hydrocephalus) and require the placement of a ventriculoperitoneal shunt, which can be lifesaving. A shunt prevents the delivery of chemotherapy via an Ommaya reservoir, and should never be turned off to facilitate IO drug delivery.

Prognosis

Untreated patients with LM have rapid progression of disease and die within 4 to 6 weeks.[24] With the initiation of treatment for LM, patients can see small improvements in survival that vary depending on histology, but most have continued neurologic deterioration that leads to death.[25] Patients with leukemia can obtain complete eradication of LM and have a median overall survival (mOS) of 11.3 months.[25] Those with breast cancer who respond to IT chemotherapy have an mOS greater than 1 year.[15] Patients with melanoma have a mOS of 4.7 months, and lung cancer a mOS of only 1.8 months.[25] Survival at 1 year is seen in 48% of patients with lymphoreticular and breast cancers, 26% in melanoma, and 18% in lung cancer.[25]

Favorable prognostic factors for response to IT treatment include controlled systemic disease at diagnosis, low initial CSF protein (likely a surrogate for good CSF flow), and concomitant systemic chemotherapy.[14] Poor prognostic factors include having a lung or melanoma primary, 12 months or less from diagnosis of primary to LM, Karnofsky Performance Score (KPS) ≤70, age ≥50, lack of cytologic response in CSF, and lack of concurrent systemic chemotherapy.[17] In a few studies, the use of systemic chemotherapy has been associated with increased OS on multivariable analysis.[17,25]

INTRAMEDULLARY METASTASES
Pathophysiology

Intramedullary metastases (IMM) primarily arise by direct hematogenous dissemination or by direct extension from LM in the subarachnoid space.[1] IMM tends to be evenly distributed along the cervical, thoracic, and lumbar spine,[26] although some studies have shown the thoracic or lumbar spine to be more involved.[27–29] When accounting for the length of spinal segments, the lumbar spine is disproportionally involved in IMM.[30] Up to 33% of patients with IMM have multifocal intramedullary disease.[27]

Clinical Presentation

At least one-half of patients have brain metastases,[26,29,31,32] and it is common for LM to be present.[31,32] The most common presenting symptoms are pain, sensory changes, and weakness.[32] Pain can be localized or radicular,[30,32] and weakness can be bilateral or unilateral.[32] Although bladder and bowel dysfunction may occur later, several studies show that more than 50% of patients had bladder/bowel dysfunction at presentation.[30,32] A sensory level and spasticity are common.[30] Brown Séquard syndrome (characterized by ipsilateral weakness and loss of vibration/proprioception, as well as contralateral loss of pain/temperature sensation) can be the presenting manifestation of IMM.[32] The clinical presentation of patients with IMM is characterized by a rapid neurologic decline resulting in paraparesis or paraplegia.[29] Symptoms can be present anywhere from 7 to 63 days before the diagnosis of IMM.[28,29]

Diagnosis

The diagnosis of IMM is made by spine MRI with contrast (**Fig. 2**). On MRI, IMM may be nodular or ring enhancing[1,27,32]; hemorrhage and intratumoral cystic changes are rare.[33] In a patient with known cancer, differentiating among IMM, LM, radiation myelopathy, and paraneoplastic myelopathy based on imaging can be difficult. However, radiation myelopathy and necrotizing myelopathy are usually painless and insidious, whereas pain occurs early in IMM and is accompanied by rapid evolution of symptoms.[34] CSF studies are not helpful in differentiating intramedullary lesions, unless LM are confirmed in the CSF.

Treatment/Prognosis

Treatment options include steroids, RT, surgical resection, chemotherapy, or a combination of these approaches.[30,32,34] RT is effective at ameliorating symptoms.[34] Several studies have explored surgery and microsurgical approaches followed by RT with improvement in OS and function,[26,31] but were limited to patients with a high functional status. Some advocate for surgical resection in patients with a solitary IMM from a radioresistant primary with well controlled systemic disease, although this is an uncommon situation.[26,31]

The mOS of patients with IMM ranges from 12 to 31 weeks.[28,32] Some patients with breast cancer fare better,[29,32] but other reports suggest that lung or breast primary was associated with inferior survival.[35] On spinal MRI, multiple IMM, involvement of 3

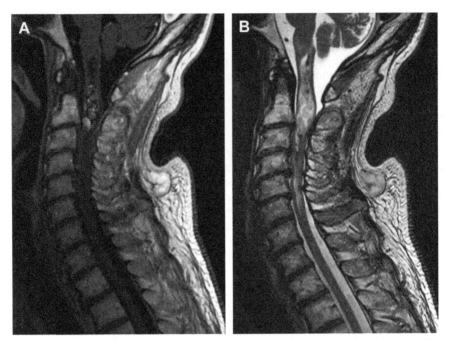

Fig. 2. IMMs. (*A*) Sagittal, T1 postcontrast imaging reveals an enhancing intramedullary metastasis at C2/C3 in a patient with adenoid cystic carcinoma of the submandibular gland. (*B*) Surrounding vasogenic edema is best appreciated on sagittal, T2.

segments or more, and visualization of any systemic involvement were associated with decreased survival.[35] The presence of LM was not associated with inferior survival.[35]

INTRACRANIAL DURAL METASTASES
Pathophysiology

Intracranial dural metastases (IDMs) are calvarial metastases with direct extension to the epidural and subdural spaces or direct involvement of the subdural space from hematogenous spread.[1] Direct extension from a skull metastasis explains the predilection of those cancers that commonly spread to bone to affect the dura.[36]

Clinical Presentation

IDMs usually present with bulky dural disease causing mass effect, edema, and compression of underlying parenchyma; rarely it can lead to a subdural hematoma (SDH) or effusion, which may require cytologic evaluation for a definitive diagnosis.[1] Alteration in mental status, visual complaints, hemiparesis, and seizures are seen frequently. Eleven percent of patients may be asymptomatic with IDM identified on imaging done for other purposes.[36]

Diagnosis

IDM is diagnosed by brain MRI with contrast, and the lesions enhance homogeneously with an associated dural tail[37] (**Fig. 3**). The main differential is a meningioma, but IDMs often have more irregular borders and underlying edema than a typical meningioma; this can be a challenging differential diagnosis, especially in women with breast cancer who have an increased incidence of meningioma.[38] Dynamic susceptibility

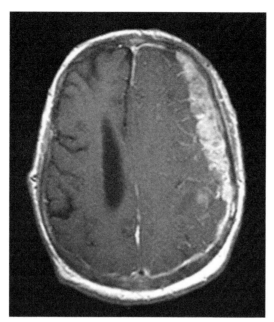

Fig. 3. Dural metastases. Enhancing, dural metastasis along the left hemisphere in a patient with metastatic prostate cancer. Note the irregular border of the lesion abutting brain and the marked mass effect.

contrast-MR/perfusion-weighted imaging can assist as relative cerebral blood volume is low in most IDMs but elevated in meningiomas.[37] Other imaging characteristics seen with IDMs include skull metastases, bony erosions, vasogenic edema, brain invasion, venous sinus compression or occlusion, and an SDH/effusion. A single lesion is most common, but diffuse dural involvement also can be seen.[36] Those with an SDH/effusion also may exhibit brisk enhancement, and there are frequently nodules along the dura or marked underlying edema to suggest this is not a benign process.

Treatment and Prognosis

There is no standard treatment for IDM, but surgical resection, RT, chemotherapy, and combinations of these 3 modalities are used depending on the clinical situation. RT has been associated with improved OS while metastatic lung cancer and low KPS were associated with worse outcomes.[36] The mOS of patients with IDM is 9.5 months with a progression-free survival of 3.7 months.[36] Chemotherapy may play an important role, as dural disease is outside the blood-brain barrier.

EPIDURAL SPINAL CORD COMPRESSION
Pathophysiology

Epidural spinal cord compression (ESCC) is caused by cancer that affects the epidural space by extension from the vertebral bodies or other bony spinal elements, infiltration through a foramen, or direct hematogenous dissemination to the epidural space.[1] Epidural disease due to direct extension from vertebral metastases occurs in 85% to 90% of ESCC.[1] The posterior vertebral body is the most common location of metastatic involvement leading to anterior cord compression.[39] In addition, metastatic involvement of the vertebral body can lead to vertebral collapse with spinal instability and potential herniation of bone, metastatic disease, and/or disk causing cord compression.[1] Paravertebral metastases can invade the epidural space via the intervertebral foramina, but this mechanism accounts for only 10% to 15% of ESCC, and is usually due to lymphoma or neuroblastoma. Compression typically occurs along the lateral cord and the bone is normal; thus, MRI is the only imaging modality that can visualize this ESCC.[1] Direct metastases to the epidural space via hematogenous spread is very rare and seen exclusively in leukemia and lymphoma.[1]

Clinical Presentation

ESCC is a neurologic emergency because of the possibility of sudden paraparesis that can occur unexpectedly, is difficult to reverse, and is likely due to a venous infarction of the spinal cord. Patients with ESCC experience back pain, weakness, sensory changes, and autonomic dysfunction (**Table 4**), but significant diagnostic delays are frequent. In one study, the median times from onset of radicular pain, weakness, sensory, and bladder problems to diagnosis were 40, 21, 13, and 3 days, respectively.[40] More striking is that in patients without a diagnosis of malignancy, the diagnosis was delayed by an additional 4 weeks.[41]

Diagnosis

The differential diagnosis for ESCC includes epidural abscess/hematoma, a primary epidural tumor, or vertebral collapse from any etiology, such as osteoporosis. MRI is the definitive imaging modality due to its high sensitivity and specificity at detecting metastatic ESCC, and it can detect multiple sites of ESCC[1] (**Fig. 4**). Multiple sites of epidural spinal metastases are seen in approximately 30% of patients, necessitating whole-spine imaging in all patients.[42] The most common location for cord compression is the thoracic spine followed by the lumbosacral, and then the cervical level.[40,42] Computed tomography (CT) myelogram is useful in cases in which MRI is contraindicated.

Table 4 Presenting complaints and physical examination findings in patients with epidural spinal cord compression	
	Frequency
Presenting complaint	
Back pain	
Local or radicular pain Exacerbated when supine, cough, sneeze, movement, or Valsalva Wakes patients at night, sleep in a seated position to alleviate pain	61%–96%[66,67]
Weakness	2%–37%[66,67]
Sensory changes	
Not a common complaint, but commonly found on examination	0%[67]
Bowel and bladder incontinence	0%–2%[66,67]
Gait disturbance/ataxia	2%[67]
Physical examination finding	
Weakness	87%–96%[67,68]
Sensory levels and deficits	78%–90%[67,68]
Autonomic dysfunction	57%–69%[67,68]
Ataxia	14%[67]

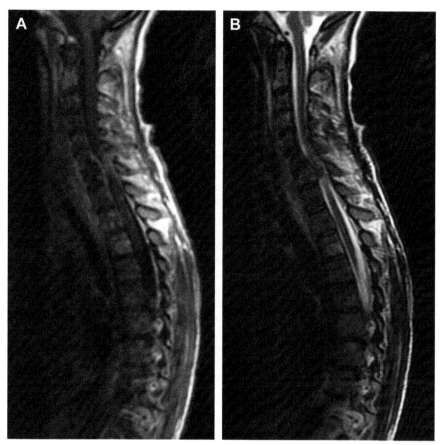

Fig. 4. Metastatic ESCC. (*A*) Sagittal, T1 postcontrast image showing extensive epidural disease arising from the vertebral body causing spinal cord compression at C6/C7 in a patient with metastatic breast cancer. (*B*) Cord compression is better visualized on T2.

Treatment

Treatment for ESCC is palliative and includes relieving pain, preserving or improving neurologic function, stabilizing the spine, and addressing the tumor.

Steroids
High-dose steroids are the first treatment in the acute management of malignant ESCC.[43] Glucocorticoids reduce local edema at the site of compression and can improve neurologic function. Although the subject of several randomized trials, there continues to be no standard dosing regimen, but in clinical practice an initial dose from 10 to 100 mg of dexamethasone is used, followed by a maintenance dose of 16 to 96 mg per day with a rapid taper following treatment.[43]

Surgery
Surgery should be directed to the site of the disease with the goal of extirpating the tumor mass. Thus, anterior and anterolateral approaches are the optimal approaches given that most disease arises from the vertebral body. A randomized trial comparing tumor resection plus RT versus RT alone for management of ESCC found that patients

who underwent surgical resection and RT were more likely to regain ambulation and retain it for a longer duration of time compared with RT alone. These patients were also more likely to maintain continence, have reduced pain and steroid use, and have improved OS.[44] Therefore, surgery should be considered in patients with ESCC who have a reasonable overall prognosis.[44] In addition, other considerations may prompt a surgical approach as the first step, such as spinal instability necessitating stabilization, deterioration during RT, need to establish a pathologic diagnosis, radioresistant tumors, and recurrence where additional RT is not an option.[39]

Radiation therapy

RT should be given to all patients who are nonsurgical candidates with ESCC and should be considered as first-line therapy in patients with highly radiosensitive tumors, such as myeloma, lymphoma, Ewing sarcoma, neuroblastoma, or seminoma.[39] RT, particularly short-course RT, is also advocated in patients with a poor prognosis, as it is noninvasive and completed rapidly in an outpatient setting.[45] RT should also follow surgery.

Currently, conventional RT is often replaced by stereotactic body RT (SBRT), especially in the postoperative setting. Conventional RT requires a relatively large treatment field encompassing 1 to 2 vertebral bodies and includes normal spinal cord. However, SBRT allows for the delivery of conformal high-dose RT in a single dose or hypofractionated doses, which allows for the safe and effective delivery of RT without spinal cord toxicity and minimal systemic toxicities.[46] Local recurrence rates of less than 5% at 1 year have been reported in patients who underwent surgery followed by high-dose hypofractionated SBRT, irrespective of tumor radiosensitivity,[46] leading to advocating for this approach in consensus guidelines.[47] SBRT also limits bone marrow toxicity compared with conventional RT, providing the opportunity for multimodality treatment with chemotherapy.

The success of SBRT in the treatment of ESCC has led to the implementation of a surgical procedure termed "separation surgery" which is followed by SBRT. This procedure allows for decompression and stabilization, but focuses on providing a separation between the spinal cord and the tumor, as opposed to achieving a gross total resection.[46] This allows for SBRT to be delivered safely and avoids the risks associated with a gross total resection while providing long-term disease control.[46]

Systemic therapies

Systemic therapies, such as chemotherapy, hormonal therapy, and immunotherapy, have a limited role in the treatment of ESCC. Most treatments directed at ESCC including surgery and RT are focal, and patients often need chemotherapy, hormonal therapy, or immunotherapy for active systemic disease. However, in certain situations in which ESCC is due to highly chemosensitive primaries, such as lymphoma or seminoma, it may be treated with systemic treatment, provided the patient has few or no neurologic signs.[46] There also may be a role for combining RT with immunotherapy, which may result in a more robust immune response leading to better clinical outcomes.[48]

Emerging therapies

A phase I study in patients with progressive epidural disease despite surgery and RT found that spinal intra-arterial chemotherapy (melphalan) was safe and feasible, and effective at stabilizing epidural disease.[49] MR-guided spinal laser interstitial thermal therapy is also being explored as a less invasive alternative to surgery for ESCC; it achieved significant decompression months after the procedure in a select patient population.[50] Percutaneous kyphoplasty does not treat ESCC, but it is safe and effective for spinal metastases,[51] and may be useful in preventing ESCC. It is also useful for vertebral body compression fractures that can occur with long-term follow-up after SBRT.

Prognosis

In patients with ESCC, the most important factor that predicts ambulatory status following treatment is the patient's ambulatory function before treatment.[44] Some patients who are nonambulatory at presentation can regain ambulation, particularly if surgery is the first intervention. With regard to survival, visceral metastases, other bony metastases, tumor type, motor function before and after treatment, rapidity of motor symptoms, interval between diagnosis and development of ESCC, sphincter dysfunction, number of epidural metastases, and number of vertebral bodies involved can all influence survival in patients with ESCC. In general, patients with lung cancer fare poorly, whereas patients with breast or prostate cancer, or myeloma/lymphoma can have prolonged survival.[1] Most of the factors influencing survival in patients with ESCC reflect the aggressive nature of the primary tumor, as most patients with ESCC die from their systemic disease.[1] The mOS in patients with ESCC is 2.9 to 10.0 months,[52,53] with significantly lower survival times in nonambulatory patients.

NERVE PLEXUSES
Brachial Plexus

Metastasis to the brachial plexus occurs primarily from lymphatic spread, but direct invasion can occur as well.[1,54] It is thought that the spread via lymphatics from the lung and breast to the lateral axillary lymph nodes leads to preferential involvement of the lower trunk (C8 and T1) due to their proximity. Compression or invasion via Pancoast tumors (apical lung tumors) are common and also lead to lower plexus involvement.[55] The upper trunk is usually involved only when tumor extends to involve the whole plexus.[54,55]

Patients with neoplastic brachial plexopathy often start with severe pain (75%) followed by sensory abnormalities and weakness of the affected arm.[54] The pain usually begins in the shoulder girdle, radiates to the elbow, down the medial forearm, and into the fourth and fifth digits.[54] Patients typically complain of hand weakness.[1] Horner syndrome is seen in approximately 50% of patients due to the close proximity of the sympathetic ganglion to the frequently involved T1 nerve root.[54] Horner syndrome often suggests there has been extension of the tumor into the cervical-thoracic epidural space, which requires this area be imaged along with the plexus itself. Weakness, atrophy, and sensory changes primarily localize to the C7, C8, and T1 nerve roots.[54]

Lumbosacral Plexus

Mechanisms of metastatic lumbosacral plexopathy include direct extension by an abdominopelvic primary (accounting for 70%), soft or bony tissue metastases causing compression, extra-abdominal metastasis directly to the plexus, lymph node or muscle involvement with compression, and tumor extension to the plexus along nerves.[1,56] The lower plexus (L5-S3) is involved in approximately one-half of cases followed by 30% involving the upper plexus (L1-L4), and 20% affecting the entire plexus.[56]

As seen in brachial plexopathies, lumbosacral plexopathies also begin with pain, followed by numbness/paresthesias, and weakness within weeks to months.[56] Pain typically has an achy or pressurelike quality that is more commonly local or radicular, but can be referred; incontinence is rare.[56] Examination demonstrates asymmetric weakness that can progress to focal paralysis.[56] Reflexes are lost and asymmetric early in the course.[56] A positive straight leg test is common and gait difficulty correlates with the level of lumbosacral plexus involvement.[56]

Diagnosis

MRI identifies plexus metastases and should include the cervical spine when a Horner syndrome is present[57] (**Fig. 5**). CT is excellent for detecting plexus involvement when MRI is not possible. PET and PET-CT may be helpful when other imaging modalities are negative, but clinical suspicion for a plexopathy is high,[57] especially with direct invasion of nerves as seen in neurolymphomatosis. Electromyography and nerve conduction studies (EMG/NCS) can localize a peripheral nerve lesion.[56] In cases in which history, examination, imaging, and EMG/NCS fail to provide a diagnosis, surgical exploration can be useful.

The most clinically relevant diagnostic dilemma is differentiating a neoplastic plexopathy from radiation plexopathy in a patient who has received prior RT that encompassed the involved plexus (**Table 5**).[54,58] The incidence of radiation plexopathy is approximately 1.2% and can develop months to years after RT.[57]

Treatment

Treatment options for malignant plexopathies include RT and rarely chemotherapy. Pain management includes analgesics, nerve blocks, cordotomy, and rhizotomy if uncontrolled.[54] Despite improvement in pain, most suffer progressive neurologic decline.[56]

SKULL BASE METASTASES
Pathophysiology

The most common mechanism of skull base metastasis is hematogenous spread, including both arterial and venous routes.[59] However, direct extension and perineural invasion of adjacent CNs can occur from head and neck primaries.[60]

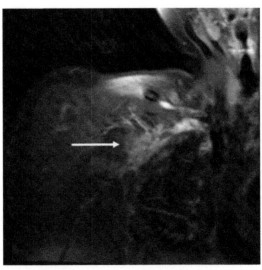

Fig. 5. Brachial plexus metastasis. Post-gadolinium MRI demonstrating a right brachial plexus metastasis (*arrow*) in a patient with breast cancer.

Table 5	
Differentiating neoplastic plexopathy from radiation induced plexopathy	
Neoplastic Plexopathy	**Radiation-Induced Plexopathy**
Brachial plexus	

Common cancers
  Breast, lung, lymphoma, melanoma, sarcoma
	Prior radiation therapy to the
	  chest, axilla (months-years)

Symptoms Pain (severe)	Numbness/Paresthesia

Signs
  Unilateral
  Lower plexus involvement (C8-T1)
  Horner syndrome
  Neck mass/supraclavicular fullness
	Unilateral
	Upper (C5-C7) or entire plexus
	  involvement
	Lymphedema

Diagnostic evaluations
  Paralyzed hemi-diaphragm on CXR
  Pancoast tumor on imaging
	Myokymic discharges on
	  EMG/NCS

Lumbosacral plexus	

Common cancers
  Breast, colorectal, genitourinary, lymphoma,
   sarcoma
	Prior radiation therapy to pelvis
	  (months-years)

Symptoms Pain (Severe)	Weakness in the lower extremities

Signs
  More commonly unilateral
  Positive straight leg test
  Palpable mass on rectal examination
	More commonly bilateral
	  (asymmetric)
	Lymphedema

Diagnostic evaluation	Myokymic discharges on EMG/NCS

Abbreviations: CXR, chest radiograph; EMG/NCS, electromyography and nerve conduction studies.

Clinical Presentation

Patients with skull base metastases present with CN deficits. Seven clinical skull base syndromes[1,59,61–63] (**Table 6**) have been identified due to their stereotyped presentations as a result of compression of CN and vascular structures that are adjacent to the associated basal foramina and sinuses that comprise the skull base.

Diagnosis

The diagnosis of skull base metastases is made with an MRI[60,64] or CT (**Fig. 6**); however, in some patients, MRI and CT are negative despite a high clinical suspicion for skull base metastases. A PET scan may be helpful. An LP cannot diagnose skull base metastases, but it is recommended to exclude coexistent LM.

Treatment/Prognosis

Treatment of skull base metastases consists of RT and rarely chemotherapy, but the treatment relies strongly on the histology of the primary.[1] Stereotactic radiosurgery has been used for both the initial treatment of a skull base metastasis and recurrence.[65] Long delays from symptom onset to treatment result in significantly inferior symptomatic improvement. In general, most patients improve following treatment.[65]

Table 6
Syndromes in skull base metastases

Location/Syndrome	Presentation
Orbital	• Supraorbital pain of the affected eye, blurred vision followed by diplopia • Ophthalmoplegia, proptosis, +/− palpable tumor, no papilledema, visual field loss, or vision loss • Prostate, lymphoma, and breast
Parasellar	• Unilateral frontal headache, diplopia • Ocular paresis (cranial nerve [CN] III, IV, VI and V1-2), no proptosis, no vision loss or visual field loss, +/− papilledema • Lymphoma
Sella turcica	• Most cases are clinically silent • When symptomatic typically present with diabetes insipidus, +/− oculomotor palsies, less likely to have vision loss and anterior pituitary insufficiency • Breast, lung, and bladder cancer
Middle cranial fossa	• Facial numbness/paresthesias and/or pain within the distribution of CN V2/V3, +/− headache and diplopia • Sensory loss of CN V, +/− pterygoid and masseter weakness, +/− ocular palsies (CN VI most common)
Jugular foramen	• Dysphagia and hoarseness, +/− glossopharyngeal neuralgia, unilateral pain behind the ear • CN X, XI, XII involvement: palatal weakness, vocal cord paralysis, and weakness/atrophy of the tongue
Occipital condyle	• Severe, unremitting unilateral occipital pain with neck stiffness, +/− dysarthria or dysphagia • Tenderness to palpation over the occiput, stiff neck, CN XII palsy
Mandible "numb-chin"	• Unilateral numbness or loss of sensation of the lower lip and chin, includes the inner lip as well, can be bilateral, pain is rare • Decreased sensation over the chin and lower lip • Breast and lymphoma

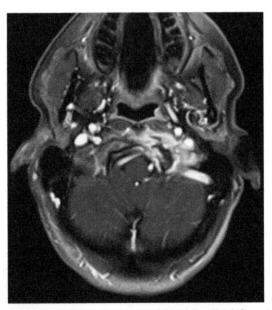

Fig. 6. Skull base metastases. Enhancing metastasis involving the left occipital condyle with hypoglossal canal involvement in a patient with breast cancer.

SUMMARY

The individual metastatic neurologic complications presented in this article are infrequent, but together they affect more than 25% of patients with metastatic tumor and can significantly affect a patient's duration and quality of life. The diagnosis is often challenging, as the differential diagnosis is extensive, but localization is possible through history, neurologic examination, and modern imaging techniques. For each of them, early diagnosis and intervention are essential to optimize outcomes and have the best opportunity for improved survival.

REFERENCES

1. DeAngelis LM, Posner JB. Neurologic complications of cancer. 2nd edition. New York: Oxford University Press; 2009.
2. Norris LK, Grossman SA, Olivi A. Neoplastic meningitis following surgical resection of isolated cerebellar metastasis: a potentially preventable complication. J Neurooncol 1997;32(3):215–23.
3. Glantz MJ, Cole BF, Glantz LK, et al. Cerebrospinal fluid cytology in patients with cancer: minimizing false-negative results. Cancer 1998;82(4):733–9.
4. Rogers LR, Duchesneau PM, Nunez C, et al. Comparison of cisternal and lumbar CSF examination in leptomeningeal metastasis. Neurology 1992;42(6):1239–41.
5. Bromberg JE, Breems DA, Kraan J, et al. CSF flow cytometry greatly improves diagnostic accuracy in CNS hematologic malignancies. Neurology 2007;68(20): 1674–9.
6. Taillibert S, Laigle-Donadey F, Chodkiewicz C, et al. Leptomeningeal metastases from solid malignancy: a review. J Neurooncol 2005;75(1):85–99.
7. Lin X, Fleisher M, Rosenblum M, et al. Cerebrospinal fluid circulating tumor cells: a novel tool to diagnose leptomeningeal metastases from epithelial tumors. Neuro Oncol 2017;(9):1248–54.
8. Patel AS, Allen JE, Dicker DT, et al. Identification and enumeration of circulating tumor cells in the cerebrospinal fluid of breast cancer patients with central nervous system metastases. Oncotarget 2011;2(10):752–60.
9. Collie DA, Brush JP, Lammie GA, et al. Imaging features of leptomeningeal metastases. Clin Radiol 1999;54(11):765–71.
10. Freilich RJ, Krol G, Deangelis LM. Neuroimaging, and cytology in the diagnosis of leptomeningeal metastasis. Ann Neurol 1995;38(1):51–7.
11. Wesley SF, Garcia-Santibanez R, Liang J, et al. Incidence of meningeal enhancement on brain MRI secondary to lumbar puncture. Neurol Clin Pract 2016;6(4): 315–20.
12. Morris PG, Reiner AS, Szenberg OR, et al. Leptomeningeal metastasis from non-small cell lung cancer: survival and the impact of whole brain radiotherapy. J Thorac Oncol 2012;7(2):382–5.
13. Shapiro WR, Young DF, Mehta BM. Methotrexate—distribution in cerebrospinal-fluid after intravenous, ventricular and lumbar injections. N Engl J Med 1975; 293(4):161–6.
14. Fizazi K, Asselain B, Vincent-Salomon A, et al. Meningeal carcinomatosis in patients with breast carcinoma. Clinical features, prognostic factors, and results of a high-dose intrathecal methotrexate regimen. Cancer 1996;77(7):1315–23.
15. Hitchins RN, Bell DR, Woods RL, et al. A prospective randomized trial of single-agent versus combination chemotherapy in meningeal carcinomatosis. J Clin Oncol 1987;5(10):1655–62.

16. Chamberlain MC. Radioisotope CSF flow studies in leptomeningeal metastases. J Neurooncol 1998;38(2–3):135–40.

17. Oechsle K, Lange-Brock V, Kruell A, et al. Prognostic factors and treatment options in patients with leptomeningeal metastases of different primary tumors: a retrospective analysis. J Cancer Res Clin Oncol 2010;136(11):1729–35.

18. Gainor JF, Sherman CA, Willoughby K, et al. Alectinib salvages CNS relapses in ALK-positive lung cancer patients previously treated with crizotinib and ceritinib. J Thorac Oncol 2015;10(2):232–6.

19. Hoffknecht P, Tufman A, Wehler T, et al. Efficacy of the irreversible ErbB family blocker afatinib in epidermal growth factor receptor (EGFR) tyrosine kinase inhibitor (TKI)-pretreated non-small-cell lung cancer patients with brain metastases or leptomeningeal disease. J Thorac Oncol 2015;10(1):156–63.

20. Grommes C, Oxnard GR, Kris MG, et al. "Pulsatile" high-dose weekly erlotinib for CNS metastases from EGFR mutant non-small cell lung cancer. Neuro Oncol 2011;13(12):1364–9.

21. Pentsova EI, Shah RH, Tang J, et al. Evaluating cancer of the central nervous system through next-generation sequencing of cerebrospinal fluid. J Clin Oncol 2016;34(20):2404–15.

22. Dudnik E, Yust-Katz S, Nechushtan H, et al. Intracranial response to nivolumab in NSCLC patients with untreated or progressing CNS metastases. Lung Cancer 2016;98:114–7.

23. Foppen MHG, Brandsma D, Blank CU, et al. Targeted treatment and immunotherapy in leptomeningeal metastases from melanoma. Ann Oncol 2016;27(6):1138–42.

24. Wasserstrom WR, Glass JP, Posner JB. Diagnosis and treatment of leptomeningeal metastases from solid tumors—experience with 90 patients. Cancer 1982;49(4):759–72.

25. Herrlinger U, Forschler H, Kuker W, et al. Leptomeningeal metastasis: survival and prognostic factors in 155 patients. J Neurol Sci 2004;223(2):167–78.

26. Sung WS, Sung MJ, Chan JH, et al. Intramedullary spinal cord metastases: a 20-year institutional experience with a comprehensive literature review. World Neurosurg 2013;79(3–4):576–84.

27. Crasto S, Duca S, Davini O, et al. MRI diagnosis of intramedullary metastases from extra-CNS tumors. Eur Radiol 1997;7(5):732–6.

28. Gasser T, Sandalcioglu IE, El Hamalawi B, et al. Surgical treatment of intramedullary spinal cord metastases of systemic cancer: functional outcome and prognosis. J Neurooncol 2005;73(2):163–8.

29. Lee SS, Kim MK, Sym SJ, et al. Intramedullary spinal cord metastases: a single-institution experience. J Neurooncol 2007;84(1):85–9.

30. Edelson RN, Deck MDF, Posner JB. Intramedullary spinal-cord metastases—clinical and radiographic findings in nine cases. Neurology 1972;22(12):1222–31.

31. Dam-Hieu P, Seizeur R, Mineo JF, et al. Retrospective study of 19 patients with intramedullary spinal cord metastasis. Clin Neurol Neurosurg 2009;111(1):10–7.

32. Schiff D, O'Neill BP. Intramedullary spinal cord metastases: clinical features and treatment outcome. Neurology 1996;47(4):906–12.

33. Rykken JB, Diehn FE, Hunt CH, et al. Intramedullary spinal cord metastases: MRI and relevant clinical features from a 13-year institutional case series. AJNR Am J Neuroradiol 2013;34(10):2043–9.

34. Winkelman MD, Adelstein DJ, Karlins NL. Intramedullary spinal-cord metastasis—diagnostic and therapeutic considerations. Arch Neurol 1987;44(5):526–31.

35. Diehn FE, Rykken JB, Wald JT, et al. Intramedullary spinal cord metastases: prognostic value of MRI and clinical features from a 13-year institutional case series. AJNR Am J Neuroradiol 2015;36(3):587–93.

36. Nayak L, Abrey LE, Iwamoto FM. Intracranial dural metastases. Cancer 2009; 115(9):1947–53.

37. Kremer S, Grand S, Remy C, et al. Contribution of dynamic contrast MR imaging to the differentiation between dural metastasis and meningioma. Neuroradiology 2004;46(8):642–8.

38. Custer BS, Koepsell TD, Mueller BA. The association between breast carcinoma and meningioma in women. Cancer 2002;94(6):1626–35.

39. Siegal T, Siegal T. Current considerations in the management of neoplastic spinal-cord compression. Spine 1989;14(2):223–8.

40. Helweglarsen S, Sorensen PS. Symptoms and signs in metastatic spinal-cord compression—a study of progression from first symptom until diagnosis in 153 patients. Eur J Cancer 1994;30a(3):396–8.

41. Schiff D, ONeill BP, Suman VJ. Spinal epidural metastasis as the initial manifestation of malignancy: clinical features and diagnostic approach. Neurology 1997;49(2):452–6.

42. Schiff D, O'Neill BP, Wang CH, et al. Neuroimaging and treatment implications of patients with multiple epidural spinal metastases. Cancer 1998;83(8):1593–601.

43. Loblaw DA, Mitera G, Ford M, et al. A 2011 updated systematic review and clinical practice guideline for the management of malignant extradural spinal cord compression. Int J Radiat Oncol Biol Phys 2012;84(2):312–7.

44. Patchell RA, Tibbs PA, Regine WF, et al. Direct decompressive surgical resection in the treatment of spinal cord compression caused by metastatic cancer: a randomised trial. Lancet 2005;366(9486):643–8.

45. Rades D, Dunst J, Schild SE. The first score predicting overall survival in patients with metastatic spinal cord compression. Cancer 2008;112(1):157–61.

46. Laufer I, Iorgulescu JB, Chapman T, et al. Local disease control for spinal metastases following "separation surgery" and adjuvant hypofractionated or high-dose single-fraction stereotactic radiosurgery: outcome analysis in 186 patients. J Neurosurg Spine 2013;18(3):207–14.

47. Redmond KJ, Lo SS, Soltys SG, et al. Consensus guidelines for postoperative stereotactic body radiation therapy for spinal metastases: results of an international survey. J Neurosurg Spine 2017;26(3):299–306.

48. Weichselbaum RR, Liang H, Deng LF, et al. Radiotherapy and immunotherapy: a beneficial liaison? Nat Rev Clin Oncol 2017;14(6):365–79.

49. Patsalides A, Yamada Y, Bilsky M, et al. Spinal intraarterial chemotherapy: interim results of a phase I clinical trial. J Neurosurg Spine 2016;24(2):217–22.

50. Tatsui CE, Lee SH, Amini B, et al. Spinal laser interstitial thermal therapy: a novel alternative to surgery for metastatic epidural spinal cord compression. Neurosurgery 2016;79(Suppl 1):S73–82.

51. Chen F, Xia YH, Cao WZ, et al. Percutaneous kyphoplasty for the treatment of spinal metastases. Oncol Lett 2016;11(3):1799–806.

52. Loblaw DA, Laperriere NJ, Mackillop WJ. A population-based study of malignant spinal cord compression in Ontario. Clin Oncol (R Coll Radiol) 2003;15(4):211–7.

53. Sioutos PJ, Arbit E, Meshulam CF, et al. Spinal metastases from solid tumors—analysis of factors affecting survival. Cancer 1995;76(8):1453–9.

54. Kori SH, Foley KM, Posner JB. Brachial-plexus lesions in patients with cancer—100 cases. Neurology 1981;31(1):45–50.

55. Gachiani J, Kim DH, Nelson A, et al. Management of metastatic tumors invading the peripheral nervous system. Neurosurg Focus 2007;22(6):E14.

56. Jaeckle KA, Young DF, Foley KM. The natural-history of lumbosacral plexopathy in cancer. Neurology 1985;35(1):8–15.

57. Jaeckle KA. Neurologic manifestations of neoplastic and radiation-induced plexopathies. Semin Neurol 2010;30(3):254–62.

58. Thomas JE, Cascino TL, Earle JD. Differential-diagnosis between radiation and tumor plexopathy of the pelvis. Neurology 1985;35(1):1–7.

59. Laigle-Donadey F, Taillibert S, Mokhtari K, et al. Dural metastases. J Neurooncol 2005;75(1):57–61.

60. Su CY, Lui CC. Perineural invasion of the trigeminal nerve in patients with naso-pharyngeal carcinoma—imaging and clinical correlations. Cancer 1996;78(10): 2063–9.

61. Greenberg HS, Deck MDF, Vikram B, et al. Metastasis to the base of the skull—clinical findings in 43 patients. Neurology 1981;31(5):530–7.

62. Lossos A, Siegal T. Numb chin syndrome in cancer-patients—etiology, response to treatment, and prognostic-significance. Neurology 1992;42(6):1181–4.

63. Max MB, Deck MDF, Rottenberg DA. Pituitary metastasis—incidence in cancer-patients and clinical-differentiation from pituitary-adenoma. Neurology 1981; 31(8):998–1002.

64. Jansen BP, Smitt PAS. Skull and dural metastases. Cancer neurology in clinical practice. Springer; 2003. p. 87–92.

65. Miller RC, Foote RL, Coffey RJ, et al. The role of stereotactic radiosurgery in the treatment of malignant skull base tumors. Int J Radiat Oncol Biol Phys 1997;39(5): 977–81.

66. Constans JP, Dedivitiis E, Donzelli R, et al. Spinal metastases with neurological manifestations—review of 600 cases. J Neurosurg 1983;59(1):111–8.

67. Gilbert RW, Kim JH, Posner JB. Epidural spinal-cord compression from metasta-tic tumor—diagnosis and treatment. Ann Neurol 1978;3(1):40–51.

68. Bach F, Larsen BH, Rohde K, et al. Metastatic spinal-cord compression—occur-rence, symptoms, clinical presentations and prognosis in 398 patients with spinal-cord compression. Acta Neurochir 1990;107(1–2):37–43.

Neurologic Complications of Radiation Therapy

Shyam K. Tanguturi, MD[a],*, Brian M. Alexander, MD, MPH[b]

KEYWORDS

- Radiation toxicity • Neurologic complications • Radiation injury • Necrosis
- Neurocognitive injury

KEY POINTS

- Cranial radiation therapy is used to treat malignant and benign conditions and carries unique set of risks and complications.
- Early complications from cranial radiation therapy include fatigue, skin reaction, alopecia, headaches, anorexia, nausea/vomiting, exacerbation of neurologic symptoms, serous otitis media, parotitis, and encephalopathy.
- Delayed complications from cranial radiation include pseudoprogression, radiation necrosis, neurocognitive changes, cerebrovascular effects, migrainelike disorders, cataracts, xerophthalmia, optic neuropathy, hearing loss, tinnitus, chronic otitis, endocrinopathy, and secondary malignancy.
- Clinicians should assess the impact of these risks and individualize treatment decisions based on specific patient factors.

INTRODUCTION

Cranial radiation therapy (CRT) is used to treat a wide range of malignant and benign conditions with both curative and palliative intent. As with all medical interventions, cranial irradiation is associated with a unique set of risks and complications. This article presents an overview of clinically relevant short-term and long-term neurologic complications for CRT and reviews some basic concepts behind the pathophysiology of radiation injury and risk factors for complications.

MECHANISM OF RADIATION INJURY

There are several modalities of radiation therapy currently in clinical use, including photons (X-rays or gamma rays, the most commonly used form of cranial radiation),

Disclosure: The authors have no relevant disclosure to make.
[a] Dana-Farber/Brigham and Women's Cancer Center, Harvard Medical School, 75 Francis Street, L2, Boston, MA 02115, USA; [b] Dana-Farber/Brigham and Women's Cancer Center, Harvard Medical School, 420 Brookline Avenue, Boston, MA 02215, USA
* Corresponding author.
E-mail address: STanguturi@LROC.harvard.edu

Neurol Clin 36 (2018) 599–625
https://doi.org/10.1016/j.ncl.2018.04.012
neurologic.theclinics.com

electrons, protons, and other particle-based radiation. CRT may be delivered from an external source (teletherapy) or through implanted or injectable radioisotopes (brachytherapy). Although these radiation modalities vary in their physical properties and dose distribution within tissue, all CRT is thought to rely on double-stranded DNA breakage as the primary mechanism of cell death in target tissues.[1]

Techniques such as stereotactic radiosurgery (SRS) or fractionated stereotactic radiotherapy (SRT) are increasingly used to minimize irradiation of adjacent normal tissues, enabling a higher dose per treatment (fraction).[2] Common doses include 12 to 24 Gy in 1 fraction for SRS and 15 to 40 Gy in 3 to 5 fractions for SRT.[1] It is now increasingly understood that SRS and SRT result in additional mechanisms of tissue injury, resulting in a more ablative effect.[3–6] As such, conventional models of cell survival after radiation, such as the linear-quadratic model, may underestimate the degree of cell damage after SRS and SRT.[7]

Several mechanisms have been hypothesized to contribute to normal tissue injury. Endothelial damage through endothelial cell apoptosis can be observed 24 hours after high doses of radiation in preclinical studies, and this process has been linked with subacute disruptions in the blood-brain barrier and with late vascular effects, including telangiectasia formation, microvascular malformations and dilatation, and histologic hyalinization of vessel walls, with a corresponding increase in the risk of ischemic stroke or intracranial hemorrhage.[8,9] Similarly, endothelial damage through fibrinoid necrosis of small vessels is associated with tissue radionecrosis through a process of capillary leakage and demyelination of the surrounding brain parenchyma.[10,11] Radionecrosis seems to be mediated by the vascular endothelial growth factor (VEGF) and by a self-perpetuating cycle of cellular and cytokine-mediated inflammation.

Risk Factors for Radiation Injury

Tissue factors

Each tissue manifests radiation injury uniquely with varying times of onset, duration, and severity of clinical symptoms. Rapidly proliferating tissues such as skin and mucosal surfaces manifest early treatment effects and associated symptoms. In contrast, slowly proliferating tissues such as neurons and microglia can take years to demonstrate tissue injury, if at all, and this injury may be irreversible. Clinical practice often relies on models of cellular death after radiation (such as the 2-compartment model[12] and the linear-quadratic model[13,14]) to estimate the risk of dose-limiting toxicities in nontarget normal tissues while maintaining doses sufficient for durable tumor control. However, as described earlier, these models may be insufficient to predict tumor kill and tissue injury in the context of higher doses per fraction, concurrent chemotherapy, and a more nuanced understanding of tissue heterogeneity and dynamic radiation resistance mechanisms.[15,16]

There is increasing evidence to suggest that complications from CRT may have an anatomic and histologic dependence as well. Neuroglial progenitor cells within several intracranial niches may have the capacity for proliferation and neurogenesis and influence response to radiation injury; accordingly, radiation-induced cytotoxicity of neuroglial progenitor may have disproportionate effects on toxicity. Neural stem cells in the hippocampus, for example, have been linked to memory formation.[17] Avoidance of this region during radiation therapy was shown to reduce cognitive decline relative to historical controls,[18] and this has become the subject of 2 ongoing randomized trials in the United States.[19,20] Similarly, radiation injury to neural stem cells in the subventricular zone and oligodendrocyte precursor cells along white matter tracts may contribute to neurocognitive impairment and reduced neural plasticity.[21,22] In addition, retrospective studies suggest an association with tumor histology, receptor status, and mutational status with radionecrosis after SRS.[23]

Radiation factors
Complications from CRT, including radiation necrosis and cognitive dysfunction, are also heavily influenced by treatment factors such as total radiation dosage, radiation fraction size and schedule, and the volume of normal brain irradiated. In one systematic literature review, rates of radiation necrosis ranged from 5% to 10% after conventionally dosed radiation with fraction sizes of less than 2.5 Gy/d; however, these rates increased steeply for twice-daily radiation schedules and were much less predictable for treatments with larger fraction sizes of greater than or equal to 2.5 Gy/d.[24] Similarly, the dose and volume of treated tissue have been linked to neurocognitive outcomes after conventional treatments in children[25–27] and to necrosis risk after single-fraction SRS.[28–32]

Patient factors
Clinical factors also seem to confound or affect the risk of radiation complications. These factors include patient comorbidities, age, genetics, prior treatment history (including prior radiation), anticipated future treatment course, and the natural course of the treated disease. Comorbidities such as diabetes and hypertension may increase the risk of vascular damage and necrosis,[33] multiple sclerosis[34,35] and collagen vascular diseases such as scleroderma may increase the risk of severe or fatal neurotoxicity,[35,36] and familial cancer syndromes such as Li-Fraumeni syndrome may increase the risk of radiation-induced malignancy.[37,38]

Patient genetics may contribute to increased radiation sensitivity and susceptibility to radiation complications.[39,40] Small studies have shown several genetic predictors for radiation complications, including radiation-induced meningiomas[41] and other organ-specific effects.[40,42,43] In contrast, among patients receiving radiation for vestibular schwannomas, those with neurofibromatosis type II seem to have a greater risk of hearing loss from treatment, suggesting an intrinsically different susceptibility to complications.[44]

Patient age is also associated with risks of neurocognitive decline and radiation complications at both ends of the spectrum. Younger age at the time of treatment (<5–7 years of age) is associated with greater relative declines in intelligence quotient (IQ), reading skills, processing speed, working memory, and broad attention,[45,46] and also with a greater risk of late endocrinopathies.[47] Similarly, older age (>60 years old) is associated with greater declines on serial neurocognitive testing after whole-brain radiation therapy (WBRT) for brain metastases[18,48] and after definitive chemotherapy and radiation therapy or primary central nervous system (CNS) lymphoma.[48–50]

Prior and future treatment history play a role in modifying the risk of CRT. Concurrent or sequential chemotherapy increases the risk of radiation-induced encephalopathy,[51] and this has been shown strikingly in primary CNS lymphoma.[48,52] Furthermore, future treatment with chemotherapy has been linked with a poorly understood phenomenon of radiation recall, an acute inflammatory reaction confined to previously irradiated areas, reported most commonly after receipt of anthracyclines, taxanes, and antimetabolite chemotherapies.[52]

The remainder of this article focuses on specific neurologic complications from CRT, organized by early and delayed onset of complications (**Table 1**). In addition, this review offers a brief discussion on evaluation and management wherever possible.

Table 1
Neurologic and medical complications of fractionated cranial radiotherapy

Early Complications	Delayed Complications
Fatigue	Pseudoprogression
Skin reaction	Radiation necrosis
Alopecia	Neurocognitive changes
Headaches	Cerebrovascular effects (vascular malformations,
Anorexia	hemorrhage, strokes, vasculopathy)
Nausea/vomiting	SMART syndrome
Exacerbation of neurologic symptoms	Cataracts
Serous otitis media (ear fullness,	Dry eyes
pain, conductive hearing loss)	Optic neuropathy
Parotitis	Hearing loss, tinnitus, chronic otitis
Encephalopathy (acute or early	Endocrinopathy
delayed)	Secondary malignancy

Abbreviation: SMART, strokelike migraine attacks after radiation therapy.

EARLY COMPLICATIONS OF CRANIAL RADIATION THERAPY
Fatigue

Incidence/severity
Fatigue may be defined as drowsiness, lethargy, and somnolence and is one of the most commonly reported complications across all cancer therapies. Among patients with primary brain tumors such as glioblastoma, 80% to 90% of patients report some degree of fatigue related to radiation therapy.[53,54] Fatigue is most commonly mild, but up to half of patients experience more noticeable symptoms in which activities are curtailed, sleep is needed through much of the day, or fatigue is unimproved after rest. Severe manifestations such as somnolence syndrome are rare. Fatigue may occur within the first 2 weeks of fractionated radiation therapy and may reach a maximum level within 2 to 4 weeks after treatment completion. Symptoms typically resolve over several months but may be reported even 6 to 12 months after treatment.

Evaluation
Patients should be evaluated for other causes of fatigue, including sleep disturbances, cardiopulmonary disorders, hematologic conditions, metabolic or endocrine disturbances, nutritional deficiencies, depression or mood disorder, and medications (including antiepileptic therapies). If fatigue is persistent after treatment, formal neurocognitive testing or sleep studies could be considered.

Management
Treatment of fatigue is largely supportive and conservative. Patient are often recommended to maintain regular sleep schedules and to allow naps as needed during the day. Light exercise and high-protein diets may also be recommended if clinically appropriate. Increasingly, patients are being introduced to complementary therapies and mind-body medicine approaches with yoga, meditation, massage therapy, polarity therapy,[55,56] reiki,[57] therapeutic touch, healing touch, and qi gong, with some evidence to support their use. Psychostimulants may be considered for bothersome or refractory fatigue.[58] However, multiple placebo-controlled randomized trials have shown evidence of a strong placebo effect with no significant benefit from methylphenidate,[59] modafinil,[60] or armodafinil.[61]

Headaches

Incidence/severity

Mild headaches may occur with cranial radiation, although typically without need for intervention. In one series, no more than 17% of patients developed mild-moderate headaches requiring medical intervention.[62]

Evaluation

Occasionally, headaches are related to underlying tumor progression or an increase in peritumoral edema, often exacerbated by treatment. Patients should be evaluated thoroughly for any progressive neurologic deficits or for other signs of increased intracranial pressure, including new or progressive nausea, vomiting, vision changes, gait instability, or incontinence.

Management

First-line pharmacologic therapy typically involves acetaminophen for more bothersome headaches. For headaches attributed to increasing peritumoral edema, corticosteroids such as dexamethasone are preferred to any analgesic or narcotic medications. Refractory or concerning symptoms should prompt further evaluation including imaging.

Exacerbation of Neurologic Symptoms

Incidence/severity

Many patients with brain tumors are symptomatic from peritumoral edema at the time of presentation before treatment. CRT can exacerbate peri-tumoral swelling, which in turn may worsen or unmask neurologic symptoms. Acute or early delayed memory disturbances may also develop, but these defects are generally transient and are not thought to portend long-term cognitive impairment. Small prospective studies of patients with low-grade tumors receiving partial brain radiation seem to show a transient decrement in verbal memory and potentially visual memory at 1.5 months post-treatment, followed by a recovery to baseline function by 1 year.[63,64]

Evaluation

Expected symptoms that are concordant with the patient's initial symptoms or tumor localization may be managed supportively. Unexpected or discordant neurologic symptoms may prompt further investigation with imaging if clinically concerning.

Management

Patients with pretreatment symptoms attributable to peritumoral edema or those at high risk for early symptomatic exacerbation may be considered for prophylactic glucocorticoids before starting radiation.[65,66] Patients with severe symptoms may be placed on dexamethasone with an initial loading dose of 10 mg followed by 16 mg/d.[67] Smaller doses per day (4–8 mg/d) are typically adequate for most patients, and doses may be given in once-daily or twice-daily schedules given the long biological half-life of dexamethasone (36–54 hours).[68] Patients may respond within hours of administration; once symptomatically improved, patients can taper their dosages by approximately 50% every 4 days. Prophylaxis for pneumocystis pneumonia may be considered for patients expected to receive prolonged courses of corticosteroid therapy (>4–6 weeks).[69]

Encephalopathy

Incidence/severity

Acute radiation encephalopathy is a rare complication characterized by severe headache, nausea, drowsiness, focal neurologic deficits, and fever from increased intracranial pressure, occurring days to weeks after irradiation.[70,71] Acute radiation encephalopathy is thought to be related to cerebral edema from disruptions in the blood-brain barrier, which in extreme cases may result in cerebral herniation and death. Early delayed encephalopathy may occur 1 to 6 months postirradiation, and is characterized by transient demyelination with somnolence. Historically, acute and early delayed encephalopathy occurred when whole-brain doses were delivered in fractions of 3 Gy or higher; however, in the modern era, WBRT is typically delivered in fractions of 3 Gy or fewer in the United States, and the risk of acute encephalopathy is exceedingly low.

Evaluation
Patients should have a comprehensive work-up to evaluate for metabolic, infectious, vascular, nutritional, or other disorders. MRI may demonstrate increased cerebral edema, but symptoms may also occur in the absence of radiographic findings.

Management
Acute and early delayed radiation encephalopathy, despite their potentially severe presentations, are typically reversible and may even resolve spontaneously. Corticosteroids are typically first-line treatment, and more invasive maneuvers to reduce intracranial hypertension may be considered in severe cases (eg, hypertonic saline, intravenous mannitol).

Edema-Related Complications of Stereotactic Radiosurgery/Stereotactic Radiotherapy

Incidence/severity
The Radiation Therapy Oncology Group (RTOG) 9005 established maximum tolerated doses of 24 Gy, 18 Gy, and 15 Gy respectively for tumors measuring less than 2 cm, 2.1 to 3.0 cm, and 3.1 to 4.0 cm in diameter.[72,73] In this study, acute severe CNS toxicities occurred in 0% to 17% across the 3 dose levels.

By 12 to 48 hours after SRS, there can be a transient increase in edema, which may contribute to symptoms within 2 weeks of treatment, including mild nausea, dizziness, vertigo, seizures, or new headaches.[74] These early effects have been reported in up to one-third of patients in a dose-dependent manner but do not seem to be predictive of subsequent late complications. Nausea may be more common for treatments near the area postrema.

Rarely, acute complications can result in severe neurologic events, including new focal deficits or seizures. In one retrospective series, severe neurologic events occurred in 18 of 835 treated patients within 7 days of SRS; 3 events were fatal.[75] Seizures may occur more commonly for treated lesions along the motor cortex,[76] and other risk factors for early SRS complications include dose, treatment volume, and concurrent systemic therapies, including chemotherapy, targeted therapy, or immunotherapy.

Evaluation
Patients and treatment plans should be evaluated thoroughly to predict for the risk of acute complications from SRS. Tumor size, treatment dosage, tumor location, and preexisting symptoms may help to inform the need for prophylactic mediations. As part of this evaluation, patients should be screened for comorbidities that may be affected by prophylactic corticosteroids. Plans for ongoing systemic therapy should also be discussed thoroughly with the primary oncologist or neuro-oncologist.

Management
Prophylactic corticosteroid and antiepileptic medications are often prescribed before and/or after SRS for seizure and symptom prevention, although there is considerable

variation in this practice and no prospective data on this topic.[77] There is similarly no consensus on the management of ongoing systemic therapies. To minimize acute and late complications, our practice is to withhold cytotoxic chemotherapy and targeted therapy for at least 4 to 5 half-lives before SRS whenever possible. Concurrent immunotherapy may be given more permissively, given the long half-life of duration, latency for effect, and indirect mechanism of action, although further investigation on this subject is needed.[78,79]

DELAYED COMPLICATIONS OF CRANIAL RADIATION THERAPY
Pseudoprogression

Incidence/severity
Pseudoprogression refers to subacute treatment-induced changes that may falsely mimic the appearance of tumor progression on MRI. This phenomenon often occurs within the first 3 months of completion of chemoradiation for gliomas[80] and is assessed retrospectively based on radiographic resolution or stabilization. Associated symptoms are seen less commonly in patients with pseudoprogression compared with those with true progression (33% vs 67%).[81]

Evaluation
MRI changes occurring in the absence of clinical symptoms and/or at early posttreatment imaging time points (especially in patients with glioblastoma with O_6-methylguanine DNA methyltransferase promoter methylation[82]) may be more suggestive of pseudoprogression than progression. Advanced imaging may reveal a lactate peak on magnetic resonance spectroscopy (MRS), decreased cerebral blood volume (CBV) on tumor perfusion imaging, or lack of hypermetabolism on PET imaging, but even these tools maintain a fair degree of uncertainty.[83]

Management
Patients with imaging features concerning for pseudoprogression should be followed closely with repeat magnetic resonance surveillance. For patients with progressive or impending symptoms or with concerning radiographic features, brain biopsy, resection, or salvage therapies may be indicated.[84]

Radiation Necrosis

Incidence/severity
Radiation necrosis is a late complication of radiation therapy, occurring 1 to 3 years after treatment (**Fig. 1**), with some late cases reported 10 years after treatment.[85] Among patients receiving conventional schedules of radiation ($\leq$4 Gy/d), necrosis seems to be dose dependent, occurring with a 5% risk at 72 Gy[10]; however, this is likely highly influenced by the number of doses per day and the presence of concurrent systemic therapies. Necrosis tends to occur at or around the treatment target, but brain and brainstem necrosis can also occur after treatment of tumors outside the brain, such as nasopharyngeal carcinoma.[86] Depending on the location, necrosis may present with focal neurologic signs or symptoms; increased intracranial pressure; or complex deficits in gait, balance, and cranial nerves, as with brainstem necrosis.

Among patients treated with SRS/SRT, radiation necrosis may occur in approximately 10%[87–92] and in 4% to 18% of patients treated with postoperative SRS at an interval of 6 months to many years after treatment.[93–96] Prior receipt of WBRT or SRS along with tumor size are the biggest risk factors for necrosis. Tumors larger than 2 cm may be treated with hypofractionated SRT to reduce the risk of necrosis.[97] Chemotherapy, targeted therapy, and immunotherapy may increase the risk of

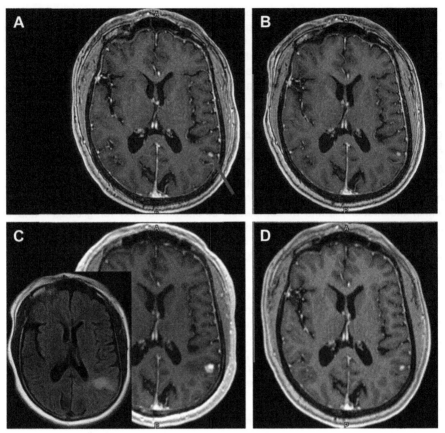

Fig. 1. Radiation necrosis. Serial MRI is shown of a patient with stage IIB lung adenocarcinoma treated with lobectomy and adjuvant cisplatin/vinorelbine chemotherapy, presenting with oligometastatic brain metastases. (*A*) Presentation of a left parietal enhancing tumor (*arrow*), presumed to be a metastasis. This tumor was treated with SRS to 20 Gy in 1 fraction. (*B*) Interval partial response, 5 months after SRS. (*C*) Increased size and more heterogeneous enhancement with surrounding T2/fluid-attenuated inversion recovery (FLAIR) hyperintensity concerning for early radiation necrosis, 13 months after SRS. (*D*) Interval self-resolution of necrotic changes without specific intervention, 20 months after SRS and 7 months after onset of necrosis.

necrosis to as high as 17%, 25%, and 38% respectively,[98–100] but these treatments may also increase the rate of intracranial tumor control.

Evaluation

Differentiating radiation necrosis from tumor progression often presents a challenge. Standard MRI may demonstrate a progressive contrast-enhancing mass with central necrosis localizing within the high-dose treatment volume; however, these imaging features are nonspecific and typically indistinguishable from tumor progression. Additional suggestions of necrosis on MRI may include the lack of a definable mass lesion on T2-weighted imaging[93] and a high edema/enhancing lesion volume ratio.[101] Ultimately, these lesions generally require serial follow-up to distinguish between tumor growth versus evolving radiation necrosis.[9] As discussed earlier, advanced imaging may reveal a lactate peak or a lipid peak on MRS,[95,96,102–105] decreased CBV on tumor perfusion imaging,[94,106] lack of restricted diffusion on diffusion-weighted MRI,[107] and lack of uptake on fluorodeoxyglucose[108–114] or methionine[115] PET or thallium chloride-201 single photon emission CT imaging.[116] Advanced imaging as described may be helpful but is often reserved for decision making before salvage therapies such as surgery or bevacizumab. For patients with progressive symptoms or with concerning radiographic features, a brain biopsy or resection may be necessary.

Management

Radiation necrosis is often a self-limited process and often subsides within 5 to 7 months after onset (see **Fig. 1**). Asymptomatic patients may be observed without intervention. Symptomatic patients may be treated with a moderate dose of corticosteroids (ie, dexamethasone 4–8 mg daily) until symptomatic improvement followed by a gradual taper. Follow-up imaging 1 to 2 months after intervention may be helpful to confirm response. Patients intolerant of corticosteroids or unable to taper their dosage can consider salvage treatments for necrosis with bevacizumab or laser interstitial thermal therapy.

Bevacizumab is thought to normalize VEGF-mediated increased capillary permeability and extracellular edema seen in radiation necrosis; its use is supported by multiple retrospective series[88,117–123] and a small randomized double-blind placebo-controlled trial that showed radiographic improvement in all patients receiving bevacizumab as initial therapy or at crossover.[120] This benefit has been drawn into question by other retrospective series.[121,122,124] The relative efficacy of bevacizumab versus steroids may be better evaluated through an ongoing phase II randomized study, Alliance A221208, for patients with brain metastases with necrosis after SRS.[125]

LITT is occasionally considered for refractory necrosis and can be combined with a biopsy. Retrospective series have shown promising results,[126–128] but there are no randomized data to support its use. Surgical resection may be required in select cases with significant mass effect or diagnostic uncertainty. Other investigational therapies include therapeutic anticoagulation, antiplatelet therapy, and hyperbaric oxygen therapy,[113,129,130] but prospective data are again lacking.

Neurocognitive Changes

Incidence/severity

Several neurocognitive effects have been described as late effects after CRT. Decline in cognitive function following CRT has been best described in children. In a Finnish cancer registry, children with brain tumors showed significantly lower scholastic achievement in all ninth-grade subjects compared with matched population controls, most notably for girls treated with radiation.[131] This finding was shown specifically among childhood survivors of acute lymphoblastic leukemia (ALL),[132] with most pronounced effects on IQ scores seen among children younger than 6 years of age who received high-dose CRT ($\geq$24 Gy) in combination with intrathecal chemotherapy.[133] In the era of reduced use of CRT in ALL, the incidence and severity of cognitive decline seems to have decreased.[134–137] Among pediatric patients with primary brain tumors treated at St Jude, Cerebrospinal irradiation (CSI) has been associated with higher rates of severe cognitive impairment (IQ<70) and with significant reductions in IQ compared with limited field or no radiation (−1.3 vs −0.5 vs +0.9 IQ points per year).[138] Among children with medulloblastoma treated in the modern era, high-risk patients treated with higher dose CSI (36–39.6 Gy) showed more pronounced declines in IQ, reading, spelling, and mathematics[45] and with process speed, attention, and working memory[46] than their standard-risk counterparts who received lower dose CSI; age at diagnosis was the most important predictor for late neurocognitive effects.

In adults, WBRT and partial brain radiation therapy similarly have been shown to be associated with neurocognitive effects. In a small randomized study investigating SRS with or without WBRT for patients with limited brain metastases, WBRT was associated a significant decline in learning and memory function as assessed by Hopkins Verbal Learning Test–Revised (HVLT-R) total recall at 4 months.[139] These results were initially questioned because of confounding from strikingly inferiorly survival outcomes in the WBRT group, but more recent studies have confirmed declines in HVLT 1 year after prophylactic cranial irradiation for locally advanced non–small cell lung cancer[140] and declines in a battery of neurocognitive testing and quality of life 3 months after WBRT.[141] In an European Organisation for Research and Treatment of Cancer (EORTC) randomized study, WBRT was associated with a greater decline in patient-reported cognitive function at 1 year compared with SRS alone.[142] Corresponding radiographic changes, including nonspecific diffuse white matter changes[143] and cerebral atrophy,[92,144] may be seen with WBRT doses of 20 Gy or higher among patients surviving beyond 1 year. The severity of these effects may correlate with the degree of symptoms.[144] Severe leukoencephalopathy, presenting with ataxia, confusion, memory loss, dementia, and rarely death, occurs in less than 5% of patients and is typically associated with large fraction size of radiation, which is now uncommonly used for WBRT.[89] When counseling patients receiving WBRT, providers should also consider the effects of systemic therapy, concurrent medications, baseline neurocognitive function, comorbidities, and overall prognosis to better assess the impact of WBRT on neurocognition and quality of life.

The impact of partial brain radiation on neurocognition is less well established and draws heavily from studies of patients with low-grade glioma with more favorable prognoses. In an observational study of 195 patients with low-grade gliomas in the Netherlands, the impact of radiation on cognition was apparent only among those patients receiving high daily doses (>2 Gy per fraction)[145]; a greater impact on cognition was estimated from the brain tumor along with antiepileptic drug use. In contrast, a later analysis of 65 patients from the cohort discussed earlier who completed formal neurocognitive testing at a mean of 12 years after diagnosis demonstrated a progressive decline in attentional functioning among patients receiving radiotherapy relative to those who did not, even among those receiving low fractional doses (≤2 Gy per fraction). These changes were also associated with radiographic white matter hyperintensity and global cortical atrophy.[146] Nonetheless, this study excluded patients with recurrent tumors from the analysis, likely underestimating the cognitive impact of tumor recurrence among those not treated with radiotherapy. In the modern era, it is possible that highly conformal and stereotactic radiotherapy may lessen the impact of radiotherapy on cognition, as suggested by a randomized study from India comparing global and performance IQ scores at 5 years among patients treated with highly conformal versus conventional radiation fields.[100] The intergroup dose-escalation study comparing 2 doses of postoperative radiotherapy (50.4 Gy and 64.8 Gy) in 203 patients with low-grade glioma identified minimal changes in either group in Folstein Mini-Mental State Examination (MMSE) testing.[147,148] The addition of PCV (procarbazine, lomustine, and vincristine) chemotherapy to radiation in this population similarly shows no significant impact on MMSE testing, as shown in a subgroup analysis of the RTOG 9801 randomized study.[149,150] Nonetheless, the lack of cognitive change in these studies may be reflective of the poor sensitivity afforded by MMSE testing.[151]

Evaluation

Among childhood survivors of CNS malignancies treated with CRT, serial neuropsychiatric examinations are recommended to assess the educational and emotional needs of children over time. These examinations may be done every 2 years or at transitions into new schools or learning environments.

Patients with a concern for neurocognitive dysfunction should undergo a formal evaluation including a thorough history, review of medications, screening for mood disorders or sleep disturbances, and so forth. Available imaging should be evaluated for reversible causes of cognitive function, including hydrocephalus or disease progression. Laboratory evaluation may include screening for vitamin deficiencies (vitamin B_{12} or folate deficiency), metabolic disturbances, and thyroid dysfunction. In adults, formal neurocognitive and neuropsychologic testing are not typically part of the standard work-up and surveillance of such patients, but these assessments may be valuable in uncovering specific cognitive domains for rehabilitation and/or underlying mood disorders to guide treatment.

Management

Reversible causes of cognitive dysfunction such as hydrocephalus are occasionally treated with a surgical procedure such as ventriculoperitoneal shunting.[90,91] For patients with persistent or progressive neurocognitive dysfunction after CRT, neurocognitive rehabilitation and pharmacologic interventions with agents such as methylphenidate, donepezil, and memantine may be considered. Given the mixed data to support such interventions, treatment decisions should be patient specific with consideration to patient comorbidities, specific domains of dysfunction, patient preference, and cost. Neurostimulants such as methylphenidate, modafinil, or armodafinil may be effective in patients seeking therapy for profound fatigue and low motivation, with positive[152] and negative studies[59,61,153] to support such treatments. Acetylcholinesterase inhibitors may also be considered, largely extrapolating from the benefits among patients with dementia. One phase II study of a 24-week course of donepezil in 34 patients with low-grade gliomas who received radiation showed improvements in cognitive functioning, mood, and health-related quality of life at 24 weeks relative to baseline.[154] A follow-up randomized study of donepezil versus placebo in 198 patients with brain tumors who received CRT showed improvements in memory and motor domains, especially for patients with lower baseline cognition. However, this study failed to show a benefit in the prespecified primary outcome of a composite score of cognitive performance, subjective confusion, and fatigue.[155]

Much effort has also been placed into strategies to prevent neurocognitive impairment from WBRT. In a randomized placebo-controlled study in patients receiving WBRT, memantine, an oral N-methyl-D-aspartate (NMDA) receptor antagonist, improved time to cognitive decline, executive function at 8 and 16 weeks, processing speed, and delayed recognition but did not improve the primary end point of HVLT-R delayed recall at 24 weeks.[156] Given the minimal added risk to patients and the lack of other options, many clinicians recommend a 6-month course of memantine with WBRT. Parallel efforts have investigated the use of hippocampal-avoidance (HA) WBRT to limit radiation exposure of neuroprogenitor stem cells in the hippocampus. A phase 2 study (RTOG 0933) comparing HA-WBRT with historical controls showed promising rates of HVLT-R total recall 4 months after radiation.[18] Based on these encouraging early results, 2 randomized trials are ongoing currently to further investigate this technique.[19,20]

Cerebrovascular Effects

Incidence/severity

Late cerebrovascular effects from radiation, including cavernous malformations, vascular disease/stroke, intracranial hemorrhage, and moyamoya disease, have been described. Risk factors for radiation-related vasculopathy include younger age at treatment, irradiation of the supraclinoid internal carotid artery and circle of Willis, radiation dose, receipt of chemotherapy, and a history of neurofibromatosis type 1.[157–159]

Cavernomas are the most common vasculopathy, occurring at a median interval of 3 to 6 years after cranial irradiation, with rates ranging from 3% to 43%.[160–162] Higher incidence has been described in series with sensitive imaging techniques[162] and among children compared with adults.[160,163] Cavernomas may grow over time and be associated with a low risk of hemorrhage.

Stroke risk has been described most thoroughly in the Childhood Cancer Survivor Study of survivors of pediatric leukemia and brain tumors, in which the risk of late strokes among brain tumor survivors was 3.4% at a median of 14 years from diagnosis, with rates as high as 6.5% among those who received radiation and alkylating chemotherapy. Uniquely, this study identified that these rates were higher than sibling controls in this cohort.[158] In a prospective randomized study of dose escalation for meningioma, stroke was noted in 20% of patients at a median of 5.6 years after therapy.[164] Radiation dose to the circle of Willis seems to be the strongest risk factor, particularly for doses higher than 40 Gy but potentially as low as 10 Gy with longer follow-up.[165] Unexplained recurrent headache also seems to predict for stroke or transient ischemic attack independent of other risk factors.[166]

Although cranial irradiation rarely results in significant cervical carotid dosage, carotid artery disease and atherosclerosis are well-known effects of high-dose head and neck radiation[167] with a corresponding increased stroke risk among these patients.[168] Radiation to the lower carotid arteries for treatment of the supraclavicular or internal mammary lymph nodes in breast cancer does not seem to carry a similar risk of stroke.[169]

Vasculopathy resembling moyamoya disease has been reported at a median of 40 months after radiation, with apparent higher rates among patients with younger age (<5 years old), neurofibromatosis type 1, or low-grade glioma.[170,171]

Collectively, these cerebrovascular effects may result in an increased risk of cerebrovascular mortality among brain tumor survivors. In a population study of Medicare data of more than 19,500 patients with brain tumors excluding glioblastoma, late cerebrovascular mortality was higher among patients receiving radiation for tumors near central arterial circulations, with rates of 0.6% and 1.1% at 10 and 20 years respectively.[172]

Management

There are no clear guidelines for primary or secondary prevention of stroke in this population. Antiplatelet therapy and mitigation of other cardiovascular risk factors can be considered on an individualized basis through multidisciplinary discussion. Patients with a history of high-dose head and neck radiation may consider screening carotid ultrasonography 5 to 10 years after treatment.[173]

Strokelike Migraine Attacks After Radiation Therapy

Incidence/severity

Strokelike migraine attacks after radiation therapy (SMART) is a rare disorder characterized by migrainelike headaches occasionally with focal neurologic signs or seizures (**Fig. 2**).[174] Symptoms typically occur late after radiation and may last for days to weeks followed by resolution. MRI may reveal focal gadolinium enhancement, often mimicking progressive tumor. Although the pathophysiology of this disorder remains unclear,[175] recent studies have suggested an association with prolonged electrographic seizures as identified on systematic continuous electroencephalogram monitoring.[176]

Management

SMART is a self-resolving condition with no specific treatment other than supportive therapy and antiepileptic therapy if indicated.

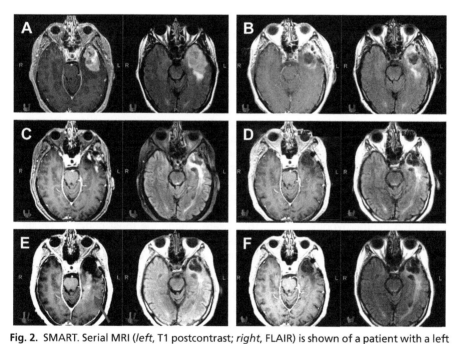

Fig. 2. SMART. Serial MRI (*left*, T1 postcontrast; *right*, FLAIR) is shown of a patient with a left temporal glioblastoma. The left temporal tumor is shown at initial presentation (*A*), after surgical resection before chemoradiation (*B*), and after completion of adjuvant chemoradiation, and 1 year of adjuvant dose-dense temozolomide (*C*). The patient remained clinically well with radiographic stability of disease 9.5 years after diagnosis (*D*). The patient presented again 10 years after diagnosis with new-onset fever, right facial droop, and right-sided weakness. MRI showed diffuse temporal enhancement and cortical thickening (*red arrow*), initially concerning for encephalitis (*E*). Lumbar puncture showed an increased protein level (107 mg/dL) and lymphocytic pleocytosis (white blood cell count 8 cells/μL) and an extensive infectious work-up was negative. Electroencephalogram revealed clinically silent seizures, which responded to levetiracetam therapy. The patient was diagnosed with SMART syndrome and clinically improved with a course of antiepileptic therapy and high-dose corticosteroids. Follow-up imaging 4 weeks later showed radiographic resolution of enhancement and cortical thickening (*F*).

Optic Neuropathy

Incidence/severity
Radiation-induced optic neuropathy (RION) typically presents with painless visual impairment (monocular or binocular depending on the location of injury) occurring between 6 and 24 months after treatment. Symptoms may progress over the course of 1 week to several weeks after onset. RION demonstrates a clear dose relationship: for conventionally fractionated treatment, severe optic neuropathy occurs rarely with doses less than 55 Gy, in 3% to 7% with doses between 55 to 60 Gy, and in 7% to 20% with doses greater than 60 Gy.[177] Larger fraction sizes (>2.5 Gy per fraction) also seem to increase the risk.[178] After SRS, RION occurs infrequently when doses to the anterior visual pathway are kept less than 10 Gy[179] or 12 Gy in 1 fraction.[180]

Evaluation
Formal neuro-ophthalmologic testing may confirm loss of vision with reduced health of the optic disc and nerve. MRI may show signal abnormality with optic nerve enhancement.

Management
However, there is no treatment proved to benefit RION. Hyperbaric oxygen,[181,182] oral corticosteroids, and anticoagulation may be considered but have limited data to support their use.

Endocrinopathy

Incidence/severity
Late endocrinopathies are common after CRT. Hypothalamic and pituitary dysfunction may occur in 80% of patients after doses as low as 20 Gy to these organs.[183–190] Endocrinopathies may be noted as early as 1 year after treatment and increase in prevalence over time. In a systematic review of patients with nonpituitary tumors treated with CRT, hypopituitarism was identified among 37% to 77% of patients, occurring between 3 and 13 years after radiation.[190] Growth hormone deficiency (50%), gonadotropin deficiency (25%), hyperprolactinemia (24%), adrenocorticotropic hormone deficiency (19%), and central hypothyroidism (16%) were among the most common pituitary axes affected. Pediatric patients with sellar or suprasellar tumors, including craniopharyngioma, may experience hypothalamic obesity after treatment.[191]

Evaluation
Patients who receive radiation to the hypothalamus or pituitary should undergo a baseline neuroendocrine evaluation within 1 year of treatment with annual follow-up. Long-term survivors should undergo periodic monitoring of thyroid-stimulating hormone and free T4 (thyroxine).

Management
Most patients with endocrinopathies are offered hormonal supplementation. Ideally, this may be managed by a neuroendocrinologist or by providers with experience titrating hormonal supplementation. Treatments for hypothalamic obesity with amphetamine derivatives, glucagonlike peptide 1 (GLP1) analogues, and oxytocin are being investigated.[191]

Secondary Malignancy

Incidence/severity
Radiation-induced malignancy is a rare but dreaded late complication. Following CRT, patients may be at increased risk for late secondary meningiomas, malignant

gliomas, nerve sheath tumors, and sarcomas, with some tumor histologies showing a dose-dependent risk. In the Childhood Cancer Survivor Study, gliomas were detected in 0.3% of patients, with an odds ratio of 6.8 among those with prior CRT.[192] Among patients with medulloblastoma treated with combined modality CSI and multiagent chemotherapy, secondary malignancies were identified in 4%.[193] Secondary malignancy may occur between 5 years and several decades after treatment, with increasing risk over time without plateau.[194] The association between narrow-field radiation, such as SRS and SRT, and secondary malignancy is less clear.[195]

Evaluation

Patients with a history of CRT should maintain long-term oncologic follow-up, possibly through a cancer survivorship program. Although routine imaging beyond standard oncologic follow-up is not recommended, work-up for unexplained symptoms should include head imaging.

Management

Patients with long-expected survival after treatment should be counseled over the risks of secondary malignancy. Proton beam radiation and other charged particle therapies can reduce the cumulative dose exposure for patients receiving treatment, which may translate to a reduction in secondary cancer risk[196,197]; however, randomized data comparing such outcomes after proton-based and photon-based therapy are currently lacking.

SUMMARY

Radiation therapy is a critical component of treatment of many brain tumors. These treatments carry risks in the short term and long term, and patients should be counseled about risks according to their expected prognosis, rationale for therapy, and individualized expectations for complications. Future efforts to mitigate risk by minimizing radiation dose and field, avoiding critical regions (ie, HA), and using proton-based/particle-based therapy are underway but randomized trials are lacking in many of these domains. In the absence of long-term comparative data on various options for treatment, clinicians assess the impact of these risks and individualize treatment decisions based on specific patient factors.

REFERENCES

1. Hall EJ, Giaccia AJ. Radiobiology for the radiologist. Philadelphia (PA): Lippincott Williams & Wilkins; 2012.
2. Potters L, Kavanagh B, Galvin JM, et al. American Society for Therapeutic Radiology and Oncology (ASTRO) and American College of Radiology (ACR) practice guideline for the performance of stereotactic body radiation therapy. Int J Radiat Oncol Biol Phys 2010;76(2):326–32.
3. Clement JJ, Tanaka N, Song CW. Tumor reoxygenation and postirradiation vascular changes. Radiology 1978;127(3):799–803.
4. Clement JJ, Song CW, Levitt SH. Changes in functional vascularity and cell number following x-irradiation of a murine carcinoma. Int J Radiat Oncol 1976; 1(7–8):671–8.
5. Song CW, Cho LC, Yuan J, et al. Radiobiology of stereotactic body radiation therapy/stereotactic radiosurgery and the linear-quadratic model. Int J Radiat Oncol Biol Phys 2013;87(1):18–9.

6. Kocher M, Treuer H, Voges J, et al. Computer simulation of cytotoxic and vascular effects of radiosurgery in solid and necrotic brain metastases. Radiother Oncol 2000;54(2):149–56.

7. Kirkpatrick JP, Meyer JJ, Marks LB. The linear-quadratic model is inappropriate to model high dose per fraction effects in radiosurgery. Semin Radiat Oncol 2008;18(4):240–3.

8. Nordal RA, Wong CS. Molecular targets in radiation-induced blood-brain barrier disruption. Int J Radiat Oncol Biol Phys 2005;62(1):279–87.

9. Dietrich J, Gondi V, Mehta M. Delayed complications of cranial irradiation. In: DeAngelis LM, editor. Waltham (MA): UpToDate; 2017. Available at: https://www.uptodate.com/contents/delayed-complications-of-cranial-irradiation?search=Dietrich%20J,%20Gondi%20V,%20Mehta%20M.%20Delayed%20complications%20of%20cranial%20irradiation.%20In:%20DeAngelis%20LM,%20editor.%20Waltham%20(MA):%20UpToDate;%202017.%20. Accessed October 28, 2017.

10. Gutin PH, Leibel SA, Sheline GE. Radiation injury to the nervous system. New York: Raven Press; 1991.

11. Burger PC, Mahley MS, Dudka L, et al. The morphologic effects of radiation administered therapeutically for intracranial gliomas: a postmortem study of 25 cases. Cancer 1979;44(4):1256–72.

12. Puck TT, Marcus PI. Action of x-rays on mammalian cells. J Exp Med 1956; 103(5):653–66.

13. Catcheside DG, Lea DE, Thoday JM. The production of chromosome structural changes in *Tradescantia* microspores in relation to dosage, intensity and temperature. J Genet 1946;47:137–49.

14. Kellerer AM, Rossi HD. Theory of dual radiation action. Curr Top Radiat Res Q 1972;8(2):85–158.

15. Attolini CS, Cheng YK, Beroukhim R, et al. A mathematical framework to determine the temporal sequence of somatic genetic events in cancer. Proc Natl Acad Sci U S A 2010;107(41):17604–9.

16. Leder K, Pitter K, Laplant Q, et al. Mathematical modeling of PDGF-driven glioblastoma reveals optimized radiation dosing schedules. Cell 2014;156(3): 603–16.

17. Rola R, Raber J, Rizk A, et al. Radiation-induced impairment of hippocampal neurogenesis is associated with cognitive deficits in young mice. Exp Neurol 2004;188(2):316–30.

18. Gondi V, Pugh SL, Tome WA, et al. Preservation of memory with conformal avoidance of the hippocampal neural stem-cell compartment during whole-brain radiotherapy for brain metastases (RTOG 0933): a phase II multi-institutional trial. J Clin Oncol 2014;32(34):3810–6.

19. Gore E, Sun A, Ramalingam SS, et al. RTOG 0937: Randomized phase II study comparing prophylactic cranial irradiation alone to prophylactic cranial irradiation and consolidative extra-cranial irradiation for extensive disease small cell lung cancer (ED-SCLC). 2016. Available at: https://www.rtog.org/ClinicalTrials/ProtocolTable/StudyDetails.aspx?study=0937. Accessed November 30, 2017.

20. Brown P. NRG-CC001: memantine hydrochloride and whole-brain radiotherapy with or without hippocampal avoidance in reducing neurocognitive decline in patients with brain metastases. Available at: https://clinicaltrials.gov/ct2/show/study/NCT02360215#contacts. Accessed November 30, 2017.

21. Monje M, Dietrich J. Cognitive side effects of cancer therapy demonstrate a functional role for adult neurogenesis. Behav Brain Res 2012;227(2):376–9.

22. Dietrich J, Monje M, Wefel J, et al. Clinical patterns and biological correlates of cognitive dysfunction associated with cancer therapy. Oncologist 2008;13(12): 1285–95.
23. Miller JA, Bennett EE, Xiao R, et al. Association between radiation necrosis and tumor biology after stereotactic radiosurgery for brain metastasis. Int J Radiat Oncol Biol Phys 2016;96(5):1060–9.
24. Lawrence YR, Li XA, el Naqa I, et al. Radiation dose-volume effects in the brain. Int J Radiat Oncol 2010;76(3):S20–7.
25. Waber DP, Turek J, Catania L, et al. Neuropsychological outcomes from a randomized trial of triple intrathecal chemotherapy compared with 18 Gy cranial radiation as CNS treatment in acute lymphoblastic leukemia: findings from Dana-Farber Cancer Institute ALL Consortium Protocol 95-01. J Clin Oncol 2007; 25(31):4914–21.
26. Smibert E, Anderson V, Godber T, et al. Risk factors for intellectual and educational sequelae of cranial irradiation in childhood acute lymphoblastic leukaemia. Br J Cancer 1996;73(6):825–30.
27. Moore IM, Kramer JH, Wara W, et al. Cognitive function in children with leukemia. Effect of radiation dose and time since irradiation. Cancer 1991;68(9): 1913–7.
28. Minniti G, Clarke E, Lanzetta G, et al. Stereotactic radiosurgery for brain metastases: analysis of outcome and risk of brain radionecrosis. Radiat Oncol 2011; 6(1):48.
29. Flickinger JC, Lunsford LD, Kondziolka D, et al. Radiosurgery and brain tolerance: an analysis of neurodiagnostic imaging changes after gamma knife radiosurgery for arteriovenous malformations. Int J Radiat Oncol Biol Phys 1992; 23(1):19–26.
30. Voges J, Treuer H, Sturm V, et al. Risk analysis of linear accelerator radiosurgery. Int J Radiat Oncol Biol Phys 1996;36(5):1055–63.
31. Korytko T, Radivoyevitch T, Colussi V, et al. 12 Gy gamma knife radiosurgical volume is a predictor for radiation necrosis in non-AVM intracranial tumors. Int J Radiat Oncol Biol Phys 2006;64(2):419–24.
32. Blonigen BJ, Steinmetz RD, Levin L, et al. Irradiated volume as a predictor of brain radionecrosis after linear accelerator stereotactic radiosurgery. Int J Radiat Oncol Biol Phys 2010;77(4):996–1001.
33. Smith MC, Ryken TC, Buatti JM. Radiotoxicity after conformal radiation therapy for benign intracranial tumors. Neurosurg Clin North Am 2006;17(2):169–80, vii.
34. Miller RC, Lachance DH, Lucchinetti CF, et al. Multiple sclerosis, brain radiotherapy, and risk of neurotoxicity: the Mayo Clinic experience. Int J Radiat Oncol Biol Phys 2006;66(4):1178–86.
35. Lowell D, Tatter SB, Bourland JD, et al. Toxicity of gamma knife radiosurgery in the treatment of intracranial tumors in patients with collagen vascular diseases or multiple sclerosis. Int J Radiat Oncol Biol Phys 2011;81(4):e519–24.
36. Ross JG, Hussey DH, Mayr NA, et al. Acute and late reactions to radiation therapy in patients with collagen vascular diseases. Cancer 1993;71(11):3744–52.
37. Hisada M, Garber JE, Li FP, et al. Multiple primary cancers in families with Li-Fraumeni syndrome. J Natl Cancer Inst 1998;90(8):606–11.
38. Suri JS, Rednam S, Teh BS, et al. Subsequent malignancies in patients with Li-Fraumeni syndrome treated with radiation therapy. Int J Radiat Oncol 2013; 87(2):S71–2.
39. Andreassen CN, Alsner J. Genetic variants and normal tissue toxicity after radiotherapy: a systematic review. Radiother Oncol 2009;92(3):299–309.

40. West CM, Barnett GC. Genetics and genomics of radiotherapy toxicity: towards prediction. Genome Med 2011;3(8):52.
41. Hosking FJ, Feldman D, Bruchim R, et al. Search for inherited susceptibility to radiation-associated meningioma by genomewide SNP linkage disequilibrium mapping. Br J Cancer 2011;104(6):1049–54.
42. Barnett GC, West CML, Dunning AM, et al. Normal tissue reactions to radiotherapy: towards tailoring treatment dose by genotype. Nat Rev Cancer 2009; 9(2):134–42.
43. Rosenstein BS. Identification of SNPs associated with susceptibility for development of adverse reactions to radiotherapy. Pharmacogenomics 2011;12(2): 267–75.
44. Combs SE, Volk S, Schulz-Ertner D, et al. Management of acoustic neuromas with fractionated stereotactic radiotherapy (FSRT): long-term results in 106 patients treated in a single institution. Int J Radiat Oncol Biol Phys 2005;63(1): 75–81.
45. Mulhern RK, Palmer SL, Merchant TE, et al. Neurocognitive consequences of risk-adapted therapy for childhood medulloblastoma. J Clin Oncol 2005; 23(24):5511–9.
46. Palmer SL, Armstrong C, Onar-Thomas A, et al. Processing speed, attention, and working memory after treatment for medulloblastoma: an international, prospective, and longitudinal study. J Clin Oncol 2013;31(28):3494–500.
47. Kortmann R-D, Timmermann B, Taylor RE, et al. Current and future strategies in radiotherapy of childhood low-grade glioma of the brain. Strahlenther Onkol 2003;179(9):585–97.
48. Abrey LE, Yahalom J, DeAngelis LM. Treatment for primary CNS lymphoma: the next step. J Clin Oncol 2000;18(17):3144–50.
49. Fisher B, Seiferheld W, Schultz C, et al. Secondary analysis of Radiation Therapy Oncology Group study (RTOG) 9310: an intergroup phase ii combined modality treatment of primary central nervous system lymphoma. J Neurooncol 2005; 74(2):201–5.
50. DeAngelis LM, Seiferheld W, Schold SC, et al, Radiation therapy oncology group study 93-10. Combination chemotherapy and radiotherapy for primary central nervous system lymphoma: Radiation Therapy Oncology Group study 93-10. J Clin Oncol 2002;20(24):4643–8.
51. Crossen JR, Garwood D, Glatstein E, et al. Neurobehavioral sequelae of cranial irradiation in adults: a review of radiation-induced encephalopathy. J Clin Oncol 1994;12(3):627–42.
52. Lai R, Abrey LE, Rosenblum MK, et al. Treatment-induced leukoencephalopathy in primary CNS lymphoma: a clinical and autopsy study. Neurology 2004;62(3): 451–6.
53. Powell C, Guerrero D, Sardell S, et al. Somnolence syndrome in patients receiving radical radiotherapy for primary brain tumours: a prospective study. Radiother Oncol 2011;100(1):131–6.
54. Faithfull S, Brada M. Somnolence syndrome in adults following cranial irradiation for primary brain tumours. Clin Oncol (R Coll Radiol) 1998;10(4):250–4.
55. Roscoe JA, Matteson SE, Mustian KM, et al. Treatment of radiotherapy-induced fatigue through a nonpharmacological approach. Integr Cancer Ther 2005;4(1): 8–13.
56. Mustian KM, Roscoe JA, Palesh OG, et al. Polarity therapy for cancer-related fatigue in patients with breast cancer receiving radiation therapy: a randomized controlled pilot study. Integr Cancer Ther 2011;10(1):27–37.

57. Tsang KL, Carlson LE, Olson K. Pilot crossover trial of Reiki versus rest for treating cancer-related fatigue. Integr Cancer Ther 2007;6(1):25–35.
58. Breitbart W, Alici Y. Psychostimulants for cancer-related fatigue. J Natl Compr Canc Netw 2010;8(8):933–42.
59. Butler JM, Case LD, Atkins J, et al. A phase III, double-blind, placebo-controlled prospective randomized clinical trial of d-threo-methylphenidate HCl in brain tumor patients receiving radiation therapy. Int J Radiat Oncol Biol Phys 2007; 69(5):1496–501.
60. Boele FW, Douw L, de Groot M, et al. The effect of modafinil on fatigue, cognitive functioning, and mood in primary brain tumor patients: a multicenter randomized controlled trial. Neuro Oncol 2013;15(10):1420–8.
61. Lee EQ, Muzikansky A, Drappatz J, et al. A randomized, placebo-controlled pilot trial of armodafinil for fatigue in patients with gliomas undergoing radiotherapy. Neuro Oncol 2016;18(6):849–54.
62. Bitterlich C, Vordermark D. Analysis of health-related quality of life in patients with brain tumors prior and subsequent to radiotherapy. Oncol Lett 2017; 14(2):1841–6.
63. Armstrong C, Ruffer J, Corn B, et al. Biphasic patterns of memory deficits following moderate-dose partial-brain irradiation: neuropsychologic outcome and proposed mechanisms. J Clin Oncol 1995;13(9):2263–71.
64. Armstrong CL, Corn BW, Ruffer JE, et al. Radiotherapeutic effects on brain function: double dissociation of memory systems. Neuropsychiatry Neuropsychol Behav Neurol 2000;13(2):101–11.
65. DeAngelis LM, Posner JB. Neurologic complications of cancer. New York: Oxford University Press; 2008. https://doi.org/10.1093/med/9780195366747.001.0001.
66. Shih HA. Acute complications of cranial irradiation. In: DeAngelis LM, editor. Waltham (MA): UpToDate; 2017. Available at: https://www.uptodate.com/contents/delayed-complications-of-cranial-irradiation?search=Dietrich%20J,%20Gondi%20V,%20Mehta%20M.%20Delayed%20complications%20of%20cranial%20irradiation.%20In:%20DeAngelis%20LM,%20editor.%20Waltham%20(MA):%20UpToDate;%202017.%20. Accessed October 28, 2017.
67. Dekker M. Use of glucocorticoids in neuro-oncology. In: Posner JB, editor. Neurological complications of cancer. New York: F.A. Davis Co; 1995. p. 199.
68. Kehlet H, Binder C, Blichert-Toft M. Glucocorticoid maintenance therapy following adrenalectomy: assessment of dosage and preparation. Clin Endocrinol (Oxf) 1976;5(1):37–41.
69. Drappatz J, Wen PY. Management of vasogenic edema in patients with primary and metastatic brain tumors. In: DeAngelis LM, editor. Waltham (MA): UpToDate; 2017. Available at: https://www.uptodate.com/contents/management-of-vasogenic-edema-in-patients-with-primary-and-metastatic-brain-tumors. Accessed October 28, 2017.
70. Greene-Schloesser D, Robbins ME, Peiffer AM, et al. Radiation-induced brain injury: a review. Front Oncol 2012;2:73.
71. Young DF, Posner JB, Chu F, et al. Rapid-course radiation therapy of cerebral metastases: results and complications. Cancer 1974;34(4):1069–76.
72. Shaw E, Scott C, Souhami L, et al. Radiosurgery for the treatment of previously irradiated recurrent primary brain tumors and brain metastases: initial report of Radiation Therapy Oncology Group protocol (90-05). Int J Radiat Oncol Biol Phys 1996;34(3):647–54.

73. Shaw E, Scott C, Souhami L, et al. Single dose radiosurgical treatment of recurrent previously irradiated primary brain tumors and brain metastases: final report of RTOG protocol 90-05. Int J Radiat Oncol Biol Phys 2000;47(2):291–8.

74. Werner-Wasik M, Rudoler S, Preston PE, et al. Immediate side effects of stereotactic radiotherapy and radiosurgery. Int J Radiat Oncol Biol Phys 1999;43(2): 299–304.

75. Chin LS, Lazio BE, Biggins T, et al. Acute complications following gamma knife radiosurgery are rare. Surg Neurol 2000;53(5):498–502 [discussion: 502].

76. Gelblum DY, Lee H, Bilsky M, et al. Radiographic findings and morbidity in patients treated with stereotactic radiosurgery. Int J Radiat Oncol Biol Phys 1998; 42(2):391–5.

77. Arvold ND, Pinnell NE, Mahadevan A, et al. Steroid and anticonvulsant prophylaxis for stereotactic radiosurgery: large variation in physician recommendations. Pract Radiat Oncol 2016;6(4):e89–96.

78. Fang P, Jiang W, Allen P, et al. Radiation necrosis with stereotactic radiosurgery combined with CTLA-4 blockade and PD-1 inhibition for treatment of intracranial disease in metastatic melanoma. J Neurooncol 2017;133(3):595–602.

79. Kotecha R, Miller JA, Venur VA, et al. Melanoma brain metastasis: the impact of stereotactic radiosurgery, BRAF mutational status, and targeted and/or immune-based therapies on treatment outcome. J Neurosurg 2017;11:1–10 [Epub ahead of print].

80. O'Brien BJ, Colen RR. Post-treatment imaging changes in primary brain tumors. Curr Oncol Rep 2014;16(8):397.

81. Taal W, Brandsma D, de Bruin HG, et al. Incidence of early pseudo-progression in a cohort of malignant glioma patients treated with chemoirradiation with temozolomide. Cancer 2008;113(2):405–10.

82. Brandes AA, Franceschi E, Tosoni A, et al. MGMT promoter methylation status can predict the incidence and outcome of pseudoprogression after concomitant radiochemotherapy in newly diagnosed glioblastoma patients. J Clin Oncol 2008;26(13):2192–7.

83. Hygino da Cruz LC, Rodriguez I, Domingues RC, et al. Pseudoprogression and pseudoresponse: imaging challenges in the assessment of posttreatment glioma. AJNR Am J Neuroradiol 2011;32(11):1978–85.

84. Pallini R, Ricci-Vitiani L, Montano N, et al. Expression of the stem cell marker CD133 in recurrent glioblastoma and its value for prognosis. Cancer 2011; 117(1):162–74.

85. Strenger V, Lackner H, Mayer R, et al. Incidence and clinical course of radionecrosis in children with brain tumors. A 20-year longitudinal observational study. Strahlenther Onkol 2013;189(9):759–64.

86. Chen J, Dassarath M, Yin Z, et al. Radiation induced temporal lobe necrosis in patients with nasopharyngeal carcinoma: a review of new avenues in its management. Radiat Oncol 2011;6(1):128.

87. Chao ST, Ahluwalia MS, Barnett GH, et al. Challenges with the diagnosis and treatment of cerebral radiation necrosis. Int J Radiat Oncol Biol Phys 2013; 87(3):449–57.

88. Sadraei NH, Dahiya S, Chao ST, et al. Treatment of cerebral radiation necrosis with bevacizumab: the Cleveland Clinic experience. Am J Clin Oncol 2015; 38(3):304–10.

89. DeAngelis LM, Delattre JY, Posner JB. Radiation-induced dementia in patients cured of brain metastases. Neurology 1989;39(6):789–96.

90. Tekkök IH, Carter DA, Robinson MG, et al. Reversal of CNS-prophylaxis-related leukoencephalopathy after CSF shunting: case histories of identical twins. Childs Nerv Syst 1996;12(6):309–14.

91. Perrini P, Scollato A, Cioffi F, et al. Radiation leukoencephalopathy associated with moderate hydrocephalus: intracranial pressure monitoring and results of ventriculoperitoneal shunting. Neurol Sci 2002;23(5):237–41.

92. Dietrich J, Klein JP. Imaging of cancer therapy-induced central nervous system toxicity. Neurol Clin 2014;32(1):147–57.

93. Kano H, Kondziolka D, Lobato-Polo J, et al. T1/T2 matching to differentiate tumor growth from radiation effects after stereotactic radiosurgery. Neurosurgery 2010;66(3):486–91.

94. Sugahara T, Korogi Y, Tomiguchi S, et al. Posttherapeutic intraaxial brain tumor: the value of perfusion-sensitive contrast-enhanced MR imaging for differentiating tumor recurrence from nonneoplastic contrast-enhancing tissue. AJNR Am J Neuroradiol 2000;21(5):901–9.

95. Henry RG, Vigneron DB, Fischbein NJ, et al. Comparison of relative cerebral blood volume and proton spectroscopy in patients with treated gliomas. AJNR Am J Neuroradiol 2000;21(2):357–66.

96. Kimura T, Sako K, Tanaka K, et al. Evaluation of the response of metastatic brain tumors to stereotactic radiosurgery by proton magnetic resonance spectroscopy, 201TlCl single-photon emission computerized tomography, and gadolinium-enhanced magnetic resonance imaging. J Neurosurg 2004;100(5): 835–41.

97. Furuse M, Kawabata S, Kuroiwa T, et al. Repeated treatments with bevacizumab for recurrent radiation necrosis in patients with malignant brain tumors: a report of 2 cases. J Neurooncol 2011;102(3):471–5.

98. Correa DD, DeAngelis LM, Shi W, et al. Cognitive functions in low-grade gliomas: disease and treatment effects. J Neurooncol 2007;81(2):175–84.

99. Kiehna EN, Mulhern RK, Li C, et al. Changes in attentional performance of children and young adults with localized primary brain tumors after conformal radiation therapy. J Clin Oncol 2006;24(33):5283–90.

100. Jalali R, Gupta T, Goda JS, et al. Efficacy of stereotactic conformal radiotherapy vs conventional radiotherapy on benign and low-grade brain tumors: a randomized clinical trial. JAMA Oncol 2017;3(10):1368–76.

101. Leeman JE, Clump DA, Flickinger JC, et al. Extent of perilesional edema differentiates radionecrosis from tumor recurrence following stereotactic radiosurgery for brain metastases. Neuro Oncol 2013;15(12):1732–8.

102. Lefebvre JL, Rolland F, Tesselaar M, et al. Phase 3 randomized trial on larynx preservation comparing sequential vs alternating chemotherapy and radiotherapy. J Natl Cancer Inst 2009;101(3):142–52.

103. Quan D, Hackney DB, Pruitt AA, et al. Transient MRI enhancement in a patient with seizures and previously resected glioma: use of MRS. Neurology 1999; 53(1):211–3.

104. Davidson A, Tait DM, Payne GS, et al. Magnetic resonance spectroscopy in the evaluation of neurotoxicity following cranial irradiation for childhood cancer. Br J Radiol 2000;73(868):421–4.

105. Lin A, Bluml S, Mamelak AN. Efficacy of proton magnetic resonance spectroscopy in clinical decision making for patients with suspected malignant brain tumors. J Neurooncol 1999;45(1):69–81.

106. Mitsuya K, Nakasu Y, Horiguchi S, et al. Perfusion weighted magnetic resonance imaging to distinguish the recurrence of metastatic brain tumors from radiation necrosis after stereotactic radiosurgery. J Neurooncol 2010;99(1):81–8.

107. Asao C, Korogi Y, Kitajima M, et al. Diffusion-weighted imaging of radiation-induced brain injury for differentiation from tumor recurrence. AJNR Am J Neuroradiol 2005;26(6):1455–60.

108. Valk PE, Budinger TF, Levin VA, et al. PET of malignant cerebral tumors after interstitial brachytherapy. Demonstration of metabolic activity and correlation with clinical outcome. J Neurosurg 1988;69(6):830–8.

109. Thiel A, Pietrzyk U, Sturm V, et al. Enhanced accuracy in differential diagnosis of radiation necrosis by positron emission tomography-magnetic resonance imaging coregistration: technical case report. Neurosurgery 2000;46(1):232–4.

110. Barker FG, Chang SM, Valk PE, et al. 18-Fluorodeoxyglucose uptake and survival of patients with suspected recurrent malignant glioma. Cancer 1997; 79(1):115–26.

111. Doyle WK, Budinger TF, Valk PE, et al. Differentiation of cerebral radiation necrosis from tumor recurrence by [18F]FDG and 82Rb positron emission tomography. J Comput Assist Tomogr 1987;11(4):563–70.

112. Janus TJ, Kim EE, Tilbury R, et al. Use of [18F]fluorodeoxyglucose positron emission tomography in patients with primary malignant brain tumors. Ann Neurol 1993;33(5):540–8.

113. Glantz MJ, Hoffman JM, Coleman RE, et al. Identification of early recurrence of primary central nervous system tumors by [18F]fluorodeoxyglucose positron emission tomography. Ann Neurol 1991;29(4):347–55.

114. Parvez K, Parvez A, Zadeh G. The diagnosis and treatment of pseudoprogression, radiation necrosis and brain tumor recurrence. Int J Mol Sci 2014;15(7): 11832–46.

115. Ross DA, Sandler HM, Balter JM, et al. Imaging changes after stereotactic radiosurgery of primary and secondary malignant brain tumors. J Neurooncol 2002;56(2):175–81.

116. Schwartz RB, Holman BL, Polak JF, et al. Dual-isotope single-photon emission computerized tomography scanning in patients with glioblastoma multiforme: association with patient survival and histopathological characteristics of tumor after high-dose radiotherapy. J Neurosurg 1998;89(1):60–8.

117. Gonzalez J, Kumar AJ, Conrad CA, et al. Effect of bevacizumab on radiation necrosis of the brain. Int J Radiat Oncol Biol Phys 2007;67(2):323–6.

118. Torcuator R, Zuniga R, Mohan YS, et al. Initial experience with bevacizumab treatment for biopsy confirmed cerebral radiation necrosis. J Neurooncol 2009;94(1):63–8.

119. Liu AK, Macy ME, Foreman NK. Bevacizumab as therapy for radiation necrosis in four children with pontine gliomas. Int J Radiat Oncol Biol Phys 2009;75(4): 1148–54.

120. Levin VA, Bidaut L, Hou P, et al. Randomized double-blind placebo-controlled trial of bevacizumab therapy for radiation necrosis of the central nervous system. Int J Radiat Oncol Biol Phys 2011;79(5):1487–95.

121. Deibert CP, Ahluwalia MS, Sheehan JP, et al. Bevacizumab for refractory adverse radiation effects after stereotactic radiosurgery. J Neurooncol 2013; 115(2):217–23.

122. Boothe D, Young R, Yamada Y, et al. Bevacizumab as a treatment for radiation necrosis of brain metastases post stereotactic radiosurgery. Neuro Oncol 2013; 15(9):1257–63.

123. Delishaj D, Ursino S, Pasqualetti F, et al. Bevacizumab for the treatment of radiation-induced cerebral necrosis: a systematic review of the literature. J Clin Med Res 2017;9(4):273–80.

124. Jeyaretna DS, Curry WT, Batchelor TT, et al. Exacerbation of cerebral radiation necrosis by bevacizumab. J Clin Oncol 2011;29(7):e159–62.

125. Chung C. A221208: Corticosteroids + bevacizumab vs. corticosteroids + placebo (BEST) for radionecrosis after radiosurgery for brain metastases. Available at: https://clinicaltrials.gov/show/NCT02490878. Accessed November 30, 2017.

126. Eisele SC, Dietrich J. Cerebral radiation necrosis: diagnostic challenge and clinical management. Rev Neurol 2015;61(5):225–32.

127. Rao MS, Hargreaves EL, Khan AJ, et al. Magnetic resonance-guided laser ablation improves local control for postradiosurgery recurrence and/or radiation necrosis. Neurosurgery 2014;74(6):658–67 [discussion: 667].

128. Smith CJ, Myers CS, Chapple KM, et al. Long-term follow-up of 25 cases of biopsy-proven radiation necrosis or post-radiation treatment effect treated with magnetic resonance-guided laser interstitial thermal therapy. Neurosurgery 2016;79(Suppl 1):S59–72.

129. Chuba PJ, Aronin P, Bhambhani K, et al. Hyperbaric oxygen therapy for radiation-induced brain injury in children. Cancer 1997;80(10):2005–12.

130. Cihan YB, Uzun G, Yildiz S, et al. Hyperbaric oxygen therapy for radiation-induced brain necrosis in a patient with primary central nervous system lymphoma. J Surg Oncol 2009;100(8):732–5.

131. Lähteenmäki PM, Harila-Saari A, Pukkala EI, et al. Scholastic achievements of children with brain tumors at the end of comprehensive education: a nationwide, register-based study. Neurology 2007;69(3):296–305.

132. Harila-Saari AH, Lähteenmäki PM, Pukkala E, et al. Scholastic achievements of childhood leukemia patients: a nationwide, register-based study. J Clin Oncol 2007;25(23):3518–24.

133. von der Weid N, Swiss Pediatric Oncology Group (SPOG). Late effects in long-term survivors of ALL in childhood: experiences from the SPOG late effects study. Swiss Med Wkly 2001;131(13–14):180–7.

134. Krull KR, Zhang N, Santucci A, et al. Long-term decline in intelligence among adult survivors of childhood acute lymphoblastic leukemia treated with cranial radiation. Blood 2013;122(4):550–3.

135. Conklin HM, Krull KR, Reddick WE, et al. Cognitive outcomes following contemporary treatment without cranial irradiation for childhood acute lymphoblastic leukemia. J Natl Cancer Inst 2012;104(18):1386–95.

136. Iyer NS, Balsamo LM, Bracken MB, et al. Chemotherapy-only treatment effects on long-term neurocognitive functioning in childhood ALL survivors: a review and meta-analysis. Blood 2015;126(3):346–53.

137. Jacola LM, Krull KR, Pui C-H, et al. Longitudinal assessment of neurocognitive outcomes in survivors of childhood acute lymphoblastic leukemia treated on a contemporary chemotherapy protocol. J Clin Oncol 2016;34(11):1239–47.

138. Fouladi M, Gilger E, Kocak M, et al. Intellectual and functional outcome of children 3 years old or younger who have CNS malignancies. J Clin Oncol 2005; 23(28):7152–60.

139. Chang EL, Wefel JS, Hess KR, et al. Neurocognition in patients with brain metastases treated with radiosurgery or radiosurgery plus whole-brain irradiation: a randomised controlled trial. Lancet Oncol 2009;10(11):1037–44.

140. Sun A, Bae K, Gore EM, et al. Phase III trial of prophylactic cranial irradiation compared with observation in patients with locally advanced non-small-cell

lung cancer: neurocognitive and quality-of-life analysis. J Clin Oncol 2011;29(3): 279–86.

141. Brown PD, Jaeckle K, Ballman KV, et al. Effect of radiosurgery alone vs radiosurgery with whole brain radiation therapy on cognitive function in patients with 1 to 3 brain metastases: a randomized clinical trial. JAMA 2016;316(4):401–9.

142. Soffietti R, Kocher M, Abacioglu UM, et al. A European Organisation for Research and Treatment of Cancer phase III trial of adjuvant whole-brain radiotherapy versus observation in patients with one to three brain metastases from solid tumors after surgical resection or radiosurgery: quality-of-life results. J Clin Oncol 2013;31(1):65–72.

143. Monaco EA, Faraji AH, Berkowitz O, et al. Leukoencephalopathy after whole-brain radiation therapy plus radiosurgery versus radiosurgery alone for metastatic lung cancer. Cancer 2013;119(1):226–32.

144. Constine LS, Konski A, Ekholm S, et al. Adverse effects of brain irradiation correlated with MR and CT imaging. Int J Radiat Oncol Biol Phys 1988;15(2):319–30.

145. Klein M, Heimans JJ, Aaronson NK, et al. Effect of radiotherapy and other treatment-related factors on mid-term to long-term cognitive sequelae in low-grade gliomas: a comparative study. Lancet 2002;360(9343):1361–8.

146. Douw L, Klein M, Fagel SS, et al. Cognitive and radiological effects of radiotherapy in patients with low-grade glioma: long-term follow-up. Lancet Neurol 2009;8(9):810–8.

147. Shaw E, Arusell R, Scheithauer B, et al. Prospective randomized trial of low-versus high-dose radiation therapy in adults with supratentorial low-grade glioma: initial report of a North Central Cancer Treatment Group/Radiation Therapy Oncology Group/Eastern Cooperative Oncology Group study. J Clin Oncol 2002;20(9):2267–76.

148. Brown PD, Buckner JC, O'Fallon JR, et al. Effects of radiotherapy on cognitive function in patients with low-grade glioma measured by the Folstein mini-mental state examination. J Clin Oncol 2003;21(13):2519–24.

149. Prabhu RS, Won M, Shaw EG, et al. Effect of the addition of chemotherapy to radiotherapy on cognitive function in patients with low-grade glioma: secondary analysis of RTOG 98-02. J Clin Oncol 2014;32(6):535–41.

150. Movsas B, Scott C, Langer C, et al. Randomized trial of amifostine in locally advanced non–small-cell lung cancer patients receiving chemotherapy and hyperfractionated radiation: Radiation Therapy Oncology Group trial 98-01. J Clin Oncol 2005;23(10):2145–54.

151. Meyers CA, Wefel JS. The use of the mini-mental state examination to assess cognitive functioning in cancer trials: no ifs, ands, buts, or sensitivity. J Clin Oncol 2003;21(19):3557–8.

152. Mulhern RK, Khan RB, Kaplan S, et al. Short-term efficacy of methylphenidate: a randomized, double-blind, placebo-controlled trial among survivors of childhood cancer. J Clin Oncol 2004;22(23):4795–803.

153. Page BR, Shaw EG, Lu L, et al. Phase II double-blind placebo-controlled randomized study of armodafinil for brain radiation-induced fatigue. Neuro Oncol 2015;17(10):1393–401.

154. Shaw EG, Rosdhal R, D'Agostino RB, et al. Phase II study of donepezil in irradiated brain tumor patients: effect on cognitive function, mood, and quality of life. J Clin Oncol 2006;24(9):1415–20.

155. Rapp SR, Case LD, Peiffer A, et al. Donepezil for irradiated brain tumor survivors: a phase III randomized placebo-controlled clinical trial. J Clin Oncol 2015;33(15):1653–9.

156. Brown PD, Pugh S, Laack NN, et al. Memantine for the prevention of cognitive dysfunction in patients receiving whole-brain radiotherapy: a randomized, double-blind, placebo-controlled trial. Neuro Oncol 2013;15(10):1429–37.

157. Campen CJ, Kranick SM, Kasner SE, et al. Cranial irradiation increases risk of stroke in pediatric brain tumor survivors. Stroke 2012;43(11):3035–40.

158. Bowers DC, Liu Y, Leisenring W, et al. Late-occurring stroke among long-term survivors of childhood leukemia and brain tumors: a report from the Childhood Cancer Survivor Study. J Clin Oncol 2006;24(33):5277–82.

159. Murphy ES, Xie H, Merchant TE, et al. Review of cranial radiotherapy-induced vasculopathy. J Neurooncol 2015;122(3):421–9.

160. Strenger V, Sovinz P, Lackner H, et al. Intracerebral cavernous hemangioma after cranial irradiation in childhood. Incidence and risk factors. Strahlenther Onkol 2008;184(5):276–80.

161. Burn S, Gunny R, Phipps K, et al. Incidence of cavernoma development in children after radiotherapy for brain tumors. J Neurosurg 2007;106(5 Suppl): 379–83.

162. Lew SM, Morgan JN, Psaty E, et al. Cumulative incidence of radiation-induced cavernomas in long-term survivors of medulloblastoma. J Neurosurg 2006; 104(2 Suppl):103–7.

163. Heckl S, Aschoff A, Kunze S. Radiation-induced cavernous hemangiomas of the brain: a late effect predominantly in children. Cancer 2002;94(12): 3285–91.

164. Sanford NN, Yeap BY, Larvie M, et al. Prospective, randomized study of radiation dose escalation with combined proton-photon therapy for benign meningiomas. Int J Radiat Oncol Biol Phys 2017;99(4):787–96.

165. El-Fayech C, Haddy N, Allodji RS, et al. Cerebrovascular diseases in childhood cancer survivors: role of the radiation dose to Willis circle arteries. Int J Radiat Oncol Biol Phys 2017;97(2):278–86.

166. Kranick SM, Campen CJ, Kasner SE, et al. Headache as a risk factor for neurovascular events in pediatric brain tumor patients. Neurology 2013;80(16): 1452–6.

167. Thalhammer C, Husmann M, Glanzmann C, et al. Carotid artery disease after head and neck radiotherapy. Vasa 2015;44(1):23–30.

168. Gujral DM, Chahal N, Senior R, et al. Radiation-induced carotid artery atherosclerosis. Radiother Oncol 2014;110(1):31–8.

169. Hooning MJ, Dorresteijn LDA, Aleman BMP, et al. Decreased risk of stroke among 10-year survivors of breast cancer. J Clin Oncol 2006;24(34):5388–94.

170. Desai SS, Paulino AC, Mai WY, et al. Radiation-induced moyamoya syndrome. Int J Radiat Oncol Biol Phys 2006;65(4):1222–7.

171. Ullrich NJ, Robertson R, Kinnamon DD, et al. Moyamoya following cranial irradiation for primary brain tumors in children. Neurology 2007;68(12):932–8.

172. Aizer AA, Du R, Wen PY, et al. Radiotherapy and death from cerebrovascular disease in patients with primary brain tumors. J Neurooncol 2015;124(2): 291–7.

173. NCCN. Hodgkin lymphoma. NCCN Guidelines Version 3 2018, April 16, 2018;(1):MS-26 Available at: https://www.nccn.org/professionals/physician_gls/pdf/hodgkins.pdf. Accessed May 2, 2018.

174. Kerklaan JP, Lycklama á Nijeholt GJ, Wiggenraad RG, et al. SMART syndrome: a late reversible complication after radiation therapy for brain tumours. J Neurol 2011;258(6):1098–104.

175. Farid K, Meissner WG, Samier-Foubert A, et al. Normal cerebrovascular reactivity in stroke-like migraine attacks after radiation therapy syndrome. Clin Nucl Med 2010;35(8):583–5.

176. Fan EP, Heiber G, Gerard EE, et al. Stroke-like migraine attacks after radiation therapy: a misnomer? Epilepsia 2018;59(1):259–68.

177. Mayo C, Martel MK, Marks LB, et al. Radiation dose-volume effects of optic nerves and chiasm. Int J Radiat Oncol Biol Phys 2010;76(3 Suppl):S28–35.

178. Harris JR, Levene MB. Visual complications following irradiation for pituitary adenomas and craniopharyngiomas. Radiology 1976;120(1):167–71.

179. Leavitt JA, Stafford SL, Link MJ, et al. Long-term evaluation of radiation-induced optic neuropathy after single-fraction stereotactic radiosurgery. Int J Radiat Oncol Biol Phys 2013;87(3):524–7.

180. Pollock BE, Link MJ, Leavitt JA, et al. Dose-volume analysis of radiation-induced optic neuropathy after single-fraction stereotactic radiosurgery. Neurosurgery 2014;75(4):456–60 [discussion: 460].

181. Borruat FX, Schatz NJ, Glaser JS, et al. Visual recovery from radiation-induced optic neuropathy. The role of hyperbaric oxygen therapy. J Clin Neuroophthalmol 1993;13(2):98–101.

182. Malik A, Golnik K. Hyperbaric oxygen therapy in the treatment of radiation optic neuropathy. J Neuroophthalmol 2012;32(2):128–31.

183. Constine LS, Woolf PD, Cann D, et al. Hypothalamic-pituitary dysfunction after radiation for brain tumors. N Engl J Med 1993;328(2):87–94.

184. Taphoorn MJ, Heimans JJ, van der Veen EA, et al. Endocrine functions in long-term survivors of low-grade supratentorial glioma treated with radiation therapy. J Neurooncol 1995;25(2):97–102.

185. Collet-Solberg PF, Sernyak H, Satin-Smith M, et al. Endocrine outcome in long-term survivors of low-grade hypothalamic/chiasmatic glioma. Clin Endocrinol (Oxf) 1997;47(1):79–85.

186. Arlt W, Hove U, Müller B, et al. Frequent and frequently overlooked: treatment-induced endocrine dysfunction in adult long-term survivors of primary brain tumors. Neurology 1997;49(2):498–506.

187. Lam KS, Tse VK, Wang C, et al. Effects of cranial irradiation on hypothalamic-pituitary function–a 5-year longitudinal study in patients with nasopharyngeal carcinoma. Q J Med 1991;78(286):165–76.

188. Pai HH, Thornton A, Katznelson L, et al. Hypothalamic/pituitary function following high-dose conformal radiotherapy to the base of skull: demonstration of a dose-effect relationship using dose-volume histogram analysis. Int J Radiat Oncol Biol Phys 2001;49(4):1079–92.

189. Minniti G, Jaffrain-Rea M-L, Osti M, et al. The long-term efficacy of conventional radiotherapy in patients with GH-secreting pituitary adenomas. Clin Endocrinol (Oxf) 2005;62(2):210–6.

190. Appelman-Dijkstra NM, Kokshoorn NE, Dekkers OM, et al. Pituitary dysfunction in adult patients after cranial radiotherapy: systematic review and meta-analysis. J Clin Endocrinol Metab 2011;96(8):2330–40.

191. Müller HL, Merchant TE, Puget S, et al. New outlook on the diagnosis, treatment and follow-up of childhood-onset craniopharyngioma. Nat Rev Endocrinol 2017; 13(5):299–312.

192. Neglia JP, Robison LL, Stovall M, et al. New primary neoplasms of the central nervous system in survivors of childhood cancer: a report from the Childhood Cancer Survivor Study. J Natl Cancer Inst 2006;98(21):1528–37.

193. Packer RJ, Gajjar A, Vezina G, et al. Phase III study of craniospinal radiation therapy followed by adjuvant chemotherapy for newly diagnosed average-risk medulloblastoma. J Clin Oncol 2006;24(25):4202–8.

194. Bowers DC, Nathan PC, Constine L, et al. Subsequent neoplasms of the CNS among survivors of childhood cancer: a systematic review. Lancet Oncol 2013;14(8):e321–8.

195. Pollock BE, Link MJ, Stafford SL, et al. The risk of radiation-induced tumors or malignant transformation after single-fraction intracranial radiosurgery: results based on a 25-year experience. Int J Radiat Oncol Biol Phys 2017; 97(5):919–23.

196. Mizumoto M, Murayama S, Akimoto T, et al. Long-term follow-up after proton beam therapy for pediatric tumors: a Japanese national survey. Cancer Sci 2017;108(3):444–7.

197. Brodin NP, Munck Af Rosenschöld P, Aznar MC, et al. Radiobiological risk estimates of adverse events and secondary cancer for proton and photon radiation therapy of pediatric medulloblastoma. Acta Oncol 2011;50(6):806–16.

Neurologic Complications of Systemic Anticancer Therapy

Kien-Ninh Ina Ly, MD, Isabel C. Arrillaga-Romany, MD, PhD*

KEYWORDS

- Neurologic complications • Neurotoxicity • Chemotherapy • Targeted agents
- Immunotherapy

KEY POINTS

- Neurologic complications of systemic cancer therapy represent an increasing problem for practitioners, as survival of cancer patients is improving, and new therapeutic agents are being developed.
- It is important to differentiate treatment-related neurologic complications from disease recurrence in the nervous system and paraneoplastic disease.
- Although neurologic complications are relatively rare with newer agents such as monoclonal antibodies and immunotherapy, their presence can be associated with significant morbidity and/or mortality.

INTRODUCTION

Neurologic complications secondary to cancer treatment-related toxicity arise either as a result of direct toxic effects on the nervous system or as an indirect consequence of treatment-induced metabolic, vascular, autoimmune, or infectious abnormalities. Symptoms can range from mild and transient to severe and permanent. When permanent, symptoms can be greatly debilitating to patients and compromise their quality of life. Both neurologists and neuro-oncologists are likely to encounter an increase in the number of patients with treatment-induced neurotoxic complications in their practice, given the increasing number of cancer survivors in the era of novel therapeutics, including targeted agents and immunotherapy. Differentiation between treatment-related toxicity, disease recurrence in the form of nervous system metastases, and paraneoplastic phenomena is important to guide appropriate management. This article focuses on the chemotherapy agents most likely to cause neurologic complications

Disclosure Statement: The authors have nothing to disclose.
Stephen E. and Catherine Pappas Center for Neuro-Oncology, Massachusetts General Hospital, Harvard Medical School, Yawkey 9E, 55 Fruit Street, Boston, MA 02114, USA
* Corresponding author.
E-mail address: iarrillaga@mgh.harvard.edu

Neurol Clin 36 (2018) 627–651
https://doi.org/10.1016/j.ncl.2018.04.013
0733-8619/18/© 2018 Elsevier Inc. All rights reserved.

(**Table 1**), as well as novel targeted and immunotherapeutic agents that have transformed the landscape of cancer treatment in recent years (**Table 2**).

Cytotoxic Chemotherapy Agents

Antimetabolites

Methotrexate Methotrexate (MTX) is a dihydrofolate reductase inhibitor that reduces the amount of tetrahydrofolate available for DNA synthesis, which eventually leads to cell death.[1] It is used in the treatment of leukemia, primary and secondary central nervous system (CNS) lymphoma, choriocarcinoma, and osteosarcoma. In addition, it is frequently administered via the intrathecal (IT) route for leptomeningeal metastases. Given its effect on folate metabolism, MTX is typically administered with leucovorin to prevent folate depletion in noncancerous cells. MTX can cause a wide range of acute, subacute, and chronic neurologic complications.

Aseptic meningitis occurs most commonly in the setting of IT MTX administration and affects approximately 10% to 30% of patients,[2,3] although incidence rates as high as 61% have been reported.[4] Symptoms are indistinguishable from those of other noninfectious and infectious causes of meningitis and include headache, nuchal rigidity, back pain, nausea, vomiting, fever, and lethargy. Symptoms typically start 2 to 4 hours after administration and can persist for 2 to 6 days.[4,5] Interestingly, the inflammatory response may be attenuated in the setting of concomitant brain irradiation.[4]

IT MTX can also lead to a transverse myelopathy; the cumulative incidence is approximately 3% for IT MTX and cytarabine (Ara-C), which are the most frequently administered drugs via the IT route.[6] Patients typically experience lower extremity sensory loss, paraplegia, and, to a variable degree, sphincter dysfunction.[6–8] Time to onset of neurologic symptoms can be highly variable, ranging from 2 days to 7 months after starting IT chemotherapy.[6,7] The occurrence of symptoms is not dose-dependent, suggesting that individual patient factors may predispose to the myelopathy.[7] Notably, spine MRI can reveal abnormal T2 hyperintensity of the dorsal column in some cases,[7] although a normal MRI should not exclude the diagnosis of transverse myelopathy. Improvement of symptoms is variable after administration of steroids, intravenous immunoglobulin, or radiation therapy.[6,7]

Both acute and subacute encephalopathy syndromes have been observed after high-dose intravenous and IT MTX.[9–11] Symptoms include confusion, disorientation, seizures, and focal neurologic deficits and usually emerge 5 to 13 days after drug administration. Brain MRI is characteristically normal.[9] In most cases, these deficits resolve spontaneously within 1 to 3 days, and patients are able to receive further courses of MTX without modifications in dose or route of administration.[9] It has been proposed that downstream methionine depletion and accumulation of homocysteine via inhibition of dihydrofolate reductase contribute to the pathogenesis of MTX encephalopathy.[1,12] Genome-wide association studies in childhood ALL patients have not revealed any definitive genetic markers that predict the likelihood of neurotoxicity.[13]

A debilitating chronic neurotoxic effect of intravenous and IT MTX is leukoencephalopathy, which begins months to years after completion of treatment. Characteristic features include progressive cognitive dysfunction, ranging from mild cognitive impairment to severe dementia, somnolence, seizures, ataxia, and hemiparesis.[14] The effects of MTX-induced white matter damage are potentiated by concurrent brain irradiation and related to the cumulative dose of MTX.[14,15] Brain MRI typically demonstrates cerebral atrophy and T2/FLAIR-hyperintense changes affecting the white matter (**Fig. 1**).

Table 1

Cytotoxic chemotherapy agents with well-established neurotoxic effects on the central nervous system and/or peripheral nervous system

Class of Drugs	Specific Drug	Central Nervous System Neurotoxicity	Peripheral Nervous System Neurotoxicity
Antimetabolites	Methotrexate	• Aseptic meningitis • Transverse myelopathy • Acute/subacute encephalopathy (acute/sub-acute) with stroke-like symptoms • Chronic leukoencephalopathy Rare: • Necrotizing leukoencephalopathy	
	5-fluorouracil (5-FU)	• Acute cerebellar syndrome • Acute encephalopathy (secondary to hyperammonemia) Rare: • Optic neuropathy • Focal dystonia • Parkinsonian symptoms • Seizures	Rare: • Peripheral neuropathy
	Capecitabine	• Cerebellar syndrome • Encephalopathy • Multifocal leukoencephalopathy • Cerebellar syndrome	
	Ara-C (cytarabine)	Rare: • Seizures • Encephalopathy • Leukoencephalopathy • Cranial neuropathy • Extrapyramidal symptoms • Spinal cord myelopathy	Rare: • Peripheral neuropathy

(continued on next page)

Table 1
(continued)

Class of Drugs	Specific Drug	Central Nervous System Neurotoxicity	Peripheral Nervous System Neurotoxicity
Platinum-based agents	Cisplatin	• Ototoxicity • Lhermitte sign Rare: • Encephalopathy (seizures and focal deficits) • Taste disturbance • Myasthenic syndrome	• Symmetric sensory neuropathy ("coasting" possible)
	Carboplatin Oxaliplatin	• Ototoxicity • Ototoxicity (less compared to cisplatin and carboplatin)	• Symmetric sensory neuropathy • Acute neuropathy (dysesthesias, paresthesias of extremities, perioral and oral region, cold sensitivity, throat discomfort, muscle cramps) • Symmetric sensory neuropathy
Taxanes	Paclitaxel	Rare: • Seizures • Encephalopathy Rare: • Lhermitte's sign	• Large-fiber sensory neuropathy • Acute pain syndrome (myalgias, arthralgias)
	Docetaxel		• Sensory neuropathy
Vinca alkaloids	Vincristine	• Cranial neuropathy • SIADH Rare: • Fatal ascending myeloencephalopathy (with inadvertent IT administration)	• Sensory > motor neuropathy • Autonomic neuropathy
	Vinblastine, vinolrebine	Similar peripheral neuropathy as vincristine but less severe	
Thalidomide, lenolidomide			• Sensory neuropathy ± motor involvement (thalidomide > lenolidomide)
Proteasome inhibitors	Bortezomib		• Painful sensory neuropathy
Alkylating agents	Ifosfamide	• Acute encephalopathy (secondary to chloroacetylaldehyde)	
	Busulfan	• Seizures	

Table 2
Neurotoxic effects of commonly used targeted agents and immunotherapy

Class of Drugs	Specific Drug	CNS Neurotoxicity	PNS Neurotoxicity
Targeted agents			
Tyrosine kinase inhibitors	Imatinib	• Subdural hematomas	• Myalgias (rare: rhabdomyolysis)
	Sunitinib	Rare:	
	Sorafenib	• PRES	
Antibodies	Bevacizumab	• Ischemic stroke	
		• Hemorrhagic stroke (bevacizumab)	
	Rituximab	Rare:	Rare:
	Alemtuzumab	• Headaches	• Myalgias
		• Dizziness	• Paresthesias
		• Progressive multifocal leukoencephalopathy (secondary to JC virus reactivation)	
	Brentuximab		• Peripheral neuropathy
	Blinatumomab	• Dizziness	• Paresthesia
		• Confusion	• Tremor
		• Headaches	
		Rare:	
		• Seizures	
		• Aphasia	
Immunotherapy			
Immune checkpoint inhibitors	Ipilimumab	• Neuroendocrine toxicity	Rare:
		Rare:	• Guillain-Barre syndrome
		• Encephalopathy	• CIDP
		• Aseptic meningitis	• Myositis
		• Tolosa-Hunt syndrome	• Myasthenia gravis
		• Transverse myelitis	• Autonomic neuropathy
	Nivolumab	• Neuroendocrine toxicity	Rare:
		Rare:	• Myasthenia gravis
		• CNS demyelination	
	Pembrolizumab	• Neuroendocrine toxicity	Rare:
		Rare:	• Myasthenia gravis
		• Intracranial vasculitis	• Guillain-Barre syndrome
		• Limib encephalitis	• Polyneuropathy
		• PRES	
CAR T cells		• Encephalopathy	
		• Headache	
		• Facial nerve palsy	
		• Tremors, myoclonus	
		• Seizures	

In rare cases, IT MTX causes disseminated necrotizing leukoencephalopathy, a condition characterized by progressive and irreversible neurologic deterioration that leads to death in most cases. The histopathologic hallmarks are multifocal areas of coagulative necrosis, demyelination, and axonal damage.[15] Brain MRI reveals diffuse confluent areas of T2-hyperintensity and patchy or mass-like areas of enhancement.[16]

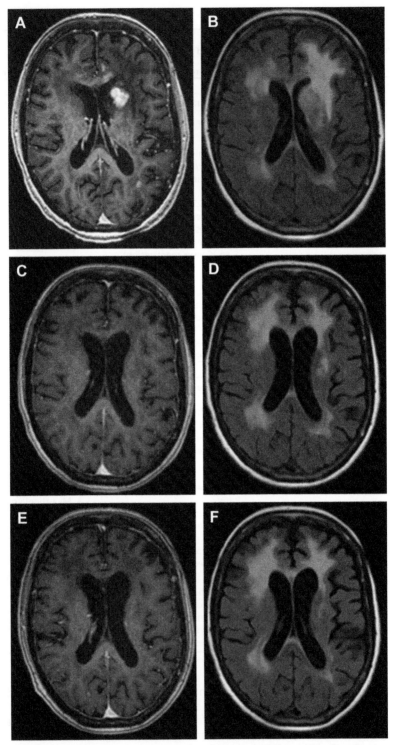

Fig. 1. Example of methotrexate (MTX)-induced leukoencephalopathy after treatment for primary CNS lymphoma. Axial brain MR images of a 68-year-old woman at the time of

Fluoropyrimidines (5-fluorouracil and capecitabine) 5-fluorouracil (5-FU) is a fluorinated pyrimidine used in the treatment of many solid organ malignancies, including colon and breast cancer. It readily crosses the blood-brain barrier and reaches highest concentrations in the cerebellum. Patients lacking dihydropyrimidine dehydrogenase, the rate-limiting enzyme in the catabolism of 5-FU, are at higher risk of developing 5-FU-induced toxicity.[17–19] In 2% to 5% of patients, 5-FU causes an acute cerebellar syndrome weeks to months after treatment initiation.[20–22] Symptoms resolve after discontinuation of therapy, and treatment can occasionally be reinstated afterward.[20,21]

In addition, an acute encephalopathy syndrome has been reported,[23–27] which can present with severe stupor or coma.[26] Mechanistically, it is thought to be caused by hyperammonemia in the absence of underlying hepatic dysfunction.[28] Rare neurologic complications of 5-FU are optic neuropathy,[17] focal dystonia,[29] a Parkinsonian syndrome,[30] peripheral neuropathy,[31,32] and seizures.[33] Ischemic stroke has been reported in patients receiving concurrent 5-FU and cisplatin.[34]

Capecitabine is a prodrug that is metabolized to its active moiety, 5-FU, by thymidine phosphorylase. Its neurotoxic effects are similar to those of 5-FU, including cerebellar toxicity,[35,36] encephalopathy, and multifocal leukoencephalopathy.[37,38] A rare complication is oromandibular dystonia leading to progressive airway obstruction.[39,40] Treatment with an anticholinergic drug can reverse these symptoms.

Cytosine arabinoside (cytarabine, Ara-C) Ara-C is a pyrimidine analog used in the management of leukemias, lymphomas, and leptomeningeal metastases. Toxicity is relatively rare when given at standard doses. However, at high intravenous or intrathecal (cumulative) doses, it causes CNS complications in approximately 12% to 29% of patients.[41] Most commonly, a cerebellar syndrome can occur that is characterized by gait ataxia, oculomotor impairment, incoordination, and dysarthria.[42] Confusion, drowsiness, and impaired attention and verbal fluency as a result of cerebellar involvement have also been reported.[42] Risk factors include age of at least 50 years, hepatic and renal compromise, and a history of neurologic dysfunction.[43,44] In 1 case series of adult leukemia patients treated with intravenous high-dose Ara-C, symptoms usually emerged during or within 24 hours after drug infusion, and most patients had a complete recovery within 2 days to a few weeks.[41] However, permanent deficits have been reported.[45]

Other less common neurologic complications seen with Ara-C include seizures, encephalopathy, leukoencephalopathy,[41] peripheral neuropathies,[46] lateral rectus palsy,[47] and extrapyramidal syndromes.[48] Progressive ascending paralysis secondary to spinal cord demyelination has been described that begins 4 to 5 months after initiation of IT Ara-C.[49] Brain MRI is typically normal at early time points, but cerebellar atrophy can be seen months later, largely reflecting loss of cerebellar Purkinje cells.[50]

---

diagnosis demonstrate areas of multifocal periventricular enhancement on T1-weighted postcontrast sequences (A) and associated T2/FLAIR hyperintensity (B). After 8 doses of MTX, there is resolution of contrast enhancement (C), consistent with a complete response. Although the FLAIR hyperintensity associated with the initial enhancing lesion in the anterior limb of the left internal capsule has improved, the degree of periventricular FLAIR hyperintensity in other areas has increased (D). There is also increased cerebral atrophy as evidenced by more prominent cerebral sulci. Seven months later, the patient remains in disease remission (E), but there is further progression of the periventricular white matter abnormality and cerebral atrophy (F).

Platinum-based agents

Platinum-based chemotherapeutics form intrastrand adducts and interstrand cross-links leading to alterations in the tertiary structure of nuclear and mitochondrial DNA,[51] which subsequently result in apoptosis.[52] These agents accumulate in the dorsal root ganglia, and, to a lesser extent, peripheral neurons. From a pharmacokinetic standpoint, cisplatin produces approximately 3 times more intrastrand adducts in the dorsal root ganglia compared with oxaliplatin, which is reflected by cisplatin's higher degree of neurotoxicity.[52] Interestingly, patient-specific single-nucleotide polymorphisms (SNPs) may play an important role in the development of neurotoxicity. Implicated genes include glutathione transferases (which are involved in detoxification), voltage-gated sodium channels, and genes affecting the activity of metal transporters.[52] However, validation studies in larger patient cohorts are required to determine the relative contributions of these genes to platinum-induced neurotoxicity. Clinically, the best known neurotoxic effects of platinum agents are peripheral neuropathy and ototoxicity, both of which are dose-limiting toxicities.

Neuroprotective strategies against platinum-induced neurotoxicity have been an area of intense research. Despite initial promising in vitro and small-scale clinical data, the American Society of Clinical Oncology does not recommend routine preventative use of amifostine for platinum-associated neurotoxicity or ototoxicity.[53] Other agents, including intratympanic dexamethasone,[54] vitamin E,[55] and sodium thiosulfate,[56] have demonstrated some benefit but require more robust testing in larger cohorts.

Treatment of platinum-induced neurotoxicity should focus on symptom relief, particularly neuropathy-associated pain. Duloxetine is the only agent that has shown a statistically significant effect on reduction of pain in a randomized placebo-controlled trial.[57] Patients who do not respond to duloxetine may be candidates for tricyclic antidepressants, gabapentin, pregabalin, or opioids, but robust evidence for the efficacy of these agents is lacking.[58,59]

Cisplatin Cisplatin is used in the treatment of medulloblastoma and head and neck, ovarian, germ cell, cervical, lung, and bladder cancers. Cisplatin-induced peripheral neuropathy presents as a symmetric sensory neuropathy that typically involves large myelinated sensory fibers at the level of the dorsal root ganglion and, to a lesser degree, peripheral nerve fibers. The clinical manifestations of cisplatin-induced peripheral neuropathy include proprioceptive loss, numbness, paresthesias in the fingers and/or toes, hyporeflexia, and eventually sensory gait ataxia.[60] The total cumulative dose is important, and symptoms typically emerge at doses of 300 mg/m^2 or higher.[60,61] The neuropathy usually improves after cessation of therapy. However, symptoms can also worsen or continue after cessation of therapy, which is referred to as coasting.[62,63] From a pathogenesis standpoint, coasting may be linked to cisplatin-induced inhibition of mitochondrial DNA replication, which leads to gradual energy failure and prolonged neurotoxicity even after cisplatin is stopped.[51] Patients often have persistent symptoms even after completion of therapy; in 1 study, approximately 20% of survivors had residual neuropathy at long-term follow-up.[61] In addition, Lhermitte sign (a shocklike sensation radiating from the neck to the feet provoked by neck flexion) has been reported, which is thought to imply involvement of the centripetal branch of the sensory pathways in the spinal cord.[64] Sural nerve biopsy reveals both demyelination and axonal loss.

Of all platinum-based drugs, cisplatin is the most ototoxic.[65] Ototoxicity presents with bilateral sensorineural hearing loss and tinnitus in up to 80% and 40% of patients,[66] respectively, which can begin during or years after treatment.[67] Mechanistically, it is related to apoptosis of auditory sensory cells secondary to abnormal protein and enzyme synthesis.[68] Otoxicity can be exacerbated by concurrent radiation.[69] All patients undergoing platinum-based therapy should thus have a baseline audiogram prior to starting treatment.

Rare complications of cisplatin neurotoxicity are encephalopathy, seizures, and focal neurologic deficits,[70,71] taste disturbance, and a myasthenic syndrome.[72]

Carboplatin Carboplatin is a second-generation platinum agent that has traditionally been regarded as less neurotoxic than cisplatin.[73] However, a recent Cochrane review comparing cisplatin and carboplatin combined with a third-generation drug in nonsmall cell lung cancer patients suggested that carboplatin had an approximately 1.5 times higher risk of causing neurotoxicity than cisplatin.[74] Carboplatin can cause a predominant sensory neuropathy at high doses,[75] as well as ototoxicity.[76]

Oxaliplatin Oxaliplatin, a third-generation platinum agent, is a standard component in the treatment of in metastatic colorectal cancer in conjunction with 5-FU and folinic acid (known as the FOLFOX regimen). Unlike cisplatin and carboplatin, it can cause an acute neuropathy-like syndrome, manifesting with dysesthesias and paresthesias affecting the fingers, toes, perioral, and oral regions.[77] In addition, cold sensitivity, sensitivity to swallowing cold items, throat discomfort, and muscle cramps may occur.[77] In a recent randomized controlled study of patients treated with FOLFOX, almost 90% reported acute neuropathic symptoms with the first treatment cycle. These emerged within a day after the first dose of oxaliplatin, peaked at day 3, and resolved thereafter.[77] As with other platinum agents, a chronic predominantly sensory neuropathy is a well-established consequence of oxaliplatin. Similar to cisplatin, the phenomenon of coasting[77] and Lhermitte sign[78] have been reported with oxaliplatin. Oxaliplatin is the least ototoxic of all platinum agents,[79,80] possibly because of pharmacokinetic differences in cochlear drug uptake compared with cisplatin.

Taxanes Taxanes bind and stabilize microtubules, resulting in mitotic arrest and apoptosis in dividing cells.[81] They are administered for numerous solid tumors, including nonsmall cell lung, ovarian, and breast cancer. The most frequently reported neurotoxic effect is a sensory peripheral neuropathy, which is more common and severe with paclitaxel than docetaxel.[82]

Paclitaxel Paclitaxel causes a predominantly large-fiber sensory axonal neuropathy that develops at high cumulative doses (1000 mg/m^2) and presents with paresthesia and pain in the hands and feet.[83,84] Axonal degeneration, secondary demyelination, and nerve fiber loss can be seen in severe cases.[85] Motor neuropathy and autonomic involvement are rare.[86,87] The neurotoxicity is exacerbated by pre-existing peripheral neuropathy, concurrent use of a platinum agent, older age, and presence of diabetes.[88] Given minimal blood-brain barrier penetration, CNS complications are much less common. These include rare reports of seizures[89] and self-resolving encephalopathy.[90,91] Both paclitaxel and docetaxel have been associated with an acute pain syndrome, characterized by myalgias and arthralgias that start 24 to 48 hours after drug administration and last for 5 to 7 days. A slightly higher incidence has been reported with paclitaxel than docetaxel (median 13.1% vs 10.3%).[92]

Recent research has focused on identifying SNPs that may predispose to taxane-induced peripheral neuropathy and found potential associations with numerous genes involved in drug metabolism and transport pathways, including the CYP2C8, CYP3A4 and ABCB1 genes.[93,94] If validated in larger cohorts, knowledge of the presence of certain SNPs may help guide selection of alternative chemotherapy agents with a more favorable adverse effect profile.

Docetaxel Docetaxel is a semisynthetic analogue of paclitaxel and produces a similar predominantly sensory neuropathy. Its neurotoxic threshold is lower than that of paclitaxel (400 mg/m^2).[84] Lhermitte sign has been observed in rare instances.[95,96]

Vinca alkaloids

Vincristine Vincristine is an antimicrotubule agent that induces arrest of dividing cells at the metaphase stage.[97] It is used in the treatment of leukemias, lymphomas, neuroblastomas, sarcomas, and brain tumors (including CNS lymphoma and malignant gliomas). Compared with vinblastine and vinolrebine, vincristine is the most neurotoxic vinca alkaloid[98] and causes some degree of neuropathy in almost all patients.[99] The neuropathy affects both sensory and motor nerves but has a predominant effect on small sensory fibers, which results in paresthesia in the fingertips and toes, pain, muscle cramps, and/or distal weakness.[100,101] Symptoms typically disappear a few months after stopping therapy, although persistence up to 40 months after treatment cessation has been observed.[102]

Autonomic and cranial neuropathies have also been reported. Autonomic neuropathy can manifest with orthostatic hypotension, paralytic ileus, constipation, bladder atony, and erectile dysfunction.[103–105] Cranial neuropathies can involve the oculomotor, abducens, recurrent laryngeal, optic, facial, and auditory nerve.[106–108] Vincristine can also have direct neurotoxic effects on the hypothalamus, neurohypophyseal tract, or the posterior pituitary gland and cause syndrome of inappropriate antidiuretic hormone secretion (SIADH).[109]

Of note, vincristine neurotoxicity has been observed at higher frequency in patients receiving concurrent azoles such as itraconazole, ketoconazole, posaconazole, and voriconazole. These agents inhibit vincristine metabolism through CYP3A4 and, to some extent, its transport by the efflux transporter P-glycoprotein.[110] In a literature review of adverse drug interactions with vincristine and azole antiantifungals, neuropathies of any type were reported in as many as 60% of patients.[110] Because azoles are frequently given prophylactically or therapeutically in certain cancer populations, the use of a nonazole antifungal agent should be considered in these cases.[110,111] Vincristine neurotoxicity is also potentiated in patients with Charcot-Marie Tooth syndrome, and its use is generally contraindicated in affected patients.[112,113]

Lastly, vincristine should never be administered intrathecally, as this can cause a severe ascending myeloencephalopathy and has resulted in fatal outcomes.[114]

Agents used in the treatment of plasma cell dyscrasias (thalidomide, lenolidomide, bortezomib)

Thalidomide and its second-generation derivative, lenolidomide, have numerous mechanisms, including immunomodulation (by means of increasing interleukin-2 production in T cells and decreasing proinflammatory cytokines) and binding to a ubiquitin ligase complex, which results in proteasomal degradation of disease-related proteins.[115] Bortezomib is a proteasome inhibitor; in addition to its inhibitory effects on transcriptional modulators, cytokine secretion, adhesion molecules, and angiogenesis, its efficacy is also based on the cancer cell's relatively higher dependence on the proteasome to clear abnormal proteins compared with normal cells.[116] All 3 agents are used in the treatment of newly diagnosed and relapsed multiple myeloma. Treatment-related peripheral neuropathy is a well-documented neurotoxic effect of thalidomide, with a reported incidence as high as 83%. It primarily causes a length-dependent sensory axonal neuropathy that emerges a few months after starting therapy.[117] Symptoms can be mild and sometimes subclinical[117] but tend to worsen with duration and dose of therapy (>200–400 mg/d).[118–120] Concurrent motor involvement has also been reported.[117,121] Lenolidomide is considered less neurotoxic than thalidomide; in 1 study, up to 27% of myeloma patients developed electrophysiologic evidence of a sensory axonal neuropathy 5 years after continuous lenolidomide therapy, but clinical symptoms were minimal.[122] Bortezomib causes a predominantly painful sensory neuropathy in up to 52% of patients.[123–126] Concurrent administration of dexamethasone may decrease this risk.[127]

Alkylating agents
Ifosfamide Ifosfamide is a nitrogen mustard alkylating agent used in the treatment of sarcomas and lymphomas. It causes an acute encephalopathy in approximately 15% to 30% of cases, presenting as somnolence, confusion, blurred vision, and progressing at times to seizures and coma.[128–130] Symptoms typically develop hours to days after ifosfamide administration and resolve 48 to 72 hours after drug discontinuation.[131] The encephalopathy is thought to be mediated by elevated levels of chloroacetylaldehyde, a neurotoxic metabolite of ifosfamide that readily crosses the blood-brain barrier.[128] Methylene blue, thiamine, and albumin can accelerate recovery but do not appear to have a prophylactic role.[132]

Busulfan At high doses, as seen in conditioning regimens for hematopoietic stem cell transplantation, busulfan can cause generalized seizures in approximately 10% of patients. These typically occur between day 2 after busulfan administration and within 24 hours after the last dose.[133] Some authors thus advocate for seizure prophylaxis in this patient population with benzodiazepines or levetiracetam.[134,135]

Targeted Agents

Unlike cytotoxic chemotherapy, targeted agents interfere with molecular pathways that are essential for the development and growth of tumor cells. Although the common assumption is that targeted agents are more selective for neoplastic cells in which aberrant pathways are upregulated, receptor cross-reactivity between tumor and normal cells can result in off-target toxicities.[136] The 2 main types of targeted agents are kinase inhibitors and monoclonal antibodies.

Tyrosine kinase inhibitors
Imatinib Imatinib inhibits the constitutively active fusion product of the BCR-ABL translocation in Philadelphia chromosome-positive chronic myelogenous leukemia and c-KIT in gastrointestinal stromal tumors.[137–139] Most commonly, mild and transient muscle cramping and myalgias occur with imatinib (incidence 49% and 20%, respectively), which are usually responsive to treatment with calcium, magnesium, or quinine.[140,141] Progression to rhabdomyolysis with concomitant creatinine kinase elevation and myoglobinuria is rare but has been reported.[142] Notably, spontaneous subdural hematomas in the absence of concurrent trauma or anticoagulation are seen in 2% to 7% of patients receiving imatinib.[143–146] Any patient with new-onset neurologic symptoms on imatinib should thus be evaluated for intracranial hemorrhage.

Sunitinib and sorafenib Sunitinib and sorafenib are both multikinase inhibitors that target the vascular endothelial growth factor (VEGF) receptor among other receptor families.[147,148] Both are approved for advanced renal cell carcinoma; sunitinib is additionally indicated in GIST and sorafenib for unresectable hepatocellular carcinoma.[149,150] In addition to hypertensive encephalopathy, sunitinib has been associated with hallucinations, confusion, and extrapyramidal symptoms in patients over 70 years with pre-existing arteriosclerotic leukoencephalopathy.[151]

Monoclonal antibodies

Antivascular endothelial growth factor agents (bevacizumab, sunitinib, sorafenib) Bevacizumab is a humanized monoclonal antibody against VEGF and approved for the treatment of renal, colorectal, lung, and cervical cancer, as well as recurrent glioblastoma.[152] Most VEGF-targeting agents, including sunitinib and sorafenib, cause hypertension and thus predispose to the PRES.[153–159] However, this appears to be a rare adverse effect, and fewer than 30 cases have been reported in the literature.[160] Blood pressure control is a crucial part of management in these cases. In addition, anti-VEGF agents increase the risk of ischemic strokes.[161] Based on meta-analyses, the incidence for arterial thromboembolic events (ATEs) was 1.4% and the relative risk of ATE 3.03 with sorafenib and sunitinib.[161] With bevacizumab, the incidence was 2.6% and relative risk 1.46 without any significant risk differences between types of malignancy.[162]

Bevacizumab has also been associated with intratumoral hemorrhage, although this risk is considered negligible. In 2 large randomized, placebo-controlled, phase 3 trials that compared bevacizumab plus standard first-line therapy (consisting of chemoradiation and adjuvant temozolomide) with standard therapy alone in patients with newly diagnosed glioblastoma,[163,164] the risk of cerebral hemorrhage was slightly higher in the bevacizumab than in the placebo group (3.3% vs 2.0% in 1 study[163]), but this did not reach statistical significance. Similarly, the overall risk of intracranial bleeding in patients with brain metastases treated with bevacizumab is low (<3%).[165–167]

Other monoclonal antibodies (rituximab, alemtuzumab, brentuximab) Other commonly used monoclonal antibodies are rarely associated with neurologic adverse effects. Rituximab is a humanized monoclonal antibody against CD20 on B lymphocytes and forms an integral part in the treatment of various B cell malignancies. Alemtuzumab neutralizes the CD25 receptor and is approved for chronic lymphocytic leukemia. Neurotoxicity is rare, but nonspecific symptoms such as headaches, myalgias, dizziness, and paresthesias can occur.[168,169] Both rituximab and alemtuzumab have been associated with reactivation of JC virus and progressive multifocal leukoencephalopathy (PML).[170]

Brentuximub vedotin, a CD30-directed antibody-drug conjugate used for CD30-positive lymphomas, has been associated with a primarily sensory peripheral neuropathy in 36% to 69% of patients.[171–173] In 1 study, more than 80% of patients experienced either resolution or improvement in their symptoms after cessation or completion of treatment.[174]

Bispecific antibodies

Blinatumomab Blinatumomab is a novel CD19-directed CD3 T cell engager approved for relapsed and refractory B-precursor acute lymphoblastic leukemia.[175] Neurotoxicity is seen in 47% to 52% of patients, most commonly paresthesia, tremor, dizziness, and confusion; of these, grade 3 or 4 toxicity has been observed in 0% to 13% of cases.[176,177] Headaches can affect approximately one-third of patients.[177] Seizures and aphasia have been reported but are not common (2%–4%).[176,177] Given these observations, blinatumomab carries a boxed warning for neurotoxicities.[178]

Immunotherapy Agents

Immune checkpoint inhibitors

Immune checkpoint inhibitors have transformed the field of medical oncology in recent years, particularly the management of metastatic melanoma and nonsmall cell lung cancer. They neutralize inhibitory T-cell signaling and increase tumor antigen-specific T-cell immunity, thereby enabling recognition and destruction of tumor cells by the immune system.[179] Immune-related adverse events (irAEs) are observed in 10% to 30% of patients treated with a single agent and as many as 55% receiving combined ipilimumab and nivolumab.[180,181] In general, irAEs tend to occur less frequently with nivolumab and pembrolizumab (5%–10%) compared with ipilimumab (22%–24%).[182] irAEs can affect virtually any organ system but most commonly involve the gastrointestinal, dermatologic, hepatic, endocrine, and pulmonary systems.[183] Neurologic toxicity occurs in only 1% to 3% of patients[183] but carries significant morbidity and can be potentially life-threatening. Most neurologic adverse events associated with checkpoint inhibitors are nonspecific grade 1 and 2 symptoms such as headaches (55%), changes in taste (13%), dizziness (10%),[184] lethargy, and asthenia.[185]

Anticytotoxic T-lymphocyte antigen-4 antibodies (ipilimumab) Ipilimumab is a recombinant human monoclonal antibody against cytotoxic T-lymphocyte antigen-4 (CTLA-4), which attained US Food and Drug Administration (FDA) approval for the treatment of stage 3 melanoma in 2011. The median time of onset of adverse effects is typically 6 weeks after initiation of therapy (ie, after 2 doses of ipilimumab).[184] Up to 17% of patients develop neuroendocrine complications as a result of hypophysitis, especially at higher doses (10 mg/kg). This is characterized by an enlarged and contrast-enhancing pituitary gland and infundibulum as well as endocrine abnormalities.[186] Among CNS-related toxicities, reports of encephalopathy with transient diffusion restriction in the splenium of the corpus callosum,[187] posterior reversible encephalopathy syndrome,[188] aseptic meningitis,[185,186,189] Tolosa-Hunt syndrome, granulomatous inflammation of the CNS, and transverse myelitis[190] exist. Peripheral nervous system complications include rare cases of Guillain-Barre syndrome,[186,191] sensory and motor neuropathies (including chronic inflammatory demyelinating polyneuropathy [CIDP]), myositis,[190] and myasthenia gravis.[192] Autonomic dysfunction such as neurogenic bladder[187] and enteric neuropathy[191,193] have also been reported. Management includes prompt discontinuation of ipilimumab, and, with grade 3 and 4 irAEs, initiation of high-dose corticosteroids, typically methylprednisolone. Plasmapheresis has also been tried with variable response rates.[190]

Anti-PD1 antibodies (pembrolizumab and nivolumab) Pembrolizumab and nivolumab are humanized monoclonal antibodies that block ligand activation of the PD-1 receptor on activated T-cells. They are both approved for selected patients with metastatic melanoma, recurrent metastatic NSCLC, recurrent or metastatic squamous carcinoma of the head and neck, and refractory classical Hodgkin lymphoma.[194,195] In addition, pembrolizumab attained accelerated approval as first line-treatment in combination with pemetrexed and carboplatin for metastatic nonsquamous NSCLC,[194] while nivolumab is also indicated for advanced renal cell carcinoma and recurrent metastatic urothelial carcinoma.[195] As with ipilimumab, anti-PD1 antibodies can cause hypophysitis. Pembrolizumab has been associated with rare reports of intracranial vasculitis,[196] limbic encephalitis after prolonged treatment for 12 months,[197] PRES,[198] a myasthenia gravis-like syndrome, and polyneuropathy.[182] Similarly, myasthenia gravis is rare with nivolumab.[199] GBS has been reported with nivolumab.[200] One patient had progressive apathy, mental status changes, and focal neurologic deficits despite immunosuppressive therapy and eventually died. Autopsy revealed widespread CNS demyelination.[201]

Chimeric antigen receptor T-cells

Chimeric antigen receptor (CAR) T cells are genetically engineered T-cells produced by manipulating a patient's own T-cells ex vivo to express the antigen-binding domain from a B-cell receptor fused to the intracellular domain of a CD3 T-cell receptor. This leads to recognition of a specific cell surface antigen on malignant cells and activation of a T-cell response.[202] CAR T-cells targeting the B-cell antigen CD19 have been studied extensively in leukemias and lymphomas[203] and are currently undergoing evaluation in clinical trials in leukemia patients. CAR T-cell-mediated tissue damage can occur via several mechanisms: (1) the tissue expresses the same targeted antigen as the cancer cell; (2) the tissue expresses an antigen that is similar to the antigen on the cancer cell (cross-reactivity); (3) an allergic reaction; and (4) tumor lysis syndrome.[203] The most common acute toxicity is a systemic inflammatory response (known as cytokine release syndrome [CRS]), which ranges in severity from mild to life-threatening. Neurotoxicity can occur concomitantly with CRS or in isolation, implying a separate mechanism responsible for the emergence of neurologic symptoms.[203] The reported incidence of neurotoxicity varies from 0% to 50%.[203] Clinically, patients present with headaches, delirium, global encephalopathy with associated aphasia and hallucinations, ataxia, apraxia, facial nerve palsy, tremors, myoclonus, and seizures.[204–210] Severe cases may necessitate intubation and mechanical ventilation. In some instances, CSF analysis reveals the presence of anti-CD19 CAR T-cells[204–208] and increased interleukin (IL)-6 levels.[211] Although systemic toxicities are typically treated with tocilizumab, an IL-6 receptor antagonist, it may have little impact on neurologic toxicity, partly due to its limited blood-brain barrier penetration and the different pathophysiologic mechanism associated with neurologic toxicity. The NCI Experimental Transplantation and Immunology Branch recommends dexamethasone as first-line therapy for CAR T-cell-induced neurotoxicity, given its excellent blood-brain barrier penetration and rapid onset of action.[203] Indications for steroid use include grade 3 toxicities for at least 24 hours, grade 4 toxicities of any duration, and any seizure. The proposed dosing is 10 mg intravenously every 6 hours until toxicities have improved to grade 1 or resolved or until 8 doses have been provided.[203] All patients with neurologic sequelae should be evaluated by the neurology service and undergo brain MRI. Lumbar puncture is indicated to exclude infectious etiologies.[203]

SUMMARY

Neurologic complications of cancer therapy can present a significant challenge in the management of oncologic patients. Prompt recognition and differentiation from other neurologic complications such as brain metastases, leptomeningeal disease, and paraneoplastic disorders can guide early treatment decisions. Future research should focus on identification of individual patient risk factors that may predispose to neurotoxic adverse effects from specific drugs and appropriate preventive or therapeutic measures to alleviate or resolve symptoms.

REFERENCES

1. Forster VJ, van Delft FW, Baird SF, et al. Drug interactions may be important risk factors for methotrexate neurotoxicity, particularly in pediatric leukemia patients. Cancer Chemother Pharmacol 2016;78(5):1093–6.
2. Rubin RC, Ommaya AK, Henderson ES, et al. Cerebrospinal fluid perfusion for central nervous system neoplasms. Neurology 1966;16(7):680–92.
3. Sullivan MP, Vietti TJ, Haggard ME, et al. Remission maintenance therapy for meningeal leukemia: intrathecal methotrexate vs. intravenous bis-nitrosourea. Blood 1971;38(6):680–8.
4. Geiser CF, Bishop Y, Jaffe N, et al. Adverse effects of intrathecal methotrexate in children with acute leukemia in remission. Blood 1975;45(2):189–95.

5. Jacob LA, Sreevatsa A, Chinnagiriyappa LK, et al. Methotrexate-induced chemical meningitis in patients with acute lymphoblastic leukemia/lymphoma. Ann Indian Acad Neurol 2015;18(2):206–9.

6. Teh HS, Fadilah SA, Leong CF. Transverse myelopathy following intrathecal administration of chemotherapy. Singapore Med J 2007;48(2):e46–9.

7. Cachia D, Kamiya-Matsuoka C, Pinnix CC, et al. Myelopathy following intrathecal chemotherapy in adults: a single institution experience. J Neurooncol 2015;122(2):391–8.

8. Gagliano RG, Costanzi JJ. Paraplegia following intrathecal methotrexate: report of a case and review of the literature. Cancer 1976;37(4):1663–8.

9. Rubnitz JE, Relling MV, Harrison PL, et al. Transient encephalopathy following high-dose methotrexate treatment in childhood acute lymphoblastic leukemia. Leukemia 1998;12(8):1176–81.

10. Packer RJ, Grossman RI, Belasco JB. High dose systemic methotrexate-associated acute neurologic dysfunction. Med Pediatr Oncol 1983;11(3):159–61.

11. Walker RW, Allen JC, Rosen G, et al. Transient cerebral dysfunction secondary to high-dose methotrexate. J Clin Oncol 1986;4(12):1845–50.

12. Kishi S, Griener J, Cheng C, et al. Homocysteine, pharmacogenetics, and neurotoxicity in children with leukemia. J Clin Oncol 2003;21(16):3084–91.

13. Radtke S, Zolk O, Renner B, et al. Germline genetic variations in methotrexate candidate genes are associated with pharmacokinetics, toxicity, and outcome in childhood acute lymphoblastic leukemia. Blood 2013;121(26):5145–53.

14. Pizzo PA, Poplack DG, Bleyer WA. Neurotoxicities of current leukemia therapy. Am J Pediatr Hematol Oncol 1979;1(2):127–40.

15. Rubinstein LJ, Herman MM, Long TF, et al. Disseminated necrotizing leukoencephalopathy: a complication of treated central nervous system leukemia and lymphoma. Cancer 1975;35(2):291–305.

16. Oka M, Terae S, Kobayashi R, et al. MRI in methotrexate-related leukoencephalopathy: disseminated necrotising leukoencephalopathy in comparison with mild leukoencephalopathy. Neuroradiology 2003;45(7):493–7.

17. Delval L, Klastersky J. Optic neuropathy in cancer patients. Report of a case possibly related to 5 fluorouracil toxicity and review of the literature. J Neurooncol 2002;60(2):165–9.

18. Milano G, Etienne MC, Pierrefite V, et al. Dihydropyrimidine dehydrogenase deficiency and fluorouracil-related toxicity. Br J Cancer 1999;79(3–4):627–30.

19. Lu Z, Zhang R, Diasio RB. Dihydropyrimidine dehydrogenase activity in human peripheral blood mononuclear cells and liver: population characteristics, newly identified deficient patients, and clinical implication in 5-fluorouracil chemotherapy. Cancer Res 1993;53(22):5433–8.

20. Gottlieb JA, Luce JK. Cerebellar ataxia with weekly 5-fluorouracil administration. Lancet 1971;1(7690):138–9.

21. Moore DH, Fowler WC Jr, Crumpler LS. 5-Fluorouracil neurotoxicity. Gynecol Oncol 1990;36(1):152–4.

22. Riehl JL, Brown WJ. Acute cerebellar syndrome secondary to 5-fluorouracil therapy. Neurology 1964;14:961–7.

23. Greenwald ES. Letter: organic mental changes with fluorouracil therapy. JAMA 1976;235(3):248–9.

24. Lynch HT, Droszcz CP, Albano WA, et al. "Organic brain syndrome" secondary to 5-fluorouracil toxicity. Dis Colon Rectum 1981;24(2):130–1.

25. Liaw CC, Wang HM, Wang CH, et al. Risk of transient hyperammonemic encephalopathy in cancer patients who received continuous infusion of 5-fluorouracil with the complication of dehydration and infection. Anticancer Drugs 1999;10(3):275–81.

26. Yeh KH, Cheng AL. High-dose 5-fluorouracil infusional therapy is associated with hyperammonaemia, lactic acidosis and encephalopathy. Br J Cancer 1997;75(3):464–5.

27. Kim YA, Chung HC, Choi HJ, et al. Intermediate dose 5-fluorouracil-induced encephalopathy. Jpn J Clin Oncol 2006;36(1):55–9.

28. Kikuta S, Asakage T, Nakao K, et al. The aggravating factors of hyperammonemia related to 5-fluorouracil infusion–a report of two cases. Auris Nasus Larynx 2008;35(2):295–9.

29. Brashear A, Siemers E. Focal dystonia after chemotherapy: a case series. J Neurooncol 1997;34(2):163–7.

30. Bergevin PR, Patwardhan VC, Weissman J, et al. Letter: neurotoxicity of 5-fluorouracil. Lancet 1975;1(7903):410.

31. Stein ME, Drumea K, Yarnitsky D, et al. A rare event of 5-fluorouracil-associated peripheral neuropathy: a report of two patients. Am J Clin Oncol 1998;21(3):248–9.

32. Werbrouck BF, Pauwels WJ, De Bleecker JL. A case of 5-fluorouracil-induced peripheral neuropathy. Clin Toxicol (Phila) 2008;46(3):264–6.

33. Pirzada NA, Ali II, Dafer RM. Fluorouracil-induced neurotoxicity. Ann Pharmacother 2000;34(1):35–8.

34. El Amrani M, Heinzlef O, Debroucker T, et al. Brain infarction following 5-fluorouracil and cisplatin therapy. Neurology 1998;51(3):899–901.

35. Gounaris I, Ahmad A. Capecitabine-induced cerebellar toxicity in a patient with metastatic colorectal cancer. J Oncol Pharm Pract 2010;16(4):277–9.

36. Renouf D, Gill S. Capecitabine-induced cerebellar toxicity. Clin Colorectal Cancer 2006;6(1):70–1.

37. Videnovic A, Semenov I, Chua-Adajar R, et al. Capecitabine-induced multifocal leukoencephalopathy: a report of five cases. Neurology 2005;65(11):1792–4 [discussion: 1685].

38. Niemann B, Rochlitz C, Herrmann R, et al. Toxic encephalopathy induced by capecitabine. Oncology 2004;66(4):331–5.

39. van Pelt-Sprangers MJ, Geijteman EC, Alsma J, et al. Oromandibular dystonia: a serious side effect of capecitabine. BMC Cancer 2015;15:115.

40. Ngeow JY, Prakash KM, Chowbay B, et al. Capecitabine-induced oromandibular dystonia: a case report and literature review. Acta Oncol 2008;47(6):1161–5.

41. Hwang TL, Yung WK, Estey EH, et al. Central nervous system toxicity with high-dose Ara-C. Neurology 1985;35(10):1475–9.

42. Zawacki T, Friedman JH, Grace J, et al. Cerebellar toxicity of cytosine arabinoside: clinical and neuropsychological signs. Neurology 2000;55(8):1234.

43. Jolson HM, Bosco L, Bufton MG, et al. Clustering of adverse drug events: analysis of risk factors for cerebellar toxicity with high-dose cytarabine. J Natl Cancer Inst 1992;84(7):500–5.

44. Smith GA, Damon LE, Rugo HS, et al. High-dose cytarabine dose modification reduces the incidence of neurotoxicity in patients with renal insufficiency. J Clin Oncol 1997;15(2):833–9.

45. Friedman JH, Shetty N. Permanent cerebellar toxicity of cytosine arabinoside (Ara C) in a young woman. Mov Disord 2001;16(3):575–7.

46. Openshaw H, Slatkin NE, Stein AS, et al. Acute polyneuropathy after high dose cytosine arabinoside in patients with leukemia. Cancer 1996;78(9):1899–905.
47. Ventura GJ, Keating MJ, Castellanos AM, et al. Reversible bilateral lateral rectus muscle palsy associated with high-dose cytosine arabinoside and mitoxantrone therapy. Cancer 1986;58(8):1633–5.
48. Luque FA, Selhorst JB, Petruska P. Parkinsonism induced by high-dose cytosine arabinoside. Mov Disord 1987;2(3):219–22.
49. Dunton SF, Nitschke R, Spruce WE, et al. Progressive ascending paralysis following administration of intrathecal and intravenous cytosine arabinoside. A Pediatric Oncology Group study. Cancer 1986;57(6):1083–8.
50. Arrillaga-Romany IC, Dietrich J. Imaging findings in cancer therapy-associated neurotoxicity. Semin Neurol 2012;32(4):476–86.
51. Podratz JL, Knight AM, Ta LE, et al. Cisplatin induced mitochondrial DNA damage in dorsal root ganglion neurons. Neurobiol Dis 2011;41(3):661–8.
52. Avan A, Postma TJ, Ceresa C, et al. Platinum-induced neurotoxicity and preventive strategies: past, present, and future. Oncologist 2015;20(4):411–32.
53. Hensley ML, Hagerty KL, Kewalramani T, et al. American Society of Clinical Oncology 2008 clinical practice guideline update: use of chemotherapy and radiation therapy protectants. J Clin Oncol 2009;27(1):127–45.
54. Marshak T, Steiner M, Kaminer M, et al. Prevention of cisplatin-induced hearing loss by intratympanic dexamethasone: a randomized controlled study. Otolaryngol Head Neck Surg 2014;150(6):983–90.
55. Kalkanis JG, Whitworth C, Rybak LP. Vitamin E reduces cisplatin ototoxicity. Laryngoscope 2004;114(3):538–42.
56. Freyer DR, Chen L, Krailo MD, et al. Effects of sodium thiosulfate versus observation on development of cisplatin-induced hearing loss in children with cancer (ACCL0431): a multicentre, randomised, controlled, open-label, phase 3 trial. Lancet Oncol 2017;18(1):63–74.
57. Smith EM, Pang H, Cirrincione C, et al. Effect of duloxetine on pain, function, and quality of life among patients with chemotherapy-induced painful peripheral neuropathy: a randomized clinical trial. JAMA 2013;309(13):1359–67.
58. Hammack JE, Michalak JC, Loprinzi CL, et al. Phase III evaluation of nortriptyline for alleviation of symptoms of cis-platinum-induced peripheral neuropathy. Pain 2002;98(1–2):195–203.
59. Rao RD, Michalak JC, Sloan JA, et al. Efficacy of gabapentin in the management of chemotherapy-induced peripheral neuropathy: a phase 3 randomized, double-blind, placebo-controlled, crossover trial (N00C3). Cancer 2007;110(9):2110–8.
60. Argyriou AA, Bruna J, Marmiroli P, et al. Chemotherapy-induced peripheral neurotoxicity (CIPN): an update. Crit Rev Oncol Hematol 2012;82(1):51–77.
61. Glendenning JL, Barbachano Y, Norman AR, et al. Long-term neurologic and peripheral vascular toxicity after chemotherapy treatment of testicular cancer. Cancer 2010;116(10):2322–31.
62. Park SB, Lin CS, Krishnan AV, et al. Oxaliplatin-induced neurotoxicity: changes in axonal excitability precede development of neuropathy. Brain 2009;132(Pt 10):2712–23.
63. Grunberg SM, Sonka S, Stevenson LL, et al. Progressive paresthesias after cessation of therapy with very high-dose cisplatin. Cancer Chemother Pharmacol 1989;25(1):62–4.
64. Cavaletti G, Alberti P, Marmiroli P. Chemotherapy-induced peripheral neurotoxicity in the era of pharmacogenomics. Lancet Oncol 2011;12(12):1151–61.

65. McKeage MJ. Comparative adverse effect profiles of platinum drugs. Drug Saf 1995;13(4):228–44.
66. Frisina RD, Wheeler HE, Fossa SD, et al. Comprehensive audiometric analysis of hearing impairment and tinnitus after cisplatin-based chemotherapy in survivors of adult-onset cancer. J Clin Oncol 2016;34(23):2712–20.
67. Bertolini P, Lassalle M, Mercier G, et al. Platinum compound-related ototoxicity in children: long-term follow-up reveals continuous worsening of hearing loss. J Pediatr Hematol Oncol 2004;26(10):649–55.
68. Thomas JP, Lautermann J, Liedert B, et al. High accumulation of platinum-DNA adducts in strial marginal cells of the cochlea is an early event in cisplatin but not carboplatin ototoxicity. Mol Pharmacol 2006;70(1):23–9.
69. Low WK, Toh ST, Wee J, et al. Sensorineural hearing loss after radiotherapy and chemoradiotherapy: a single, blinded, randomized study. J Clin Oncol 2006; 24(12):1904–9.
70. Ito Y, Arahata Y, Goto Y, et al. Cisplatin neurotoxicity presenting as reversible posterior leukoencephalopathy syndrome. AJNR Am J Neuroradiol 1998; 19(3):415–7.
71. Lyass O, Lossos A, Hubert A, et al. Cisplatin-induced non-convulsive encephalopathy. Anticancer Drugs 1998;9(1):100–4.
72. Posner JB. Side effects of chemotherapy. In: Davis FA, editor. Neurologic complications of cancer. Philadelphia: FA Davis Company; 1995. p. 282.
73. Albers JW, Chaudhry V, Cavaletti G, et al. Interventions for preventing neuropathy caused by cisplatin and related compounds. Cochrane Database Syst Rev 2014;(3):CD005228.
74. de Castria TB, da Silva EM, Gois AF, et al. Cisplatin versus carboplatin in combination with third-generation drugs for advanced non-small cell lung cancer. Cochrane Database Syst Rev 2013;(8):CD009256.
75. Heinzlef O, Lotz JP, Roullet E. Severe neuropathy after high dose carboplatin in three patients receiving multidrug chemotherapy. J Neurol Neurosurg Psychiatry 1998;64(5):667–9.
76. Clemens E, de Vries AC, Pluijm SF, et al. Determinants of ototoxicity in 451 platinum-treated Dutch survivors of childhood cancer: a DCOG late-effects study. Eur J Cancer 2016;69:77–85.
77. Pachman DR, Qin R, Seisler DK, et al. Clinical course of oxaliplatin-induced neuropathy: results from the randomized phase III trial N08CB (alliance). J Clin Oncol 2015;33(30):3416–22.
78. Taieb S, Trillet-Lenoir V, Rambaud L, et al. Lhermitte sign and urinary retention: atypical presentation of oxaliplatin neurotoxicity in four patients. Cancer 2002; 94(9):2434–40.
79. Hijri FZ, Arifi S, Ouattassi N, et al. Oxaliplatin-induced ototoxicity in adjuvant setting for colorectal cancer: unusual side effect. J Gastrointest Cancer 2014; 45(1):106–8.
80. Vietor NO, George BJ. Oxaliplatin-induced hepatocellular injury and ototoxicity: a review of the literature and report of unusual side effects of a commonly used chemotherapeutic agent. J Oncol Pharm Pract 2012;18(3):355–9.
81. Gornstein E, Schwarz TL. The paradox of paclitaxel neurotoxicity: mechanisms and unanswered questions. Neuropharmacology 2014;76 Pt A:175–83.
82. Lee JJ, Swain SM. Peripheral neuropathy induced by microtubule-stabilizing agents. J Clin Oncol 2006;24(10):1633–42.

83. Argyriou AA, Koltzenburg M, Polychronopoulos P, et al. Peripheral nerve damage associated with administration of taxanes in patients with cancer. Crit Rev Oncol Hematol 2008;66(3):218–28.
84. Grisold W, Cavaletti G, Windebank AJ. Peripheral neuropathies from chemotherapeutics and targeted agents: diagnosis, treatment, and prevention. Neuro Oncol 2012;14(Suppl 4):iv45–54.
85. Sahenk Z, Barohn R, New P, et al. Taxol neuropathy. Electrodiagnostic and sural nerve biopsy findings. Arch Neurol 1994;51(7):726–9.
86. Freilich RJ, Balmaceda C, Seidman AD, et al. Motor neuropathy due to docetaxel and paclitaxel. Neurology 1996;47(1):115–8.
87. Winer EP, Berry DA, Woolf S, et al. Failure of higher-dose paclitaxel to improve outcome in patients with metastatic breast cancer: cancer and leukemia group B trial 9342. J Clin Oncol 2004;22(11):2061–8.
88. Hershman DL, Till C, Wright JD, et al. Comorbidities and risk of chemotherapy-induced peripheral neuropathy among participants 65 years or older in southwest oncology group clinical trials. J Clin Oncol 2016;34(25):3014–22.
89. McGuire WP, Rowinsky EK, Rosenshein NB, et al. Taxol: a unique antineoplastic agent with significant activity in advanced ovarian epithelial neoplasms. Ann Intern Med 1989;111(4):273–9.
90. Perry JR, Warner E. Transient encephalopathy after paclitaxel (Taxol) infusion. Neurology 1996;46(6):1596–9.
91. Rook J, Rosser T, Fangusaro J, et al. Acute transient encephalopathy following paclitaxel treatment in an adolescent with a recurrent suprasellar germinoma. Pediatr Blood Cancer 2008;50(3):699–700.
92. Fernandes R, Mazzarello S, Majeed H, et al. Treatment of taxane acute pain syndrome (TAPS) in cancer patients receiving taxane-based chemotherapy-a systematic review. Support Care Cancer 2016;24(4):1583–94.
93. Kus T, Aktas G, Kalender ME, et al. Polymorphism of CYP3A4 and ABCB1 genes increase the risk of neuropathy in breast cancer patients treated with paclitaxel and docetaxel. Onco Targets Ther 2016;9:5073–80.
94. de Graan AJ, Elens L, Sprowl JA, et al. CYP3A4*22 genotype and systemic exposure affect paclitaxel-induced neurotoxicity. Clin Cancer Res 2013; 19(12):3316–24.
95. van den Bent MJ, Hilkens PH, Sillevis Smitt PA, et al. Lhermitte's sign following chemotherapy with docetaxel. Neurology 1998;50(2):563–4.
96. Hilkens PH, Verweij J, Vecht CJ, et al. Clinical characteristics of severe peripheral neuropathy induced by docetaxel (Taxotere). Ann Oncol 1997;8(2):187–90.
97. Jordan MA, Wilson L. Microtubules as a target for anticancer drugs. Nat Rev Cancer 2004;4(4):253–65.
98. Moudi M, Go R, Yien CY, et al. Vinca alkaloids. Int J Prev Med 2013;4(11): 1231–5.
99. Mora E, Smith EM, Donohoe C, et al. Vincristine-induced peripheral neuropathy in pediatric cancer patients. Am J Cancer Res 2016;6(11):2416–30.
100. Purser MJ, Johnston DL, McMillan HJ. Chemotherapy-induced peripheral neuropathy among paediatric oncology patients. Can J Neurol Sci 2014;41(4): 442–7.
101. Jain P, Gulati S, Seth R, et al. Vincristine-induced neuropathy in childhood ALL (acute lymphoblastic leukemia) survivors: prevalence and electrophysiological characteristics. J Child Neurol 2014;29(7):932–7.
102. Postma TJ, Benard BA, Huijgens PC, et al. Long-term effects of vincristine on the peripheral nervous system. J Neurooncol 1993;15(1):23–7.

103. Egbelakin A, Ferguson MJ, MacGill EA, et al. Increased risk of vincristine neurotoxicity associated with low CYP3A5 expression genotype in children with acute lymphoblastic leukemia. Pediatr Blood Cancer 2011;56(3):361–7.
104. Roca E, Bruera E, Politi PM, et al. Vinca alkaloid-induced cardiovascular autonomic neuropathy. Cancer Treat Rep 1985;69(2):149–51.
105. Legha SS. Vincristine neurotoxicity. Pathophysiology and management. Med Toxicol 1986;1(6):421–7.
106. Talebian A, Goudarzi RM, Mohammadzadeh M, et al. Vincristine-induced cranial neuropathy. Iran J Child Neurol 2014;8(1):66–8.
107. Tuxen MK, Hansen SW. Neurotoxicity secondary to antineoplastic drugs. Cancer Treat Rev 1994;20(2):191–214.
108. Ngamphaiboon N, Sweeney R, Wetzler M, et al. Pyridoxine treatment of vincristine-induced cranial polyneuropathy in an adult patient with acute lymphocytic leukemia: case report and review of the literature. Leuk Res 2010; 34(8):e194–6.
109. Escuro RS, Adelstein DJ, Carter SG. Syndrome of inappropriate secretion of antidiuretic hormone after infusional vincristine. Cleve Clin J Med 1992;59(6): 643–4.
110. Moriyama B, Henning SA, Leung J, et al. Adverse interactions between antifungal azoles and vincristine: review and analysis of cases. Mycoses 2012; 55(4):290–7.
111. Teusink AC, Ragucci D, Shatat IF, et al. Potentiation of vincristine toxicity with concomitant fluconazole prophylaxis in children with acute lymphoblastic leukemia. Pediatr Hematol Oncol 2012;29(1):62–7.
112. Aghajan Y, Yoon JM, Crawford JR. Severe vincristine-induced polyneuropathy in a teenager with anaplastic medulloblastoma and undiagnosed Charcot-Marie-Tooth disease. BMJ Case Rep 2017;2017 [pii:bcr-2016-218981].
113. Nishikawa T, Kawakami K, Kumamoto T, et al. Severe neurotoxicities in a case of Charcot-Marie-Tooth disease type 2 caused by vincristine for acute lymphoblastic leukemia. J Pediatr Hematol Oncol 2008;30(7):519–21.
114. Grissinger M. Death and neurological devastation from intrathecal vinca alkaloids. P T 2016;41(8):464–525.
115. Fink EC, Ebert BL. The novel mechanism of lenalidomide activity. Blood 2015; 126(21):2366–9.
116. Hideshima T, Richardson PG, Anderson KC. Mechanism of action of proteasome inhibitors and deacetylase inhibitors and the biological basis of synergy in multiple myeloma. Mol Cancer Ther 2011;10(11):2034–42.
117. Plasmati R, Pastorelli F, Cavo M, et al. Neuropathy in multiple myeloma treated with thalidomide: a prospective study. Neurology 2007;69(6):573–81.
118. Glasmacher A, Hahn C, Hoffmann F, et al. A systematic review of phase-II trials of thalidomide monotherapy in patients with relapsed or refractory multiple myeloma. Br J Haematol 2006;132(5):584–93.
119. Ghobrial IM, Rajkumar SV. Management of thalidomide toxicity. J Support Oncol 2003;1(3):194–205.
120. Richardson P, Schlossman R, Jagannath S, et al. Thalidomide for patients with relapsed multiple myeloma after high-dose chemotherapy and stem cell transplantation: results of an open-label multicenter phase 2 study of efficacy, toxicity, and biological activity. Mayo Clin Proc 2004;79(7):875–82.
121. Mileshkin L, Stark R, Day B, et al. Development of neuropathy in patients with myeloma treated with thalidomide: patterns of occurrence and the role of electrophysiologic monitoring. J Clin Oncol 2006;24(27):4507–14.

122. Dalla Torre C, Zambello R, Cacciavillani M, et al. Lenalidomide long-term neurotoxicity: clinical and neurophysiologic prospective study. Neurology 2016;87(11): 1161–6.

123. Jagannath S, Durie BG, Wolf J, et al. Bortezomib therapy alone and in combination with dexamethasone for previously untreated symptomatic multiple myeloma. Br J Haematol 2005;129(6):776–83.

124. Richardson PG, Sonneveld P, Schuster MW, et al. Bortezomib or high-dose dexamethasone for relapsed multiple myeloma. N Engl J Med 2005;352(24): 2487–98.

125. Richardson PG, Briemberg H, Jagannath S, et al. Frequency, characteristics, and reversibility of peripheral neuropathy during treatment of advanced multiple myeloma with bortezomib. J Clin Oncol 2006;24(19):3113–20.

126. Badros A, Goloubeva O, Dalal JS, et al. Neurotoxicity of bortezomib therapy in multiple myeloma: a single-center experience and review of the literature. Cancer 2007;110(5):1042–9.

127. Kumar SK, Laubach JP, Giove TJ, et al. Impact of concomitant dexamethasone dosing schedule on bortezomib-induced peripheral neuropathy in multiple myeloma. Br J Haematol 2017;178(5):756–63.

128. Szabatura AH, Cirrone F, Harris C, et al. An assessment of risk factors associated with ifosfamide-induced encephalopathy in a large academic cancer center. J Oncol Pharm Pract 2015;21(3):188–93.

129. Lorigan P, Verweij J, Papai Z, et al. Phase III trial of two investigational schedules of ifosfamide compared with standard-dose doxorubicin in advanced or metastatic soft tissue sarcoma: a European Organisation for Research and Treatment of Cancer Soft Tissue and Bone Sarcoma Group Study. J Clin Oncol 2007; 25(21):3144–50.

130. David KA, Picus J. Evaluating risk factors for the development of ifosfamide encephalopathy. Am J Clin Oncol 2005;28(3):277–80.

131. Ajithkumar T, Parkinson C, Shamshad F, et al. Ifosfamide encephalopathy. Clin Oncol (R Coll Radiol) 2007;19(2):108–14.

132. Richards A, Marshall H, McQuary A. Evaluation of methylene blue, thiamine, and/or albumin in the prevention of ifosfamide-related neurotoxicity. J Oncol Pharm Pract 2011;17(4):372–80.

133. Eberly AL, Anderson GD, Bubalo JS, et al. Optimal prevention of seizures induced by high-dose busulfan. Pharmacotherapy 2008;28(12):1502–10.

134. Diaz-Carrasco MS, Olmos R, Blanquer M, et al. Clonazepam for seizure prophylaxis in adult patients treated with high dose busulfan. Int J Clin Pharm 2013; 35(3):339–43.

135. Soni S, Skeens M, Termuhlen AM, et al. Levetiracetam for busulfan-induced seizure prophylaxis in children undergoing hematopoietic stem cell transplantation. Pediatr Blood Cancer 2012;59(4):762–4.

136. Gharwan H, Groninger H. Kinase inhibitors and monoclonal antibodies in oncology: clinical implications. Nat Rev Clin Oncol 2016;13(4):209–27.

137. Gambacorti-Passerini C, le Coutre P, Mologni L, et al. Inhibition of the ABL kinase activity blocks the proliferation of BCR/ABL+ leukemic cells and induces apoptosis. Blood Cells Mol Dis 1997;23(3):380–94.

138. van der Kuip H, Moehring A, Wohlbold L, et al. Imatinib mesylate (STI571) prevents the mutator phenotype of Bcr-Abl in hematopoietic cell lines. Leuk Res 2004;28(4):405–8.

139. Sleijfer S, Wiemer E, Verweij J. Drug insight: gastrointestinal stromal tumors (GIST)–the solid tumor model for cancer-specific treatment. Nat Clin Pract Oncol 2008;5(2):102–11.

140. Deininger MW, O'Brien SG, Ford JM, et al. Practical management of patients with chronic myeloid leukemia receiving imatinib. J Clin Oncol 2003;21(8): 1637–47.

141. Kantarjian H, Shah NP, Hochhaus A, et al. Dasatinib versus imatinib in newly diagnosed chronic-phase chronic myeloid leukemia. N Engl J Med 2010; 362(24):2260–70.

142. Penel N, Blay JY, Adenis A. Imatinib as a possible cause of severe rhabdomyolysis. N Engl J Med 2008;358(25):2746–7.

143. Theodotou CB, Shah AH, Ivan ME, et al. Subdural hematoma in a patient taking imatinib for GIST: a case report and discussion of risk with other chemotherapeutics. Anticancer Drugs 2016;27(3):259–63.

144. Song KW, Rifkind J, Al-Beirouti B, et al. Subdural hematomas during CML therapy with imatinib mesylate. Leuk Lymphoma 2004;45(8):1633–6.

145. Pollack IF, Jakacki RI, Blaney SM, et al. Phase I trial of imatinib in children with newly diagnosed brainstem and recurrent malignant gliomas: a Pediatric Brain Tumor Consortium report. Neuro Oncol 2007;9(2):145–60.

146. Wen PY, Yung WK, Lamborn KR, et al. Phase I/II study of imatinib mesylate for recurrent malignant gliomas: North American Brain Tumor Consortium Study 99-08. Clin Cancer Res 2006;12(16):4899–907.

147. Adnane L, Trail PA, Taylor I, et al. Sorafenib (BAY 43-9006, Nexavar), a dual-action inhibitor that targets RAF/MEK/ERK pathway in tumor cells and tyrosine kinases VEGFR/PDGFR in tumor vasculature. Methods Enzymol 2006;407: 597–612.

148. Le Tourneau C, Raymond E, Faivre S. Sunitinib: a novel tyrosine kinase inhibitor. A brief review of its therapeutic potential in the treatment of renal carcinoma and gastrointestinal stromal tumors (GIST). Ther Clin Risk Manag 2007;3(2):341–8.

149. FDA. Highlights of prescribing information: Nexavar (sorafenib). 2010. Available at: https://www.accessdata.fda.gov/drugsatfda_docs/label/2010/021923s008s 009lbl.pdf. Accessed August 17, 2017.

150. FDA. Highlights of prescribing information: Sutent. 2011. Available at: https:// www.accessdata.fda.gov/drugsatfda_docs/label/2011/021938s13s17s18lbl.pdf. Accessed August 17, 2017.

151. van der Veldt AA, van den Eertwegh AJ, Hoekman K, et al. Reversible cognitive disorders after sunitinib for advanced renal cell cancer in patients with preexisting arteriosclerotic leukoencephalopathy. Ann Oncol 2007;18(10):1747–50.

152. FDA. Highlights of prescribing information: Avastin. 2014. Available at: https:// www.accessdata.fda.gov/drugsatfda_docs/label/2014/125085s301lbl.pdf. Accessed July 31, 2017.

153. Ozcan C, Wong SJ, Hari P. Reversible posterior leukoencephalopathy syndrome and bevacizumab. N Engl J Med 2006;354(9):980–2 [discussion: 980–2].

154. Allen JA, Adlakha A, Bergethon PR. Reversible posterior leukoencephalopathy syndrome after bevacizumab/FOLFIRI regimen for metastatic colon cancer. Arch Neurol 2006;63(10):1475–8.

155. Koopman M, Muller EW, Punt CJ. Reversible posterior leukoencephalopathy syndrome caused by bevacizumab: report of a case. Dis Colon Rectum 2008; 51(9):1425–6.

156. Glusker P, Recht L, Lane B. Reversible posterior leukoencephalopathy syndrome and bevacizumab. N Engl J Med 2006;354(9):980–2 [discussion: 980–2].

157. Govindarajan R, Adusumilli J, Baxter DL, et al. Reversible posterior leukoence- phalopathy syndrome induced by RAF kinase inhibitor BAY 43-9006. J Clin On- col 2006;24(28):e48.
158. Kapiteijn E, Brand A, Kroep J, et al. Sunitinib induced hypertension, thrombotic microangiopathy and reversible posterior leukencephalopathy syndrome. Ann Oncol 2007;18(10):1745–7.
159. Martin G, Bellido L, Cruz JJ. Reversible posterior leukoencephalopathy syn- drome induced by sunitinib. J Clin Oncol 2007;25(23):3559.
160. Tlemsani C, Mir O, Boudou-Rouquette P, et al. Posterior reversible encephalop- athy syndrome induced by anti-VEGF agents. Target Oncol 2011;6(4):253–8.
161. Choueiri TK, Schutz FA, Je Y, et al. Risk of arterial thromboembolic events with sunitinib and sorafenib: a systematic review and meta-analysis of clinical trials. J Clin Oncol 2010;28(13):2280–5.
162. Schutz FA, Je Y, Azzi GR, et al. Bevacizumab increases the risk of arterial ischemia: a large study in cancer patients with a focus on different subgroup outcomes. Ann Oncol 2011;22(6):1404–12.
163. Chinot OL, Wick W, Mason W, et al. Bevacizumab plus radiotherapy- temozolomide for newly diagnosed glioblastoma. N Engl J Med 2014;370(8): 709–22.
164. Gilbert MR, Dignam JJ, Armstrong TS, et al. A randomized trial of bevacizumab for newly diagnosed glioblastoma. N Engl J Med 2014;370(8):699–708.
165. Carden CP, Larkin JM, Rosenthal MA. What is the risk of intracranial bleeding during anti-VEGF therapy? Neuro Oncol 2008;10(4):624–30.
166. Sandler A, Hirsh V, Reck M, et al. An evidence-based review of the incidence of CNS bleeding with anti-VEGF therapy in non-small cell lung cancer patients with brain metastases. Lung Cancer 2012;78(1):1–7.
167. Besse B, Lasserre SF, Compton P, et al. Bevacizumab safety in patients with central nervous system metastases. Clin Cancer Res 2010;16(1):269–78.
168. Maloney DG, Grillo-Lopez AJ, Bodkin DJ, et al. IDEC-C2B8: results of a phase I multiple-dose trial in patients with relapsed non-Hodgkin's lymphoma. J Clin On- col 1997;15(10):3266–74.
169. Foran JM, Rohatiner AZ, Cunningham D, et al. European phase II study of ritux- imab (chimeric anti-CD20 monoclonal antibody) for patients with newly diag- nosed mantle-cell lymphoma and previously treated mantle-cell lymphoma, immunocytoma, and small B-cell lymphocytic lymphoma. J Clin Oncol 2000; 18(2):317–24.
170. Piccinni C, Sacripanti C, Poluzzi E, et al. Stronger association of drug-induced progressive multifocal leukoencephalopathy (PML) with biological immunomo- dulating agents. Eur J Clin Pharmacol 2010;66(2):199–206.
171. Younes A, Bartlett NL, Leonard JP, et al. Brentuximab vedotin (SGN-35) for relapsed CD30-positive lymphomas. N Engl J Med 2010;363(19):1812–21.
172. Pro B, Advani R, Brice P, et al. Brentuximab vedotin (SGN-35) in patients with relapsed or refractory systemic anaplastic large-cell lymphoma: results of a phase II study. J Clin Oncol 2012;30(18):2190–6.
173. Corbin ZA, Nguyen-Lin A, Li S, et al. Characterization of the peripheral neurop- athy associated with brentuximab vedotin treatment of mycosis fungoides and Sezary syndrome. J Neurooncol 2017;132(3):439–46.
174. Chen R, Gopal AK, Smith SE, et al. Five-year survival and durability results of brentuximab vedotin in patients with relapsed or refractory Hodgkin lymphoma. Blood 2016;128(12):1562–6.

175. Kroschinsky F, Stolzel F, von Bonin S, et al. New drugs, new toxicities: severe side effects of modern targeted and immunotherapy of cancer and their management. Crit Care 2017;21(1):89.

176. Topp MS, Gokbuget N, Stein AS, et al. Safety and activity of blinatumomab for adult patients with relapsed or refractory B-precursor acute lymphoblastic leukaemia: a multicentre, single-arm, phase 2 study. Lancet Oncol 2015;16(1): 57–66.

177. Martinelli G, Boissel N, Chevallier P, et al. Complete hematologic and molecular response in adult patients with relapsed/refractory Philadelphia chromosome-positive B-precursor acute lymphoblastic leukemia following treatment with blinatumomab: results from a phase II, single-arm, multicenter study. J Clin Oncol 2017;35(16):1795–802.

178. FDA. Highlights of prescribing information: Blincyto. 2017. Available at: https://www.accessdata.fda.gov/drugsatfda_docs/label/2017/125557s008lbl.pdf. Accessed July 31, 2017.

179. Pardoll DM. The blockade of immune checkpoints in cancer immunotherapy. Nat Rev Cancer 2012;12(4):252–64.

180. Larkin J, Chiarion-Sileni V, Gonzalez R, et al. Combined nivolumab and ipilimumab or monotherapy in untreated melanoma. N Engl J Med 2015;373(1):23–34.

181. Robert C, Schachter J, Long GV, et al. Pembrolizumab versus Ipilimumab in advanced Melanoma. N Engl J Med 2015;372(26):2521–32.

182. Zimmer L, Goldinger SM, Hofmann L, et al. Neurological, respiratory, musculoskeletal, cardiac and ocular side-effects of anti-PD-1 therapy. Eur J Cancer 2016;60:210–25.

183. Spain L, Walls G, Julve M, et al. Neurotoxicity from immune-checkpoint inhibition in the treatment of melanoma: a single centre experience and review of the literature. Ann Oncol 2017;28(2):377–85.

184. Cuzzubbo S, Javeri F, Tissier M, et al. Neurological adverse events associated with immune checkpoint inhibitors: review of the literature. Eur J Cancer 2017; 73:1–8.

185. Voskens CJ, Goldinger SM, Loquai C, et al. The price of tumor control: an analysis of rare side effects of anti-CTLA-4 therapy in metastatic melanoma from the ipilimumab network. PLoS One 2013;8(1):e53745.

186. Bot I, Blank CU, Boogerd W, et al. Neurological immune-related adverse events of ipilimumab. Pract Neurol 2013;13(4):278–80.

187. Conry RM, Sullivan JC, Nabors LB 3rd. Ipilimumab-induced encephalopathy with a reversible splenial lesion. Cancer Immunol Res 2015;3(6):598–601.

188. Maur M, Tomasello C, Frassoldati A, et al. Posterior reversible encephalopathy syndrome during ipilimumab therapy for malignant melanoma. J Clin Oncol 2012;30(6):e76–8.

189. Yang JC, Hughes M, Kammula U, et al. Ipilimumab (anti-CTLA4 antibody) causes regression of metastatic renal cell cancer associated with enteritis and hypophysitis. J Immunother 2007;30(8):825–30.

190. Liao B, Shroff S, Kamiya-Matsuoka C, et al. Atypical neurological complications of ipilimumab therapy in patients with metastatic melanoma. Neuro Oncol 2014; 16(4):589–93.

191. Wilgenhof S, Neyns B. Anti-CTLA-4 antibody-induced Guillain-Barre syndrome in a melanoma patient. Ann Oncol 2011;22(4):991–3.

192. Johnson DB, Saranga-Perry V, Lavin PJ, et al. Myasthenia gravis induced by Ipilimumab in patients with metastatic melanoma. J Clin Oncol 2015;33(33): e122–4.

193. Bhatia S, Huber BR, Upton MP, et al. Inflammatory enteric neuropathy with severe constipation after ipilimumab treatment for melanoma: a case report. J Immunother 2009;32(2):203–5.

194. FDA. Highlights of prescribing information: Keytruda. 2017. Available at: https://www.accessdata.fda.gov/drugsatfda_docs/label/2017/125514s016lbl.pdf. Accessed July 31, 2017.

195. FDA. Highlights of prescribing information: Opdivo. 2017. Available at: https://www.accessdata.fda.gov/drugsatfda_docs/label/2017/125554s024lbl.pdf. Accessed July 31, 2017.

196. Khoja L, Maurice C, Chappell M, et al. Eosinophilic fasciitis and acute encephalopathy toxicity from pembrolizumab treatment of a patient with metastatic melanoma. Cancer Immunol Res 2016;4(3):175–8.

197. Salam S, Lavin T, Turan A. Limbic encephalitis following immunotherapy against metastatic malignant melanoma. BMJ Case Rep 2016;2016 [pii:bcr2016215012].

198. LaPorte J, Solh M, Ouanounou S. Posterior reversible encephalopathy syndrome following pembrolizumab therapy for relapsed Hodgkin's lymphoma. J Oncol Pharm Pract 2017;23(1):71–4.

199. Shirai T, Sano T, Kamijo F, et al. Acetylcholine receptor binding antibody-associated myasthenia gravis and rhabdomyolysis induced by nivolumab in a patient with melanoma. Jpn J Clin Oncol 2016;46(1):86–8.

200. Schneiderbauer R, Schneiderbauer M, Wick W, et al. PD-1 antibody-induced Guillain-Barre syndrome in a patient with metastatic melanoma. Acta Derm Venereol 2017;97(3):395–6.

201. Maurice C, Schneider R, Kiehl TR, et al. Subacute CNS demyelination after treatment with nivolumab for melanoma. Cancer Immunol Res 2015;3(12):1299–302.

202. Sadelain M, Brentjens R, Riviere I. The basic principles of chimeric antigen receptor design. Cancer Discov 2013;3(4):388–98.

203. Brudno JN, Kochenderfer JN. Toxicities of chimeric antigen receptor T cells: recognition and management. Blood 2016;127(26):3321–30.

204. Brentjens RJ, Davila ML, Riviere I, et al. CD19-targeted T cells rapidly induce molecular remissions in adults with chemotherapy-refractory acute lymphoblastic leukemia. Sci Transl Med 2013;5(177):177ra38.

205. Maude SL, Frey N, Shaw PA, et al. Chimeric antigen receptor T cells for sustained remissions in leukemia. N Engl J Med 2014;371(16):1507–17.

206. Lee DW, Kochenderfer JN, Stetler-Stevenson M, et al. T cells expressing CD19 chimeric antigen receptors for acute lymphoblastic leukaemia in children and young adults: a phase 1 dose-escalation trial. Lancet 2015;385(9967):517–28.

207. Davila ML, Riviere I, Wang X, et al. Efficacy and toxicity management of 19-28z CAR T cell therapy in B cell acute lymphoblastic leukemia. Sci Transl Med 2014;6(224):224ra25.

208. Grupp SA, Kalos M, Barrett D, et al. Chimeric antigen receptor-modified T cells for acute lymphoid leukemia. N Engl J Med 2013;368(16):1509–18.

209. Turtle CJ, Hanafi LA, Berger C, et al. CD19 CAR-T cells of defined CD4+:CD8+ composition in adult B cell ALL patients. J Clin Invest 2016;126(6):2123–38.

210. Kochenderfer JN, Dudley ME, Feldman SA, et al. B-cell depletion and remissions of malignancy along with cytokine-associated toxicity in a clinical trial of anti-CD19 chimeric-antigen-receptor-transduced T cells. Blood 2012;119(12):2709–20.

211. Lee DW, Gardner R, Porter DL, et al. Current concepts in the diagnosis and management of cytokine release syndrome. Blood 2014;124(2):188–95.

Neurocognitive Function in Adult Cancer Patients

Rebecca A. Harrison, MD[a],*, Jeffrey S. Wefel, PhD[b]

KEYWORDS

- Behavioral oncology • Neurotoxicity • Cognition • Chemotherapy
- Radiation therapy • Complications of therapy

KEY POINTS

- Impaired neurocognitive function (NCF) is common among patients with brain and noncentral nervous system cancer. The malignancy itself, cancer therapies, comorbidities, and psychosocial stressors are potential contributors.
- Given its persistent neurogenesis, the hippocampus is distinctly vulnerable to systemic chemotherapy and brain radiation toxicities, consistent with the high frequency of memory impairment in patients with cancer
- Stimulants, acetylcholinesterase inhibitors, and behavioral therapies have been evaluated for treatment of cancer-associated impaired NCF, with varying success.

INTRODUCTION

Cancer and its treatments can have a broad influence on brain structure and function. Therapeutic toxicities, systemic comorbidities, structural brain lesions, and psychosocial stresses may all influence brain health. The potential implications of impaired neurocognitive function (NCF) for patients with cancer are vast as they navigate complex treatment decisions, financial challenges, and alterations in family and societal roles. When present, impaired NCF frequently persists long after cancer treatment and remission, making it a pervasive health issue among the growing population of cancer survivors.

An understanding of the neurocognitive sequelae of cancer has value beyond individual patient care because growing evidence emphasizes its importance in the

---

Disclosure Statement: R.A. Harrison has no disclosures. J.S. Wefel has served as a consultant for Angiochem, Cogstate, F.Hoffman-La Roche Ltd, June Therapeutics, and Novocure; and on advisory boards for AbbVie, Bayer, Genentech, Inc, Insys, and Threshold Pharmaceuticals.
 ^a Department of Neuro-Oncology, The University of Texas M.D. Anderson Cancer Center, 1400 Holcombe Boulevard, Unit 0431, Houston, TX 77030, USA; ^b Section of Neuropsychology, Department of Neuro-Oncology, The University of Texas M.D. Anderson Cancer Center, 1400 Holcombe Boulevard, Unit 0431, Houston, TX 77030, USA
* Corresponding author.
E-mail address: raharrison@mdanderson.org

broader context of oncology research. Therapeutic clinical trials are increasingly incorporating neurocognitive endpoints for brain and non-central nervous system (CNS) cancers, and efforts are being made to refine therapies and minimize neurocognitive toxicity. As new avenues of cancer treatment are explored, an understanding of their neurocognitive toxicities provides insight about their effect on brain biology, patient well-being, and disease trajectory.

NEUROCOGNITIVE EVALUATION IN PATIENTS WITH CANCER

Although patients in some centers are seen by neuropsychologists as a routine part of the early (ie, presurgical) multidisciplinary care, allowing for routine identification of NCF abnormalities, many patients are seen in centers where neuropsychologists are not available or consulted later to help diagnose and manage changes in NCF and behavior. In such settings, the neurologic evaluation is the point of care at which patient complaints of changes in NCF and objective signs of abnormal NCF may first be appreciated. A thorough history identifying the onset, nature, and functional impact of neurocognitive symptoms is warranted by the evaluating physician, and a detailed neurologic examination may illustrate the neurocognitive difficulties. Although short neurocognitive screening tests, such as the Mini-Mental State Examination (MMSE) and Montreal Cognitive Assessment (MoCA), are commonly used in medical practice to screen for impaired NCF, they lack sensitivity in patients with cancer.[1,2] As such, although the initial neurologic evaluation is important in the identification and screening of neurocognitive complaints and signs, it lacks sensitivity in this realm, and formal neuropsychological assessment remains integral to the diagnosis and management of impaired NCF in patients with cancer.

Neuropsychologists must choose from thousands of tests the appropriate measures for the given patient, referral question, and clinical context. Most neuropsychologists have ascribed to a flexible hypothesis-driven clinical assessment approach. Thus, no preset battery of tests is recommended. **Box 1** lists common domains of NCF that have been observed to be affected in many patients with cancer. However, individual patient's deficits (as well as background), clinical setting, and assessment purpose will vary and flexible assessments will be required. The administration and interpretation of NCF tests requires specialized training and, as such, are performed in the context of a formal neurocognitive evaluation (NCE) by a neuropsychologist. The time required to complete formal NCE varies as a function of the same factors that influence choice of tests (eg, it may take 2 hours for a routine follow-up vs 8 or more hours for a disability or comprehensive return to work evaluation). Several hours of assessment are generally well-tolerated by patients. The time and nature of assessment may need to be adjusted in patients based on symptom burden (eg, fatigue).

Box 1
Neurocognitive domains frequently assessed

Neurocognitive domain

Attention

Processing speed

Executive function

Language

Verbal learning and memory

Clinical trials with neurocognitive endpoints commonly use high-yield subsets of tests that facilitate identification of neurocognitive deficit in this population. These tests are selected for the ability to test vulnerable neurocognitive domains, be reproducibly administered, and minimize practice effects, as well as have normative data to facilitate interpretation.[3–9]

DIAGNOSTIC EVALUATION

Given the breadth of potential etiologic factors of impaired NCF in patients with cancer, a comprehensive review of the affected patient's developmental history, psychosocial history, disease history, therapeutic interventions, current mood and symptoms, and medical history is warranted. Beyond direct disease and treatment toxicities, the systemic sequelae of cancer place patients at risk of a multiplicity of other conditions that can affect NCF. As such, the patient who has cancer with impaired NCF often requires a more expansive investigation into contributing etiologic factors than would be warranted in the general population. Hypermetabolic state, reduced oral intake, gastrointestinal surgeries, and antimetabolite chemotherapies can precipitate nutritional deficiencies that are rarely seen in the general population.[10] Pathologic alterations in the coagulation cascade can lead to ischemic stroke, thrombotic microvascular disease, cerebral microbleeds, and hemorrhage.[11] Cancer and its treatments frequently incur altered immune system function. Immunodeficiency lends itself to opportunistic infections that have a tropism for the brain. Cellular and synaptic encephalitides may arise from the generation of auto-antibodies, and the host of new immune-stimulating and adoptive cell transfer treatments can promote neurologic immunotoxicity. An awareness of these complications and others is necessary when evaluating causes of impaired NCF in patients with cancer (**Table 1**).

NEUROCOGNITIVE IMPAIRMENT IN SYSTEMIC CANCER PATIENTS
Pretreatment Deficits

Neurocognitive deficits may appear before the initiation of anticancer therapy. A randomized controlled trial of subjects with breast cancer identified significant impairment in 33% of subjects before adjuvant therapy,[12] with impaired verbal learning and memory being the most affected domains. Imaging studies lend further support to an early neuroactive process, with reduced gray[13] and white matter[14] volumes, and altered white matter tract integrity[15] found in newly diagnosed subjects with cancer.

Multiple variables seem to contribute to pretreatment deficits. The potential for shared causative mechanisms of neurocognitive decline and cancer has been introduced, with impaired gene repair mechanisms and immune dysregulation potentially inciting both pathologies.[16] In preclinical study, implantation of a peripheral tumor in mice led to impaired performance on hippocampus-based memory tasks and, pathologically, to reduced hippocampal neural proliferation, lower brain derived neurotrophic factor levels, and altered expression of proinflammatory cytokines.[17]

Disentangling the influence of the cancer from the neurobehavioral impact of the diagnosis is a limitation of preclinical models exploring this subject.[18,19] Severe stress responses in individuals associated with their diagnosis may disrupt normal neurocognitive operations,[20,21] and functional MRI (fMRI) evaluations have suggested greater pretreatment executive network variance and lower network efficiency in patients with cancer with high anxiety.[22,23] However, numerous clinical studies in subjects with cancer have found nominal associations between neurocognitive dysfunction and affective distress.[24] Thus, it is likely that admixtures of multiple mechanisms interact to influence the development of neurocognitive dysfunction.

Table 1
Diagnostic evaluation of neurocognitive impairment in patients with cancer

Potential Cancer Complications	Mechanistic Considerations	Diagnostic Evaluation
CNS metastasis	Brain metastases Leptomeningeal disease	CT or MRI brain with contrast CSF evaluation
Complications of radiation	Early acute effects Early delayed effects Late effects Radiation necrosis	MRI brain
Chemotherapy toxicity	Acute, subacute, or chronic encephalopathy Leukoencephalopathy Posterior reversible encephalopathy syndrome	MRI brain Serum and CSF evaluations, depending on agent
Nutritional deficiency	Cancer cachexia Gastrointestinal surgery Therapy-induced Cancer-related malnutrition Reduced oral intake Hypermetabolic state Carcinoid syndrome Antimetabolite cytotoxic therapy	Thiamine Vitamin B12 level Folate Niacin
Endocrinopathy	Metastatic involvement of endocrine organs Direct radiation effects Immunotherapy-induced	Thyroid stimulating hormone Thyroglobulin (T4) Triiodothyronine (T3) Blood glucose, hemoglobin A1c ACTH Morning cortisol level FSH LH Growth hormone Prolactin Electrolytes
Stroke	Cancer-associated coagulopathy Treatment-induced coagulopathy Radiation vasculopathy Chemotherapy toxicity	CT or MRI brain CT or MRI angiogram CT or MRI venogram
Seizure	CNS metastasis Reduced seizure threshold (systemic infection, metabolic derangement, medications, therapy toxicity) CNS infection	Electroencephalogram (EEG) Evaluation for underlying cause
End-organ dysfunction	Systemic cancer progression Therapeutic toxicity	Liver panel Renal function studies Electrolytes Complete blood count

(continued on next page)

Table 1
(continued)

Potential Cancer Complications	Mechanistic Considerations	Diagnostic Evaluation
Supportive medication toxicities	Corticosteroids Antiemetic medications Anticonvulsant medications	Comprehensive medication review
CNS infections	Immunosuppression	CSF protein, cell count, glucose CSF bacterial gram stain and culture CSF viral culture, PCR CSF fungal culture
Immune-mediated encephalitis	Paraneoplastic Graft-versus-host disease Immunotherapy-associated	CSF protein, cell count, glucose CSF IgG index Paraneoplastic antibodies

Abbreviations: ACTH, adrenocorticotropic hormone; CSF, cerebrospinal fluid; CT, computed tomography; FSH, follicle stimulating hormone; IgG, immunoglobulin G; LH, luteinizing hormone; PCR, polymerase chain reaction.

Cytotoxic Chemotherapy

Commonly referred to as chemobrain, the relationship between chemotherapies and impaired NCF is well-established.[25] The incorporation of baseline and longitudinal assessment of neurocognitive outcomes in subjects with breast cancer established the presence of frequent declines in neurocognitive performance during adjuvant chemotherapy,[12] with 61% of subjects experiencing a significant decline in at least 1 neurocognitive domain. Only half of these subjects were found to demonstrate improvement at long-term follow-up.

Impaired NCF from chemotherapy is most often mild to moderate in severity, with domains of attention, executive function, memory, and processing speed being reproducibly impacted.[12,26,27] Certain cytotoxic agents are more strongly associated with this impairment (**Box 2**).[27–37]

Preclinical studies
Although a breadth of cytotoxic agents have been associated with impaired NCF, there is overlap in the biological processes proposed to underlie these changes, with multiple cell lines and neural structures affected (**Box 3**).[38–44]

Genetic predisposition
Differences in germline genetic background may portend an increased susceptibility to chemotherapy-induced neurocognitive changes. Carriers of the epsilon 4 (ε4) allele of apolipoprotein E (ApoE), a variant associated with impairments in neuronal membrane repair and synaptic plasticity,[45] may portend a selective vulnerability to neurotoxicity from chemotherapy.[46] Several additional genes have been postulated to play a role as well (**Table 2**).[47–52]

Imaging studies
Imaging studies reveal structural and functional brain changes with chemotherapy. Dynamic changes in gray matter volumes have been found in patients with breast cancer, with declines in gray matter volume and density after 1 month chemotherapy,

---

Box 2
Chemotherapies strongly associated with impaired neurocognitive function

Cytotoxic chemotherapy

Platinum agents
- Cisplatin

Alkylating agents
- Cyclophosphamide
- Ifosfamide

Topoisomerase inhibitors
- Etoposide

Vinca alkaloids
- Vincristine

Antimetabolites
- Methotrexate
- Cytarabine
- Fluorouracil

Anthracyclines
- Doxorubicin

Targeted therapy

Antiangiogenic
- Bevacizumab
- Sunitinib
- Sorafenib

Immunotherapy

- Interferon-α

- Chimeric antigen receptor (CAR) T cells

Data from Refs.[27–37]

Box 3
Biologic mechanisms of chemotherapy-associated neurocognitive impairment

Mechanism

Oxidative stress
- Mitochondrial dysfunction[43]
- Toxicity obviated with antioxidant administration[39]

Mitotic inhibition
- Reduced cell populations in mitotically active structures[40]
  - Subgranular zone
  - Subventricular zone
  - White matter precursors
    - oligodendrocyte-type-2 astrocyte (O2-A) progenitor cells, oligodendrocyte progenitor cells (OPCs)

Apoptosis
- Cell death in mitotically inactive regions of the nervous system

Gene expression
- Multiple epigenetic modifications[44]
- Impaired Olig2 expression, a growth factor for white matter[42]

Table 2
Genes proposed to increase vulnerability to chemotherapy-induced neurocognitive impairment

Gene	Function	Pathologic Allele or Variant	Mechanism by Which It Increases Vulnerability
ApoE[45,46]	Neuronal membrane repair Synaptic plasticity	ε4 allele	Reduced ApoE ε4 activity Reduced capacity for neuronal repair
Catechol-o-methyl-transferase (COMT) gene[47,48]	Mediates enzymatic degradation of catecholamines, including dopamine	Val allele	Reduced dopamine reaching synaptic centers Vulnerability of dopamine-dependent circuitry
Human multidrug resistance (MDR1) gene[49–51]	Encodes a p-glycoprotein that expels toxins from CSF	Polymorphisms	Increased penetrance of cytotoxic agents in nervous system
Proinflammatory cytokine genes (eg, IL6)[52]	Mediate neuro-inflammatory response	Polymorphisms for example, IL6-174 (rs1800795 G > C)	Augment inflammatory neurotoxicity associated with chemotherapy

particularly in frontal and temporal regions, followed by incomplete recovery at 1 year.[53,54] These structural changes have been found to occur in parallel with changes in NCF, particularly processing speed.[55] Functional imaging in this population has also revealed impaired executive spatial network variance,[56] as well as reduced functional connectivity in the dorsal attention and default mode networks,[57] reflective of the alterations of brain function after chemotherapy exposure.

Hormonal Therapy

Endocrine therapy is used routinely in the treatment of hormone-dependent breast cancers. Although the relationship is not fully expounded, estrogen receptors are present in both the hippocampus and prefrontal cortex, where they initiate intracellular signal transduction pathways and induce spinogenesis and synaptogenesis,[58] which may provide the biologic basis for changes in NCF associated with these treatments. Treatment with tamoxifen, a selective estrogen receptor modulator, compared with exemestane, an aromatase inhibitor, has been associated with significantly poorer verbal learning and memory, and executive function.[59] Studies with aromatase inhibitors have yielded mixed results.[60] However, neurocognitive outcomes from the Anastrozole, Tamoxifen Alone, or in Combination (ATAC) trial found subjects on either therapy have greater impairment in verbal memory and processing speed than controls.[61,62] No significant difference in NCF between agents was found.

Targeted Therapy

More novel therapeutic approaches are also potential causes of neurocognitive impairment. Several classes of targeted therapies, aimed at specific molecular pathways, are incorporated in the treatment of various cancers. Antiangiogenic agents have been associated with impaired NCF in clinical trials (see **Box 2**),[63,64] including demonstration of impaired episodic memory, processing speed, and executive function. At this time, evidence is limited regarding the neurocognitive impact of other targeted therapies.

Immunotherapy

Immunotherapies, which harness the body's immune system to augment an anticancer response, have also emerged as a focus of therapeutic development in oncology and are incorporated as standard therapy in several cancer subtypes. Interferons (INFs), used in an early form of immunotherapy, which exhibit antitumor effect in cancers such as melanoma, have been associated with psychiatric and neurocognitive sequelae.[65] In addition to neurovegetative symptoms, patients treated with INF-α display more depressive symptoms and neurocognitive disturbances, such as memory and concentration impairments.

Newer immunotherapy modalities, particularly chimeric antigen receptor (CAR)-T cells, have documented associations with central neurotoxicity.[55,66,67] A CAR-T cell–related encephalopathy syndrome (CRES) has been characterized with features including encephalopathy, seizures, sensorimotor dysfunction, and cerebral edema.[66] The pathophysiology of this syndrome is still a subject of investigation. It is thought to be distinct from the cytokine release syndrome associated with these adoptive therapies and the direct neurotoxic impact of the CAR-T cells themselves.[68] At this time, the precise impact of these therapies on NCF is not known, and persistent clinical and preclinical efforts are warranted to understand these neurologic sequelae.

Comorbidities

Neurocognitive change in the context of cancer frequently cooccurs with anxiety, mood disturbance, fatigue, and sleep changes.[69] As with other disease entities,[70] depression has been found to be predictive of subjective neurocognitive complaints.[71,72] Impairment in tasks of executive function is noted in patients with either depression or anxiety, with markedly worse performance in those with both comorbidities, suggesting a potential synergistic impact on this domain.[73] An inverse relationship between fatigue and NCF has been reproducibly demonstrated in patients with breast cancer,[74,75] and altered resting state connectivity on fMRI in patients with persistent cancer-related fatigue provides biologic evidence of this connection.[76] The connection between these entities emphasizes the importance of screening for these comorbidities when neurocognitive dysfunction is present.

Treatment of Neurocognitive Decline in Non-Central Nervous System Cancers

Cognitive behavioral therapy

Cognitive behavioral therapy (CBT) approaches the psychological response to the neurocognitive change rather than the precise cause of neurologic injury.[77] Memory and adaptation training (MAAT) is a form of CBT developed for patients with cancer[77] that aims to build adaptive skills and reduce the disparity between neurocognitive demand and perceived ability to cope with neurocognitive demands. Three clinical trials have evaluated MAAT in subjects with breast cancer.[78–80] Each of these trials demonstrated gains in both subjective and objective neurocognitive performance and quality of life measures. Improvements in neurocognitive performance have also been noted with compensatory[81] and computer-based[82] neurocognitive training. Sustained performance improvements has been demonstrated months after CBT[83,84] and transfer effects to nontrained domains have been observed.[84]

Exercise

Exercise has been found to induce alterations in hippocampal neurogenesis, dendritic density, and neurotrophic factors,[85] and several animal and human studies support the use of exercise for chemotherapy-related impairment of NCF.[86,87] One rodent model of chemotherapy-induced neurocognitive dysfunction found overnight exercise during chemotherapy administration mitigated the development of impairment on hippocampal-dependent tasks.[88] Findings in human studies support the therapeutic impact of exercise on NCF, comorbid fatigue, and mood symptoms.[89] Regular hatha yoga practice has been found to reduce neurocognitive complaints in breast-cancer survivors[90] and help perceived quality of life and fatigue.[91] Despite the evidence for improved neuroplasticity and NCF with cardiorespiratory fitness,[92,93] clinical evidence for its use in chemotherapy-induced impairment in NCF is lacking, and warrants exploration.

Pharmacotherapy

Currently, there is no established pharmacotherapy for cancer-associated neurocognitive impairment, with a paucity of pertinent clinical trials and poor participation in those that are executed. Methylphenidate, a stimulant inhibiting catecholamine reuptake, failed to demonstrate a significant effect on neurocognition or fatigue when evaluated in a trial of 57 subjects with breast cancer on adjuvant chemotherapy,[94] though this trial had poor accrual and was underpowered. Acetylcholinesterase inhibitors, such as donepezil, improve cholinergic deficiency and may support hippocampal neurogenesis.[95–97] The potential efficacy of donepezil is supported by a rodent model, in which it was found to enhance memory performance and partially reverse the hypometabolism induced by chemotherapy.[98] Although a feasibility study of donepezil in breast cancer survivors showed improvement in objective NCF,[99] a robust evaluation of its clinical efficacy is pending.

NEUROCOGNITIVE IMPAIRMENT IN PATIENTS WITH PRIMARY AND METASTATIC BRAIN TUMORS

The value of NCE in neurooncology is reflected by the increasing incorporation of neurocognitive endpoints into therapeutic clinical trials in subjects with brain tumors. Early measures of NCF serve as independent predictors of survival in patients with brain metastases[4] and primary brain tumors,[100] with domains of executive function and attention being most strongly predictive.[100] NCE is a sensitive clinical tool to follow disease trajectory. Decreased NCF precedes radiographic progression in high-grade glioma by an average of 6 weeks, and precedes worsening of functional independence and quality of life measures by even greater intervals.[101]

Pretreatment Deficits

Neurocognitive impairment is common among patients with brain tumor, with incidence estimates of up to 90% before therapeutic intervention.[102,103] Although lesion location may grossly predict the nature of impairment, the neurocognitive profiles of this population are distinct. In comparison to stroke, brain tumors are associated with more subtle and diffuse deficits,[104] and more than half of patients with brain tumor with impairment have multiple neurocognitive domains affected,[103] likely due to the more insidious chronology and infiltrative nature of many tumors.

Various tumor features contribute to the extent and nature of neurocognitive impairment. In primary brain tumors, slower growing[105] and lower histologic grade tumors[106] demonstrate less neurologic impairment than size-matched rapidly growing, higher grade tumors. The tumor's molecular topography may also contribute. A mutation in the isocitrate dehydrogenase (IDH) gene, portending a less aggressive tumor phenotype, is associated with better neurocognitive outcomes than IDH wild-type gliomas.[107] These findings invoke the concept of lesion momentum. Faster growing, higher momentum lesions are more disruptive to the brain's connectome, leading to poorer brain network organization, and lower network efficiency,[108] which is, in turn, associated with poorer NCF. In patients with brain metastases, in which multiple discrete lesions are commonplace, the severity of neurocognitive dysfunction has been found to correlate with total tumor volume, rather than with the number of brain metastases present.[4]

Surgery

Neurosurgical intervention has the potential to influence neurocognition. Although general anesthesia, perioperative stress, pericavitary ischemia, and surgical manipulation may each impart neurocognitive insults, postoperative improvement is often noted,[109,110] likely secondary to reduction in intracranial pressure and mass effect.

Radiation

Radiation therapy is a central component in the treatment regimen of many brain tumors. Preclinical animal models have been instrumental in elucidating the biologic underpinnings of radiation-induced neurologic injury. Radiation neurotoxicity is thought to be the result of multiple dynamic pathologic conditions, and a growing understanding of the underlying mechanisms has spurred new concepts to mitigate these neurologic sequelae.

Preclinical studies

Radiation incites multiple biologic events, leading to progressive neurologic injury and corresponding neurocognitive decline.[111] Radiation is preferentially toxic to actively proliferating regions of the brain, where it impedes stem cell proliferation and differentiation.[112] Radiation-induced apoptosis contributes to degeneration in nonproliferating brain cells.[113] Although oligodendrocytes are most vulnerable to this injury, subependymal cells, some neurons, and neuronal precursors are also affected. Microglial activation, alterations of inflammatory gene expression, and upregulation of intracellular adhesion molecules and cytokines are initiated within hours of radiation exposure[114] and persist for months,[115] suggesting a sustained inflammatory response may play a role in the development of late effects. Vascular contributions to the neurotoxicity are also thought to play a significant role[116] with capillary loss preceding radiation-induced neurocognitive changes.[117]

Clinical studies

Although brain tumors, not surprisingly, frequently have adverse effects on NCF, a physician's ability to modify the impact of a largely unpredictable, newly diagnosed brain tumor on NCF is limited to nil. Thus, efforts to understand potentially modifiable contributors to neurocognitive toxicity such as off-target treatment effects have been of great interest. Analyses of clinical cohorts of subjects with brain tumor have added to the understanding of radiation-induced neurotoxicity. In a study of low-grade glioma (LGG), subjects treated with intensity-modulated radiation therapy (IMRT) had worse NCF than those with LGG who were not exposed to radiation.[118] Neurocognitive performance in subjects with LGG declined further in long-term follow-up at

12 years, whereas NCF remained stable in nonirradiated subjects.[119] This finding of progressive neurocognitive decline extending years beyond the treatment period has been reproduced[120] and is a critical consideration in the management of diseases with prolonged survival, in which the potential for acquiring delayed radiation neurotoxicity can be substantial.

The indications for whole brain radiation therapy (WBRT) have narrowed in recognition of its neurocognitive impact, with increasing efforts to use less toxic strategies. In 2 trials in which subjects with 1 to 3 brain metastases were randomized to stereotactic radiosurgery (SRS) versus a combination of SRS and WBRT (MDACC [MD Anderson Cancer Center] ID00–377, NCCTG [North Central Cancer Treatment Group] N0574),[121,122] the administration of adjuvant WBRT was associated with greater deterioration in tests of memory and executive function and, despite better control of CNS disease, no extension of overall survival. As such, initial treatment with SRS followed by close monitoring is commonly used for patients with oligometastatic brain disease.

Because hippocampal dysfunction is a central feature of radiation-induced neurocognitive impairment, hippocampal-avoidant WBRT has been evaluated as a method to reduce this risk in WBRT candidates. This radiation technique was studied in a single-arm phase II cooperative group trial (RTOG 0933 [Radiation Therapy Oncology Group]), finding a relative preservation of memory in the study population, with a 7% incidence of memory decline, versus 30% in historical controls.[123] The potential for improved NCF outcomes by sparing this structure alone is subject to debate. The neural circuitry that subserves memory and other NCF extends beyond the hippocampus, suggesting the potential impact of sparing this structure alone may be limited. Conversely, hippocampal neural progenitor cells migrate to more distant areas of brain injury, suggesting hippocampal avoidance may a have more far-reaching impact in the capacity for postradiation neural regeneration and thus NCF recovery. A phase III study of this radiation technique (NRG CC003) is currently underway to address this area of equipoise.

The use of protons (intensity modulated proton therapy) in lieu of standard photon therapy has been proposed to minimize radiation dose to normal brain and eloquent fiber tracts.[124] Although theoretically this should aid in neurocognitive preservation, confirmation of this hypothesis is pending and is under active study at several centers.

Tumor Treating Fields

A novel therapeutic device, tumor-treating fields, delivers alternating low-intensity electric fields to selectively impede the mitosis of proliferating malignant cells. It has been evaluated in 2 multicenter clinical trials for the treatment of glioblastoma. Subjective neurocognitive symptoms were stable for subjects treated with recurrent glioblastoma[125] and NCF data are currently pending from the trial of newly diagnosed glioblastoma.[126,127]

Chemotherapy

Cytotoxic therapies

Temozolomide is used routinely in the management of diffuse gliomas. Established standard therapy for glioblastoma involves concurrent chemoradiation with daily temozolomide for 6 weeks, followed by a series of adjuvant temozolomide cycles.[128] Temozolomide has been found to be well-tolerated.[129] However, when NCF is serially assessed, a subset of patients demonstrate neurocognitive decline while on therapy and free of progression,[130] reflecting either subclinical treatment toxicity or subclinical disease progression.[101]

The cytotoxic combination regimen of procarbazine, CCNU/lomustine, and vincristine (PCV) is also frequently used in patients with diffuse glioma. A randomized controlled trial evaluating adjuvant chemotherapy in LGG (RTOG 9802),[131] found no difference in neurocognitive outcomes as measured by the MMSE between subjects treated with radiation alone or radiation and adjuvant PCV over the 5 years this information was collected. As noted previously, the use of the MMSE as a measure of neurocognitive impairment in brain tumors patients is inadequate. Although it is widely used as a neurocognitive screen in this population,[132] it has been demonstrated that it is insufficiently sensitive to identify and characterize the subtle and diffuse neurocognitive deficits in patients with brain tumor.[1,133] A trial evaluating preradiation PCV in anaplastic oligodendrogliomas and oligoastrocytomas (RTOG 9402)[134] failed to detect a difference in MMSE performance in the chemotherapy treatment arm, though only 10% of subjects were followed out to 5 years from enrollment.

Bevacizumab

Bevacizumab, a humanized monoclonal antibody directed at vascular endothelial growth factor A, is frequently used in the treatment of recurrent glioblastoma, radiation necrosis, and other systemic malignances. In addition to its role in angiogenesis, it has been found to have both neurotrophic[135] and neuroprotective effects,[136] and to promote neural growth.[137] Two multicenter randomized controlled trials have evaluated its efficacy in newly diagnosed glioblastoma. Both RTOG 0825[64] and AVAglio[138] found some improvement in progression-free survival with the addition of bevacizumab to standard therapy, without any significant change in overall survival. The RTOG study found declines in objective and subjective neurocognitive performance in the subjects treated with bevacizumab and without evidence of progression.

In addition to differences in subject eligibility, follow-up, treatment, and radiographic criteria, the instruments used to evaluate NCF and resulting data became a central point of discussion on publication of these trials, highlighting the role that neurocognitive endpoints play in the interpretation and application of trial results. The AVAglio trial used the MMSE to serially evaluate NCF at study visits, and found stability on this test before deterioration at disease progression. Conversely, RTOG 0825 used the Clinical Trial Battery of neurocognitive tests (HVLT-R, TMT, COWA) focused on domains commonly compromised in patients with brain tumor. Contrary to the AVAglio trial, the data from the RTOG substudy identified a statistically significant deterioration in NCF over time in the group exposed to bevacizumab. Differences in mean scores from baseline were significantly different for the Clinical Trial Battery composite score, as well as subtests of processing speed (TMT-A) and executive function (COWA). Furthermore, the NCF scale from 2 subject-reported outcomes (MDASI-BT [MD Anderson Symptom Inventory for brain tumor] and EORTC [European Organisation for Research and Treatment of Cancer] QLQ-C30 [Quality of Life Questionnaire-Core 30] and QLQ-BN20 [Quality of Life Questionnaire- Brain Cancer Modules]) also found greater subject-reported neurocognitive complaints over time in subjects receiving bevacizumab.

BCNU wafers

BCNU wafers are a surgically implanted local chemotherapy that diffuses carmustine into the surrounding tumor and brain parenchyma. Their placement in newly diagnosed glioblastoma has been associated with improved survival,[139,140] though no formal NCE was incorporated in these trials. One study in subjects with 1 to 3 brain metastases found stable to improved NCF in subjects treated with BCNU wafers.[141] Despite these results, significant morbidity has been associated with BCNU wafers, including malignant edema and infectious complications,[142,143] which are potential secondary causes of impaired NCF.

Comorbidities

Multiple interacting comorbidities and consequences of impaired NCF occur in patients with brain tumor. Comorbid seizures occur in up to 78% of this population.[144,145] Although seizures and treatment with older-generation antiseizure medications negatively impact NCF,[146] newer agents such as levetiracetam may in fact have a beneficial effect on verbal memory[147] and warrant further study. Corticosteroids are frequently used to curtail tumor-associated vasogenic edema. Although reduction in edema may improve neurologic performance, steroids have been shown to impair hippocampal neurogenesis in vitro, with a dose-dependent decrease in neurotrophic growth factors.[148] The translation of these pathologic changes into clinical symptoms is unclear, and the chronology of these changes in humans is unknown.

Treatment of Neurocognitive Decline in Patients with Brain Tumor

Pharmacotherapy

Similar to non-CNS cancers, the data for pharmacotherapies in neurocognitively impaired patients with brain tumor is limited. Methylphenidate improved functional gains and neurocognitive performance in a small cohort of subjects with diffuse glioma.[149] In a pilot trial of methylphenidate and modafinil, objective improvement was noted in processing speed and attention with each agent, and a general benefit was found in measures of fatigue, mood, and quality of life.[150] Dexmethylphenidate prophylaxis before radiation therapy for brain metastases was evaluated in a randomized trial.[151] Although results were negative, poor accrual and high attrition rates limit their interpretation. A small randomized placebo-controlled study of 6 weeks of modafinil in subjects with primary brain tumor failed to demonstrate improved symptom management compared with placebo.[152]

Memantine, a glutamate antagonist, has been evaluated as a neuroprotective agent in subjects undergoing whole brain radiation. A placebo-controlled trial of memantine during WBRT found beneficial effects on memory function at 4 months, the primary outcome; however, this result did not reach statistical significance.[153] Time to neurocognitive decline, however, was greater in subjects who received memantine compared with placebo. The small subject numbers in the analysis render the interpretation of these results challenging and, as such, incorporation of prophylactic memantine into clinical practice is variable.

Benefit has been noted in a pilot and a phase II trial of donepezil in primary subjects with brain tumor,[154,155] with multidomain improvement in NCF and quality of life. A phase III trial evaluating its use in subjects receiving prophylactic cranial irradiation, subjects with brain metastases, and those with primary brain tumors found no benefit compared with placebo on the primary outcome variable (neurocognitive composite score). However, exploratory analyses revealed modest improvements in memory and dominant-hand fine motor dexterity.[156]

Cognitive therapy

Cognitive training may impart a benefit in select patients, particularly those with prolonged survival, such as LGG patients. A multiinstitutional randomized controlled trial allocated subjects with low-grade and anaplastic gliomas to a computer-based attention retraining and compensatory skills training of attention, memory, and executive function intervention versus a waitlist control condition.[157] No immediate postintervention improvement in performance was observed but a delayed improvement after 6 months was observed in memory and subject reports of reduced mental fatigue.

SUMMARY

Neurocognitive dysfunction is an increasingly recognized consequence of cancer and its treatments. It serves as a valuable biomarker, reflecting treatment effects, disease status, psychological well-being, and overall brain health. Its merit is reflected by its increased incorporation as an outcome measure in clinical trials for both systemic and brain cancers, and efforts to facilitate and standardize its implementation have also been undertaken. The biologic underpinnings of neurocognitive impairment in patients with cancer are complex, however, and there is a paucity of interventions proven to reduce its incidence. Persistent academic and clinical investment in this area is crucial to the development of effective treatments to prevent and mitigate this injury.

REFERENCES

1. Meyers CA, Wefel JS. The use of the mini-mental state examination to assess cognitive functioning in cancer trials: no ifs, ands, buts, or sensitivity. J Clin Oncol 2003;21:3557–8.
2. Robinson GA, Biggs V, Walker DG. Cognitive screening in brain tumors: short but sensitive enough? Front Oncol 2015;5:60.
3. Wefel JS, Saleeba AK, Buzdar AU, et al. Acute and late onset cognitive dysfunction associated with chemotherapy in women with breast cancer. Cancer 2010; 116:3348–56.
4. Meyers CA, Smith JA, Bezjak A, et al. Neurocognitive function and progression in patients with brain metastases treated with whole-brain radiation and motexafin gadolinium: results of a randomized phase III trial. J Clin Oncol 2004;22: 157–65.
5. Wefel JS, Vardy J, Ahles T, et al. International Cognition and Cancer Task Force recommendations to harmonise studies of cognitive function in patients with cancer. Lancet Oncol 2011;12:703–8.
6. Reardon DA, Galanis E, DeGroot JF, et al. Clinical trial end points for high-grade glioma: the evolving landscape. Neuro Oncol 2011;13:353–61.
7. Lin NU, Wefel JS, Lee EQ, et al, Response Assessment in Neuro-Oncology (RANO) Group. Challenges relating to solid tumour brain metastases in clinical trials, part 2: neurocognitive, neurological, and quality-of-life outcomes. A report from the RANO group. Lancet Oncol 2013;14:e407–16.
8. Camidge DR, Lee EQ, Lin NU, et al. Clinical trial design for systemic agents in patients with brain metastases from solid tumours: a guideline by the Response Assessment in Neuro-Oncology Brain Metastases working group. The Lancet Oncology 2018;19:e20–32.
9. Alexander BM, Brown P, Ahluwalia MS, et al, Response Assessment in Neuro-Oncology (RANO) Group. Clinical trial design for local therapies for brain metastases: a guideline by the Response Assessment in Neuro-Oncology Brain Metastases working group. Lancet Oncol 2018;19(1):e33–42.
10. Dreizen S, McCredie KB, Keating MJ, et al. Nutritional deficiencies in patients receiving cancer chemotherapy. Postgrad Med 1990;87:163–7, 170.
11. DeAngelis LM, Posner JB. Neurologic complications of cancer. 2nd edition. New York: Oxford University Press; 2009.
12. Wefel JS, Lenzi R, Theriault RL, et al. The cognitive sequelae of standard-dose adjuvant chemotherapy in women with breast carcinoma: results of a prospective, randomized, longitudinal trial. Cancer 2004;100:2292–9.
13. Amidi A, Agerbæk M, Wu LM, et al. Changes in cognitive functions and cerebral grey matter and their associations with inflammatory markers, endocrine

markers, and APOE genotypes in testicular cancer patients undergoing treatment. Brain Imaging Behav 2017;11:769–83.

14. Scherling C, Collins B, MacKenzie J, et al. Structural brain differences in breast cancer patients compared to matched controls prior to chemotherapy. Int J Biol 2012;4:3–25.

15. Menning S, de Ruiter MB, Veltman DJ, et al. Multimodal MRI and cognitive function in patients with breast cancer prior to adjuvant treatment–the role of fatigue. Neuroimage Clin 2015;7:547–54.

16. Ahles TA, Saykin AJ. Candidate mechanisms for chemotherapy-induced cognitive changes. Nat Rev Cancer 2007;7:192–201.

17. Yang M, Kim J, Kim JS, et al. Hippocampal dysfunctions in tumor-bearing mice. Brain Behav Immun 2014;36:147–55.

18. Schrepf A, Lutgendorf SK, Pyter LM. Pre-treatment effects of peripheral tumors on brain and behavior: neuroinflammatory mechanisms in humans and rodents. Brain Behav Immun 2015;49:1–17.

19. Dantzer R, Meagher MW, Cleeland CS. Translational approaches to treatment-induced symptoms in cancer patients. Nat Rev Clin Oncol 2012;9:414–26.

20. Hermelink K, Voigt V, Kaste J, et al. Elucidating pretreatment cognitive impairment in breast cancer patients: the impact of cancer-related post-traumatic stress. J Natl Cancer Inst 2015;107 [pii:djv099].

21. Reid-Arndt SA, Cox CR. Stress, coping and cognitive deficits in women after surgery for breast cancer. J Clin Psychol Med Settings 2012;19:127–37.

22. Berman MG, Askren MK, Jung M, et al. Pretreatment worry and neurocognitive responses in women with breast cancer. Health Psychol 2014;33:222–31.

23. Askren MK, Jung M, Berman MG, et al. Neuromarkers of fatigue and cognitive complaints following chemotherapy for breast cancer: a prospective fMRI investigation. Breast Cancer Res Treat 2014;147:445–55.

24. Schagen SB, Wefel JS. Post-traumatic stress as the primary cause for cognitive decline-not the whole story, and perhaps no story at all. J Natl Cancer Inst 2017;109(10):djx091.

25. Ouimet LA, Stewart A, Collins B, et al. Measuring neuropsychological change following breast cancer treatment: an analysis of statistical models. J Clin Exp Neuropsychol 2009;31:73–89.

26. Wefel JS, Kesler SR, Noll KR, et al. Clinical characteristics, pathophysiology, and management of noncentral nervous system cancer-related cognitive impairment in adults. CA Cancer J Clin 2015;65:123–38.

27. Wefel JS, Schagen SB. Chemotherapy-related cognitive dysfunction. Curr Neurol Neurosci Rep 2012;12:267–75.

28. Janelsins MC, Heckler CE, Thompson BD, et al. A clinically relevant dose of cyclophosphamide chemotherapy impairs memory performance on the delayed spatial alternation task that is sustained over time as mice age. Neurotoxicology 2016;56:287–93.

29. Seigers R, Loos M, Van Tellingen O, et al. Neurobiological changes by cytotoxic agents in mice. Behav Brain Res 2016;299:19–26.

30. Shabani M, Larizadeh MH, Parsania S, et al. Profound destructive effects of adolescent exposure to vincristine accompanied with some sex differences in motor and memory performance. Can J Physiol Pharmacol 2012;90:379–86.

31. Ramalho M, Fontes F, Ruano L, et al. Cognitive impairment in the first year after breast cancer diagnosis: a prospective cohort study. Breast 2017;32:173–8.

32. Quesnel C, Savard J, Ivers H. Cognitive impairments associated with breast cancer treatments: results from a longitudinal study. Breast Cancer Res Treat 2009;116:113–23.

33. Falleti MG, Sanfilippo A, Maruff P, et al. The nature and severity of cognitive impairment associated with adjuvant chemotherapy in women with breast cancer: a meta-analysis of the current literature. Brain Cogn 2005;59:60–70.

34. Simo M, Root JC, Vaquero L, et al. Cognitive and brain structural changes in a lung cancer population. J Thorac Oncol 2015;10:38–45.

35. Schagen SB, Boogerd W, Muller MJ, et al. Cognitive complaints and cognitive impairment following BEP chemotherapy in patients with testicular cancer. Acta Oncol 2008;47:63–70.

36. Perry A, Schmidt RE. Cancer therapy-associated CNS neuropathology: an update and review of the literature. Acta Neuropathol 2006;111:197–212.

37. Rieger C, Fiegl M, Tischer J, et al. Incidence and severity of ifosfamide-induced encephalopathy. Anticancer Drugs 2004;15:347–50.

38. Seigers R, Fardell JE. Neurobiological basis of chemotherapy-induced cognitive impairment: a review of rodent research. Neurosci Biobehav Rev 2011;35:729–41.

39. Konat GW, Kraszpulski M, James I, et al. Cognitive dysfunction induced by chronic administration of common cancer chemotherapeutics in rats. Metab Brain Dis 2008;23:325–33.

40. Monje M, Dietrich J. Cognitive side effects of cancer therapy demonstrate a functional role for adult neurogenesis. Behav Brain Res 2012;227:376–9.

41. Wick A, Wick W, Hirrlinger J, et al. Chemotherapy-induced cell death in primary cerebellar granule neurons but not in astrocytes: in vitro paradigm of differential neurotoxicity. J Neurochem 2004;91:1067–74.

42. Han R, Yang YM, Dietrich J, et al. Systemic 5-fluorouracil treatment causes a syndrome of delayed myelin destruction in the central nervous system. J Biol 2008;7:12.

43. Vichaya EG, Chiu GS, Krukowski K, et al. Mechanisms of chemotherapy-induced behavioral toxicities. Front Neurosci 2015;9:131.

44. Kovalchuk A, Kolb B. Chemo brain: from discerning mechanisms to lifting the brain fog—An aging connection. Cell Cycle 2017;16:1345–9.

45. White F, Nicoll JA, Roses AD, et al. Impaired neuronal plasticity in transgenic mice expressing human apolipoprotein E4 compared to E3 in a model of entorhinal cortex lesion. Neurobiol Dis 2001;8:611–25.

46. Ahles TA, Saykin AJ, Noll WW, et al. The relationship of APOE genotype to neuropsychological performance in long-term cancer survivors treated with standard dose chemotherapy. Psychooncology 2003;12:612–9.

47. Goldberg TE, Weinberger DR. Genes and the parsing of cognitive processes. Trends Cogn Sci 2004;8:325–35.

48. Small BJ, Rawson KS, Walsh E, et al. Catechol-O-methyltransferase genotype modulates cancer treatment-related cognitive deficits in breast cancer survivors. Cancer 2011;117:1369–76.

49. Higgins CF, Callaghan R, Linton KJ, et al. Structure of the multidrug resistance P-glycoprotein. Semin Cancer Biol 1997;8:135–42.

50. Ling V. P-glycoprotein: its role in drug resistance. Am J Med 1995;99:31S–4S.

51. Gottesman MM, Pastan I. Biochemistry of multidrug resistance mediated by the multidrug transporter. Annu Rev Biochem 1993;62:385–427.

52. Chae J-W, Ng T, Yeo HL, et al. Impact of TNF-α (rs1800629) and IL-6 (rs1800795) polymorphisms on cognitive impairment in Asian breast cancer patients. PLoS One 2016;11:e0164204.
53. McDonald BC, Conroy SK, Ahles TA, et al. Gray matter reduction associated with systemic chemotherapy for breast cancer: a prospective MRI study. Breast Cancer Res Treat 2010;123:819–28.
54. Lepage C, Smith AM, Moreau J, et al. A prospective study of grey matter and cognitive function alterations in chemotherapy-treated breast cancer patients. Springerplus 2014;3:444.
55. Turtle CJ, Hay KA, Gust J, et al. Cytokine release syndrome (CRS) and neurotoxicity (NT) after CD19-specific chimeric antigen receptor- (CAR-) modified T cells. J Clin Oncol 2017;35:3020.
56. Jung MS, Zhang M, Askren MK, et al. Cognitive dysfunction and symptom burden in women treated for breast cancer: a prospective behavioral and fMRI analysis. Brain Imaging Behav 2017;11:86–97.
57. Dumas JA, Makarewicz J, Schaubhut GJ, et al. Chemotherapy altered brain functional connectivity in women with breast cancer: a pilot study. Brain Imaging Behav 2013;7:524–32.
58. Hara Y, Waters EM, McEwen BS, et al. Estrogen effects on cognitive and synaptic health over the lifecourse. Physiol Rev 2015;95:785–807.
59. Schilder CM, Seynaeve C, Beex LV, et al. Effects of tamoxifen and exemestane on cognitive functioning of postmenopausal patients with breast cancer: results from the neuropsychological side study of the tamoxifen and exemestane adjuvant multinational trial. J Clin Oncol 2010;28:1294–300.
60. Batalo M, Nagaiah G, Abraham J. Cognitive dysfunction in postmenopausal breast cancer patients on aromatase inhibitors. Expert Rev Anticancer Ther 2011;11:1277–82.
61. Shilling V, Jenkins V, Fallowfield L, et al. The effects of hormone therapy on cognition in breast cancer. J Steroid Biochem Mol Biol 2003;86:405–12.
62. Jenkins V, Shilling V, Fallowfield L, et al. Does hormone therapy for the treatment of breast cancer have a detrimental effect on memory and cognition? A pilot study. Psychooncology 2004;13:61–6.
63. Mulder SF, Bertens D, Desar IME, et al. Impairment of cognitive functioning during Sunitinib or Sorafenib treatment in cancer patients: a cross sectional study. BMC Cancer 2014;14:219.
64. Gilbert MR, Dignam JJ, Armstrong TS, et al. A randomized trial of bevacizumab for newly diagnosed glioblastoma. N Engl J Med 2014;370:699–708.
65. Capuron L, Gumnick JF, Musselman DL, et al. Neurobehavioral effects of interferon-alpha in cancer patients: phenomenology and paroxetine responsiveness of symptom dimensions. Neuropsychopharmacology 2002;26:643–52.
66. Neelapu SS, Tummala S, Kebriaei P, et al. Chimeric antigen receptor T-cell therapy - assessment and management of toxicities. Nat Rev Clin Oncol 2018;15(1):47–62.
67. Brudno JN, Kochenderfer JN. Toxicities of chimeric antigen receptor T cells: recognition and management. Blood 2016;127:3321–30.
68. Hu Y, Sun J, Wu Z, et al. Predominant cerebral cytokine release syndrome in CD19-directed chimeric antigen receptor-modified T cell therapy. J Hematol Oncol 2016;9:70.
69. Vardy J, Dhillon HM, Pond GR, et al. Cognitive function and fatigue after diagnosis of colorectal cancer. Ann Oncol 2014;25:2404–12.

70. Shin SY, Katz P, Julian L. The relationship between perceived cognitive dysfunction and objective neuropsychological performance in persons with rheumatoid arthritis. Arthritis Care Res 2013;65:481–6.

71. Kinsinger SW, Lattie E, Mohr DC. Relationship between depression, fatigue, subjective cognitive impairment, and objective neuropsychological functioning in patients with multiple sclerosis. Neuropsychology 2010;24:573–80.

72. Bender CM, Pacella ML, Sereika SM, et al. What do perceived cognitive problems reflect? J Support Oncol 2008;6:238–42.

73. Snyder HR. Major depressive disorder is associated with broad impairments on neuropsychological measures of executive function: a meta-analysis and review. Psychol Bull 2013;139:81–132.

74. Sampson JH, Vlahovic G, Sahebjam S, et al. Preliminary safety and activity of nivolumab and its combination with ipilimumab in recurrent glioblastoma (GBM): CHECKMATE-143. J Clin Oncol 2015;33:3010.

75. Castellon SA, Ganz PA, Bower JE, et al. Neurocognitive performance in breast cancer survivors exposed to adjuvant chemotherapy and tamoxifen. J Clin Exp Neuropsychol 2004;26:955–69.

76. Hampson JP, Zick SM, Khabir T, et al. Altered resting brain connectivity in persistent cancer related fatigue. Neuroimage Clin 2015;8:305–13.

77. Kucherer S, Ferguson RJ. Cognitive behavioral therapy for cancer-related cognitive dysfunction. Curr Opin Support Palliat Care 2017;11:46–51.

78. Ferguson RJ, Sigmon ST, Pritchard AJ, et al. A randomized trial of videoconference-delivered cognitive behavioral therapy for survivors of breast cancer with self-reported cognitive dysfunction. Cancer 2016;122:1782–91.

79. Ferguson RJ, McDonald BC, Rocque MA, et al. Development of CBT for chemotherapy-related cognitive change: results of a waitlist control trial. Psychooncology 2012;21:176–86.

80. Ferguson RJ, Ahles TA, Saykin AJ, et al. Cognitive-behavioral management of chemotherapy-related cognitive change. Psychooncology 2007;16:772–7.

81. Park J-H, Jung YS, Kim KS, et al. Effects of compensatory cognitive training intervention for breast cancer patients undergoing chemotherapy: a pilot study. Support Care Cancer 2017;25:1887–96.

82. Bail J, Meneses K. Computer-based cognitive training for chemotherapy-related cognitive impairment in breast cancer survivors. Clin J Oncol Nurs 2016;20:504–9.

83. Damholdt MF, Mehlsen M, O'Toole MS, et al. Web-based cognitive training for breast cancer survivors with cognitive complaints-a randomized controlled trial. Psychooncology 2016;25:1293–300.

84. Von Ah D, Carpenter JS, Saykin A, et al. Advanced cognitive training for breast cancer survivors: a randomized controlled trial. Breast Cancer Res Treat 2012;135:799–809.

85. Voss MW, Vivar C, Kramer AF, et al. Bridging animal and human models of exercise-induced brain plasticity. Trends Cogn Sci 2013;17:525–44.

86. Zimmer P, Baumann FT, Oberste M, et al. Effects of exercise interventions and physical activity behavior on cancer related cognitive impairments: a systematic review. Biomed Res Int 2016;2016:1820954.

87. Hotting K, Roder B. Beneficial effects of physical exercise on neuroplasticity and cognition. Neurosci Biobehav Rev 2013;37:2243–57.

88. Fardell JE, Vardy J, Shah JD, et al. Cognitive impairments caused by oxaliplatin and 5-fluorouracil chemotherapy are ameliorated by physical activity. Psychopharmacology 2012;220:183–93.

89. Mustian KM, Sprod LK, Janelsins M, et al. Exercise recommendations for cancer-related fatigue, cognitive impairment, sleep problems, depression, pain, anxiety, and physical dysfunction: a review. Oncol Hematol Rev 2012;8: 81–8.

90. Derry HM, Jaremka LM, Bennett JM, et al. Yoga and self-reported cognitive problems in breast cancer survivors: a randomized controlled trial. Psychooncology 2015;24:958–66.

91. Janelsins MC, Peppone LJ, Heckler CE, et al. YOCAS yoga, fatigue, memory difficulty, and quality of life: results from a URCC CCOP randomized, controlled clinical trial among 358 cancer survivors. J Clin Oncol 2012;30:9142.

92. Hayes SM, Hayes JP, Cadden M, et al. A review of cardiorespiratory fitness-related neuroplasticity in the aging brain. Front Aging Neurosci 2013;5:31.

93. Chapman SB, Aslan S, Spence JS, et al. Shorter term aerobic exercise improves brain, cognition, and cardiovascular fitness in aging. Front Aging Neurosci 2013;5:75.

94. Mar Fan HG, Clemons M, Xu W, et al. A randomised, placebo-controlled, double-blind trial of the effects of d-methylphenidate on fatigue and cognitive dysfunction in women undergoing adjuvant chemotherapy for breast cancer. Support Care Cancer 2008;16:577–83.

95. Salmond CH, Chatfield DA, Menon DK, et al. Cognitive sequelae of head injury: involvement of basal forebrain and associated structures. Brain 2005;128: 189–200.

96. Itou Y, Nochi R, Kuribayashi H, et al. Cholinergic activation of hippocampal neural stem cells in aged dentate gyrus. Hippocampus 2011;21:446–59.

97. Narimatsu N, Harada N, Kurihara H, et al. Donepezil improves cognitive function in mice by increasing the production of insulin-like growth factor-I in the hippocampus. J Pharmacol Exp Ther 2009;330:2–12.

98. Lim I, Joung HY, Yu AR, et al. PET evidence of the effect of donepezil on cognitive performance in an animal model of chemobrain. Biomed Res Int 2016;2016: 6945415.

99. Lawrence JA, Griffin L, Balcueva EP, et al. A study of donepezil in female breast cancer survivors with self-reported cognitive dysfunction 1 to 5 years following adjuvant chemotherapy. J Cancer Surviv 2016;10:176–84.

100. Johnson DR, Sawyer AM, Meyers CA, et al. Early measures of cognitive function predict survival in patients with newly diagnosed glioblastoma. Neuro Oncol 2012;14:808–16.

101. Meyers CA, Hess KR. Multifaceted end points in brain tumor clinical trials: cognitive deterioration precedes MRI progression. Neuro Oncol 2003;5:89–95.

102. Tucha O, Smely C, Preier M, et al. Cognitive deficits before treatment among patients with brain tumors. Neurosurgery 2000;47:324–33.

103. Zucchella C, Bartolo M, Di Lorenzo C, et al. Cognitive impairment in primary brain tumors outpatients: a prospective cross-sectional survey. J Neurooncol 2013;112:455–60.

104. Anderson SW, Damasio H, Tranel D. Neuropsychological impairments associated with lesions caused by tumor or stroke. Arch Neurol 1990;47:397–405.

105. Hom J, Reitan RM. Neuropsychological correlates of rapidly vs. slowly growing intrinsic cerebral neoplasms. J Clin Neuropsychol 1984;6:309–24.

106. Noll KR, Sullaway C, Ziu M, et al. Relationships between tumor grade and neurocognitive functioning in patients with glioma of the left temporal lobe prior to surgical resection. Neuro Oncol 2015;17:580–7.

107. Wefel JS, Noll KR, Rao G, et al. Neurocognitive function varies by IDH1 genetic mutation status in patients with malignant glioma prior to surgical resection. Neuro Oncol 2016;18:1656–63.
108. Kesler SR, Noll K, Cahill DP, et al. The effect of IDH1 mutation on the structural connectome in malignant astrocytoma. J Neurooncol 2017;131:565–74.
109. Meskal I, Gehring K, Rutten G-JM, et al. Cognitive functioning in meningioma patients: a systematic review. J Neurooncol 2016;128:195–205.
110. Habets EJ, Kloet A, Walchenbach R, et al. Tumour and surgery effects on cognitive functioning in high-grade glioma patients. Acta Neurochir (Wien) 2014;156: 1451–9.
111. Makale MT, McDonald CR, Hattangadi-Gluth JA, et al. Mechanisms of radiotherapy-associated cognitive disability in patients with brain tumours. Nat Rev Neurol 2017;13:52–64.
112. Monje ML, Mizumatsu S, Fike JR, et al. Irradiation induces neural precursor-cell dysfunction. Nat Med 2002;8:955–62.
113. Shinohara C, Gobbel GT, Lamborn KR, et al. Apoptosis in the subependyma of young adult rats after single and fractionated doses of X-rays. Cancer Res 1997; 57:2694–702.
114. Hwang SY, Jung JS, Kim TH, et al. Ionizing radiation induces astrocyte gliosis through microglia activation. Neurobiol Dis 2006;21:457–67.
115. Lee WH, Sonntag WE, Mitschelen M, et al. Irradiation induces regionally specific alterations in pro-inflammatory environments in rat brain. Int J Radiat Biol 2010; 86:132–44.
116. Coderre JA, Morris GM, Micca PL, et al. Late effects of radiation on the central nervous system: role of vascular endothelial damage and glial stem cell survival. Radiat Res 2006;166:495–503.
117. Brown WR, Blair RM, Moody DM, et al. Capillary loss precedes the cognitive impairment induced by fractionated whole-brain irradiation: a potential rat model of vascular dementia. J Neurol Sci 2007;257:67–71.
118. Klein M, Heimans JJ, Aaronson NK, et al. Effect of radiotherapy and other treatment-related factors on mid-term to long-term cognitive sequelae in low-grade gliomas: a comparative study. Lancet 2002;360:1361–8.
119. Douw L, Klein M, Fagel SSAA, et al. Cognitive and radiological effects of radiotherapy in patients with low-grade glioma: long-term follow-up. Lancet Neurol 2009;8:810–8.
120. Surma-aho O, Niemela M, Vilkki J, et al. Adverse long-term effects of brain radiotherapy in adult low-grade glioma patients. Neurology 2001;56:1285–90.
121. Brown P, Asher A, Ballman K, et al. BMET-05NCCTG N0574 (ALLIANCE): a phase III randomized trial of whole brain radiation therapy (WBRT) in addition to radiosurgery (SRS) in patients with 1 to 3 brain metastases. Neuro Oncol 2015;17:v45–6.
122. Chang EL, Wefel JS, Hess KR, et al. Neurocognition in patients with brain metastases treated with radiosurgery or radiosurgery plus whole-brain irradiation: a randomised controlled trial. Lancet Oncol 2009;10:1037–44.
123. Gondi V, Pugh SL, Tome WA, et al. Preservation of memory with conformal avoidance of the hippocampal neural stem-cell compartment during whole-brain radiotherapy for brain metastases (RTOG 0933): a phase II multi-institutional trial. J Clin Oncol 2014;32:3810–6.
124. Munck AF, Rosenschold P, Engelholm S, et al. Photon and proton therapy planning comparison for malignant glioma based on CT, FDG-PET, DTI-MRI and fiber tracking. Acta Oncol 2011;50:777–83.

125. Stupp R, Wong ET, Kanner AA, et al. NovoTTF-100A versus physician's choice chemotherapy in recurrent glioblastoma: a randomised phase III trial of a novel treatment modality. Eur J Cancer 2012;48:2192–202.

126. Stupp R, Taillibert S, Kanner AA, et al. Maintenance therapy with tumor-treating fields plus temozolomide vs temozolomide alone for glioblastoma: a randomized clinical trial. JAMA 2015;314:2535–43.

127. Stupp R, Idbaih A, Steinberg DM, et al. LTBK-01: prospective, multi-center phase III trial of tumor treating fields together with temozolomide compared to temozolomide alone in patients with newly diagnosed glioblastoma. Neuro Oncol 2016;18:i1.

128. Stupp R, Mason WP, van den Bent MJ, et al. Radiotherapy plus concomitant and adjuvant temozolomide for glioblastoma. N Engl J Med 2005;352:987–96.

129. Hilverda K, Bosma I, Heimans JJ, et al. Cognitive functioning in glioblastoma patients during radiotherapy and temozolomide treatment: initial findings. J Neurooncol 2010;97:89–94.

130. Armstrong TS, Wefel JS, Wang M, et al. Net clinical benefit analysis of radiation therapy oncology group 0525: a phase III trial comparing conventional adjuvant temozolomide with dose-intensive temozolomide in patients with newly diagnosed glioblastoma. J Clin Oncol 2013;31:4076–84.

131. Prabhu RS, Won M, Shaw EG, et al. Effect of the addition of chemotherapy to radiotherapy on cognitive function in patients with low-grade glioma: secondary analysis of RTOG 98-02. J Clin Oncol 2014;32:535–41.

132. Brown PD, Buckner JC, O'Fallon JR, et al. Effects of radiotherapy on cognitive function in patients with low-grade glioma measured by the folstein minimental state examination. J Clin Oncol 2003;21:2519–24.

133. Klein M, Heimans JJ. The measurement of cognitive functioning in low-grade glioma patients after radiotherapy. J Clin Oncol 2004;22:966–7.

134. Wang M, Cairncross G, Shaw E, et al. Cognition and quality of life after chemotherapy plus radiotherapy (RT) vs. RT for pure and mixed anaplastic oligodendrogliomas: radiation therapy oncology group trial 9402. Int J Radiat Oncol Biol Phys 2010;77:662–9.

135. Rosenstein JM, Mani N, Khaibullina A, et al. Neurotrophic effects of vascular endothelial growth factor on organotypic cortical explants and primary cortical neurons. J Neurosci 2003;23:11036–44.

136. Jin KL, Mao XO, Greenberg DA. Vascular endothelial growth factor: direct neuroprotective effect in in vitro ischemia. Proc Natl Acad Sci U S A 2000;97:10242–7.

137. Khaibullina AA, Rosenstein JM, Krum JM. Vascular endothelial growth factor promotes neurite maturation in primary CNS neuronal cultures. Brain Res Dev Brain Res 2004;148:59–68.

138. Chinot OL, Wick W, Mason W, et al. Bevacizumab plus radiotherapy-temozolomide for newly diagnosed glioblastoma. N Engl J Med 2014;370:709–22.

139. Brem H, Piantadosi S, Burger PC, et al. Placebo-controlled trial of safety and efficacy of intraoperative controlled delivery by biodegradable polymers of chemotherapy for recurrent gliomas. The Polymer-brain Tumor Treatment Group. Lancet 1995;345:1008–12.

140. Westphal M, Hilt DC, Bortey E, et al. A phase 3 trial of local chemotherapy with biodegradable carmustine (BCNU) wafers (Gliadel wafers) in patients with primary malignant glioma. Neuro Oncol 2003;5:79–88.

141. Brem S, Meyers CA, Palmer G, et al. Preservation of neurocognitive function and local control of 1 to 3 brain metastases treated with surgery and carmustine wafers. Cancer 2013;119:3830–8.

142. Kuramitsu S, Motomura K, Natsume A, et al. Double-edged Sword in the Placement of Carmustine (BCNU) Wafers along the Eloquent area: a case report. NMC Case Rep J 2015;2:40–5.

143. Kleinberg LR, Weingart J, Burger P, et al. Clinical course and pathologic findings after Gliadel and radiotherapy for newly diagnosed malignant glioma: implications for patient management. Cancer Invest 2004;22:1–9.

144. Hildebrand J, Lecaille C, Perennes J, et al. Epileptic seizures during follow-up of patients treated for primary brain tumors. Neurology 2005;65:212–5.

145. Glantz MJ, Cole BF, Forsyth PA, et al. Practice parameter: anticonvulsant prophylaxis in patients with newly diagnosed brain tumors. Report of the Quality Standards Subcommittee of the American Academy of Neurology. Neurology 2000;54:1886–93.

146. Klein M, Engelberts NH, van der Ploeg HM, et al. Epilepsy in low-grade gliomas: the impact on cognitive function and quality of life. Ann Neurol 2003;54:514–20.

147. de Groot M, Douw L, Sizoo EM, et al. Levetiracetam improves verbal memory in high-grade glioma patients. Neuro Oncol 2013;15:216–23.

148. Yu IT, Lee SH, Lee YS, et al. Differential effects of corticosterone and dexamethasone on hippocampal neurogenesis in vitro. Biochem Biophys Res Commun 2004;317:484–90.

149. Meyers CA, Weitzner MA, Valentine AD, et al. Methylphenidate therapy improves cognition, mood, and function of brain tumor patients. J Clin Oncol 1998;16:2522–7.

150. Gehring K, Patwardhan SY, Collins R, et al. A randomized trial on the efficacy of methylphenidate and modafinil for improving cognitive functioning and symptoms in patients with a primary brain tumor. J Neurooncol 2012;107:165–74.

151. Butler JM Jr, Case LD, Atkins J, et al. A phase III, double-blind, placebo-controlled prospective randomized clinical trial of d-threo-methylphenidate HCl in brain tumor patients receiving radiation therapy. Int J Radiat Oncol Biol Phys 2007;69:1496–501.

152. Boele FW, Douw L, de Groot M, et al. The effect of modafinil on fatigue, cognitive functioning, and mood in primary brain tumor patients: a multicenter randomized controlled trial. Neuro Oncol 2013;15:1420–8.

153. Brown PD, Pugh S, Laack NN, et al. Memantine for the prevention of cognitive dysfunction in patients receiving whole-brain radiotherapy: a randomized, double-blind, placebo-controlled trial. Neuro Oncol 2013;15:1429–37.

154. Correa DD, Kryza-Lacombe M, Baser RE, et al. Cognitive effects of donepezil therapy in patients with brain tumors: a pilot study. J Neurooncol 2016;127:313–9.

155. Shaw EG, Rosdhal R, D'Agostino RB Jr, et al. Phase II study of donepezil in irradiated brain tumor patients: effect on cognitive function, mood, and quality of life. J Clin Oncol 2006;24:1415–20.

156. Rapp SR, Case LD, Peiffer A, et al. Donepezil for irradiated brain tumor survivors: a phase III randomized placebo-controlled clinical trial. J Clin Oncol 2015;33:1653–9.

157. Gehring K, Sitskoorn MM, Gundy CM, et al. Cognitive rehabilitation in patients with gliomas: a randomized, controlled trial. J Clin Oncol 2009;27:3712–22.

Paraneoplastic Neurologic Syndromes

Myrna R. Rosenfeld, MD, PhD[a], Josep Dalmau, MD, PhD[b],*

KEYWORDS

- Paraneoplastic • Autoimmune encephalitis • Antibody • Neurologic • Cancer

KEY POINTS

- Paraneoplastic neurologic syndromes are immune mediated.
- Paraneoplastic neurologic syndromes can affect any part of the nervous system.
- Paraneoplastic neurologic syndromes often present acutely and before the cancer diagnosis is known.
- Some paraneoplastic neurologic syndromes are highly responsive to treatment.

INTRODUCTION

Paraneoplastic neurologic syndromes (PNS) are mostly immune-mediated disorders that occur in patients with cancer. For some PNS, the immune pathogenesis has been confirmed, whereas in others there is strong evidence supporting underlying immune mechanisms. Once considered medical oddities, it is now known that some PNS are common. Furthermore, contrary to the past concept that PNS predominate in older individuals (neuroblastoma-associated opsoclonus was a rare exception), some recently identified disorders predominately occur in younger age groups. The identification of the paraneoplastic origin of a patient's symptoms is important for several reasons. PNS often develop before the cancer diagnosis is known and recognition of PNS can lead to early cancer identification. Additionally, it has been shown that early initiation of treatment (immunotherapy and tumor treatment, when present) can improve PNS outcomes. In this article, we provide general concepts regarding

Disclosure Statement: M.R. Rosenfeld and J. Dalmau receive royalties from Athena Diagnostics for the use of Ma2 as an autoantibody test and from Euroimmun for the use of NMDA receptor as an autoantibody test. J. Dalmau received royalties from Euroimmun for the use of GABAB receptor, DPPX, GABAA receptor, and IgLON5 as autoantibody tests and has received an unrestricted research grant from Euroimmun.

[a] Neuroimmunology, Institut d'Investigació Biomèdica August Pi i Sunyer (IDIBAPS), Casanova 143, Barcelona, Spain 08036; Neurology, University of Pennsylvania, 3400 Spruce Street, Philadelphia, PA 19107, USA; [b] Neurology, Hospital Clínic and Neuroimmunology, Institut d'Investigació Biomèdica August Pi i Sunyer (IDIBAPS), Casanova 143, Barcelona, Spain 08036; University of Pennsylvania, 3400 Spruce Street, Philadelphia, PA 19107, USA
* Corresponding author.
E-mail address: jdalmau@clinic.ub.es

PNS; for detailed descriptions of the clinical features of individual PNS detailed reviews are available.[1–4]

EPIDEMIOLOGY

In general, the classic PNS are rare and occur in approximately 1 in 10,000 patients with cancer.[5] An exception is the Lambert-Eaton myasthenic syndrome (LEMS), which has been reported in about 1% of all patients with small-cell lung cancer (SCLC). In contrast, anti-N-methyl-D-aspartate receptor (NMDAR) encephalitis, which has an age-related tumor association, is considered the second most common cause of autoimmune encephalitis after acute demyelinating encephalomyelitis.[6]

DIAGNOSING PARANEOPLASTIC NEUROLOGIC SYNDROMES

Initial clues that a patient has a PNS are found in the history and symptom presentation and include the patient's age, cancer risk factors, or known cancer history (**Table 1**). Most PNS develop acutely or subacutely and may resemble a viral process. Although the same neurologic syndromes seen in PNS also occur without a cancer association, some syndromes, such as LEMS or limbic encephalitis, are so commonly cancer associated they are referred to as classical PNS and a paraneoplastic cause should be suspected when one of these syndromes is seen.[7] Other disorders have a more variable association with cancer and for some this association is age and sex dependent. It is important to keep in mind that the co-occurrence of a neurologic syndrome and cancer may simply be coincidental. The presence of cerebrospinal fluid (CSF) pleocytosis, elevated protein concentration, intrathecal synthesis of immunoglobulin, and/or oligoclonal bands is supportive of paraneoplasia, although normal CSF studies do not rule out PNS. Neuroimaging is helpful to exclude other nonparaneoplastic causes but may be normal. An exception is limbic encephalitis in which MRI often shows unilateral or bilateral mesial temporal lobe abnormalities best seen on T2-weighted and fluid-attenuated inversion recovery images (**Fig. 1**).[8]

TUMOR SCREENING

If PNS is suspected tumor screening should proceed.[9] The search may initially be focused to those tumor types more commonly associated with the patient's syndrome or type of antineuronal antibody, but should be expanded if no tumor is found because unexpected cancer-antibody associations may occur. Similarly, if the tumor found is not a histologic type that typically associates with the syndrome or antibody, a search for a second neoplasm should be undertaken. Because PNS onset often precedes the cancer diagnosis or occurs when the tumor is small and difficult to detect, a multidisciplinary approach to cancer diagnosis is warranted. The investigating team should be informed that PNS is suspected and that questionable or inconclusive results of tumor screening should be thoroughly investigated. If no cancer is found but PNS remains the likely diagnosis, cancer screening should be repeated periodically up to 4 years. The frequency of cancer screening depends on the type of disorder. For example, for classical paraneoplastic syndromes (anti-Hu usually related to SCLC and similar), cancer screening every 6 months seems reasonable, but for other disorders (eg, anti-NMDAR encephalitis) less frequent and shorter duration of screening is reasonable (evaluation for ovarian teratoma yearly for 2 years). In greater than 90% of patients with solid tumors and PNS, the tumor is found within 1 year of PNS presentation.

Table 1
Antibodies, neurologic syndromes, cancer associations, and treatment response

Predominant Syndrome	Antibody	Main Cancer Associations	Response to Treatment[b]
Classic paraneoplastic syndromes (often or almost always are cancer associated)			
Encephalomyelitis (~25% of patients with autonomic dysfunction including cardiac dysrhythmias and respiratory failure)	Anti-Hu	SCLC, others	Poor
Subacute sensory neuronopathy	Anti-Hu when SCLC present	SCLC, others	Poor
Encephalomyelitis, chorea, optic neuritis, uveitis, peripheral neuropathy	Anti-CV2/CRMP5	SCLC, thymoma	Poor
Limbic, brainstem, and/or hypothalamic encephalitis	Anti-Ma2	Testicular germ cell tumors in men <40 y, lung cancer in older patients	About 30% respond
Cerebellar degeneration	Anti-Yo	Gynecologic or breast cancers	Poor
Cerebellar degeneration, opsoclonus, brainstem encephalitis	Anti-Ri	Gynecologic or breast cancers	Poor; laryngospasm and trismus may respond to botulinum toxin
Cerebellar degeneration	Anti-Tr (DNER)	Hodgkin lymphoma	About 20% respond
Opsoclonus-myoclonus	Multiple antibodies reported, none are specific markers for the opsoclonus-myoclonus or paraneoplasia other than anti-Ri (see above)	Children: neuroblastoma Adults: various solid tumors	Children often respond but may have residual behavioral and cognitive deficits; for adults, tumor treatment decreases risk for progression to severe encephalopathy and death
Stiff person syndrome, encephalomyelitis	Anti-amphiphysin	Breast, SCLC	Variable

(continued on next page)

Table 1
(continued)

Predominant Syndrome	Antibody	Main Cancer Associations	Response to Treatment[b]
Retinopathy (CAR)	Anti-recoverin and to other retinal proteins	SCLC	Isolated reports of stabilization and rarely improvement with immunotherapy, response seems independent of tumor treatment
Retinopathy (MAR)	Anti-retinal bipolar cells and to other retinal proteins	Melanoma	Isolated reports of response to immunotherapy and/or cytoreductive surgery
Syndromes that associate with cancer but also occur without cancer			
LEMS ± cerebellar degeneration	Anti-VGCC	Paraneoplastic in ~60% of cases; SCLC	Good for LEMS, poor for cerebellar degeneration
Myasthenia gravis	Anti-muscle AChR	Paraneoplastic in ~10% of cases; thymoma	Good
Autonomic neuropathy	Anti-ganglionic AChR	More commonly not paraneoplastic; SCLC	Good
Encephalitis ± neuromyotonia (Morvan syndrome)	Anti-Caspr2	Paraneoplastic in ~25% of cases (particularly patients with Morvan syndrome; thymoma)	Almost all patients respond but about 25% have relapses
Limbic encephalitis	Anti-LGI1 (60% with hyponatremia, faciobrachial seizures are common)	<10% of cases are paraneoplastic; thymoma	Good
Anti-NMDAR encephalitis	Anti-NMDA receptor	Teratoma (age-related association; 45% females >18 y, 9% females <14 y; rare in children; 23% of patients >45 y have other types of tumors [lung, ovarian, breast])	Often respond but may require aggressive immunotherapy; recovery may be prolonged

Limbic encephalitis	Anti-AMPA receptor (often with psychiatric features and a tendency to relapse)	~60% of cases are paraneoplastic; frequently lung, thymoma, breast, teratoma	Good
Limbic encephalitis with predominant seizures	Anti-GABA(B) receptor	50% of cases are paraneoplastic; SCLC or other neuroendocrine lung cancer	Good
Encephalitis with refractory seizures, status epilepticus, and frequent multifocal MRI abnormalities	Anti-GABA(A) receptor	~30% are paraneoplastic (mostly thymoma)	Often responds
Cerebellar ataxia, encephalomyelitis, cerebellar degeneration	Anti-GAD65	Thymoma	Patients with subacute onset have more responses than those with chronic course
Limbic encephalitis; often with severe temporal lobe seizures	Anti-GAD65	Lung, thymic (cancer risk increases with age, male sex, and presence of coexisting neuronal cell-surface antibodies)	Limited response
Limbic encephalitis	Anti-mGluR5	Hodgkin lymphoma[a]	Good response
Cognitive deficits, psychiatric symptoms, CNS hyperexcitability (including hyperekplexia, myoclonus, tremor, seizures, among others)	Anti-DPPX	Often preceded by diarrhea, other gastrointestinal symptoms, and weight loss with cachexia suggesting paraneoplasia; a few cases with lymphoma	Substantial or moderate improvement in 60%; about 25% of patients have relapses
Basal ganglia encephalitis	Anti-dopamine-2 receptor in a small number of patients	The neuropsychiatric syndrome often with abnormal movements can suggest other potentially cancer-associated autoimmune encephalitis	Only a small number of patients reported with variable responses to immunotherapy
Vasculitic neuropathy (symmetric or asymmetric painful sensorimotor neuropathy or less commonly mononeuritis multiplex)	No specific antibodies reported	Solid tumors and lymphoma	Often responds to immunosuppression

(continued on next page)

Table 1
(continued)

Predominant Syndrome	Antibody	Main Cancer Associations	Response to Treatment[b]
Cerebellar degeneration	Anti-mGluR1	Hodgkin lymphoma	Reported to improve
Stiff-person syndrome, PERM	Anti-GlyR	Rarely lung, thymoma lymphoma	Reported to improve
Dermatomyositis	A variety of antibodies have been reported; antibodies to the TIF-1 family of proteins may associate with an increased risk of paraneoplasia	Age-dependent; frequently paraneoplastic in patients >50 y	Treatment is the same as idiopathic dermatomyositis with patients often responding to immunotherapy
Acute necrotizing myopathy	Anti-SRP and anti-HMGCR are found in two-thirds of patients; seronegativity or the presence of anti-HMGCR antibodies may increase risk for a cancer association	Lung, bladder, breast, and gastrointestinal tract	May respond to corticosteroids combined with immunosuppressants

Abbreviations: AChR, acetylcholine receptor; AMPA, α-amino-3-hydroxy-5-methylisoxazole-4-propionic acid receptor; CAR, cancer-associated retinopathy; Caspr2, connectin-associated protein 2; CNS, central nervous system; CRMP, collapsing response-mediator protein; DNER, delta/notch-like epidermal growth factor-related receptor; DPPX, dipeptidyl-peptidase-like protein 6; GABA(B), γ-aminobutyric acid type B; GAD, glutamic acid decarboxylase; GluR1, metabotropic glutamate receptor 1; GlyR, glycine receptor; HMGCR, 3-hydroxy-3-methylglutaryl-coenzyme A reductase; LGI1, leucine-rich glioma inactivated 1; MAR, melanoma-associated retinopathy; mGluR5, metabotropic glutamate receptor 5; PERM, progressive encephalomyelitis with myoclonus; SRP, signal recognition particle; TIF1, human transcription intermediary factor−1; VGCC, voltage-gated potassium channel.

[a] The co-occurrence of Hodgkin lymphoma and limbic encephalitis is known as Ophelia syndrome.

[b] Includes treatment of the tumor when present, immunotherapy, and supportive care (eg, anticonvulsants).

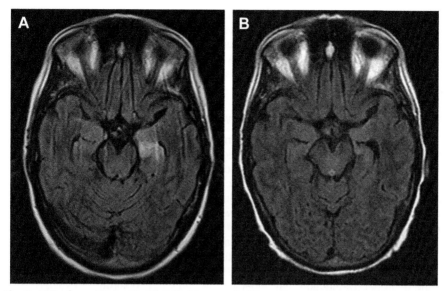

Fig. 1. MRI of a patient with SCLC, limbic encephalitis, and γ-aminobutyric acid type B antibodies. This 60-year-old woman presented with confusion, short-term memory loss, and treatment-refractory seizures (tonic-clonic and partial complex). Cranial nerves, strength, sensation, and reflexes were normal. CSF revealed nine white blood cells, normal protein and glucose, and negative cytology. Infectious evaluation was negative. (A) Axial fluid-attenuated inversion recovery MRI showed increased signal in the medial temporal lobes. Combined computed tomography/fluorodeoxyglucose-PET revealed mediastinal lymphadenopathy; biopsy demonstrated SCLC. She was treated with intravenous immunoglobulins and corticosteroids and chemotherapy and had improvement of memory function. (B) Axial fluid-attenuated inversion recovery MRI after 1 month of treatment shows improvement that remained stable over 9 months. This patient was found to have serum and CSF antibodies to the γ-aminobutyric acid type B receptor. (*From* Lancaster E, Lai M, Peng X, et al. Antibodies to the GABA(B) receptor in limbic encephalitis with seizures: case series and characterisation of the antigen. Lancet Neurol 2010;9:71; Reprinted with permission from Elsevier.)

ANTIBODIES AND PARANEOPLASTIC NEUROLOGIC SYNDROMES

Although detection of some antineuronal antibodies can confirm the diagnosis of PNS, it is important to understand the role of the antibodies in the disease, the limitations of antibody testing, and the danger of a reliance on test results more than clinical judgment.[10] Clinically useful antineuronal antibodies are divided into two groups: antibodies that are markers of PNS, and antibodies that are markers of specific neurologic syndromes.

Antibodies That Are Markers of Paraneoplastic Neurologic Syndromes

These antibodies (often called paraneoplastic or onconeuronal antibodies) are almost exclusively found in the serum and CSF of patients with PNS. When present, they confirm the paraneoplastic cause of the neurologic syndrome and may suggest the most likely underlying cancer type. The target antigens of these antibodies reside inside the neuron (with the exception of anti-Tr). Because antibodies cannot enter live cells these antibodies are unable to interfere with the function of their targets. In PNS associated with antibodies against intracellular antigens, neuronal dysfunction and death is mediated by cytotoxic T cells with data suggesting that the antibodies participate in inducing or enhancing the T-cell response.[11] These antibodies are measured by a variety of techniques and false-positive or -negative results are rare. A caveat is that these antibodies may be found at low titers in serum of some patients with cancer or without neurologic syndromes.

Antibodies That Are Markers of Specific Neurologic Syndromes

These antibodies associate with specific neurologic syndromes and are found in patients with or without cancer. The suspicion that the syndrome is paraneoplastic as opposed to nonparaneoplastic relies on clinical and paraclinical grounds, including knowledge of how often the disorder is cancer related (eg, about 60% of cases of LEMS with P/Q type voltage-gated calcium channel antibodies are paraneoplastic but only 10% of cases of encephalitis with anti-leucine-rich glioma-inactivated–1 protein antibodies are tumor related). The target antigens of these antibodies reside on or are at times exposed to the neuronal cell surface and are therefore accessible to the antibodies. For many of these antibodies there are data demonstrating that antibody binding alters the structure and/or function of the target antigens resulting in the neuronal dysfunction that underlies the neurologic disorder.[12] Evaluation for these antibodies should include serum and CSF, because some antibodies in this group are preferentially found in CSF and may be absent in serum.[13] Additionally, false-positive results are more common with serum testing.

Caveats and Limitations of Antibody Studies

The absence of specific antibodies does not rule out that a syndrome is paraneoplastic. In patients in whom no antibodies are found, the suspicion for paraneoplasia is based on presentation, syndrome type, risk factors for cancer, and ancillary tests supportive of an immune process. Guidelines that can assist in diagnosing PNS and are particularly useful for antibody-negative patients are available.[7]

Reports of antibody associations with unexpected clinical settings, often presented as widening the spectrum of the antibody-associated disease, are frequently based on the detection of low titer antibodies in serum. If an antibody is found that does not fit the well-characterized antibody-syndrome association, one should question the clinical relevance of the result, test for the antibody using a different technique, and if only serum was tested, CSF testing should be undertaken. In other cases, it may be that the antibody measured is not clinically relevant. For example, IgG antibodies against the GluN1 subunit of the NMDA receptor are specific for anti-NMDAR encephalitis.[14] Antibodies to linear epitopes of the GluN2 or GluR ε2 subunits of the NMDA receptor or IgM or IgA antibodies against the NMDA receptor are unrelated to anti-NMDAR encephalitis. These antibodies have been reported in the serum of healthy control subjects and patients with a variety of disorders (including some that are not immune mediated) and have no proven clinical significance.

A limitation inherent to any serologic test is the test turnaround time. Considering the importance of early initiation of therapy, waiting for antibody results before starting therapy can lead to worse outcomes. Clinical judgment should prevail and if PNS is suspected and other reasonable alternative etiologies ruled out, prompt initiation of immunotherapy should be considered.[15] Treatment course can be modified on review of antibody testing results when available, along with information obtained from the ongoing clinical observations.

TRIGGERS OF PARANEOPLASTIC (AUTOIMMUNE) NEUROLOGIC SYNDROMES

The mechanisms that trigger PNS are not fully understood. Generally, it is thought that the ectopic expression of neuronal proteins (called onconeuronal proteins) by systemic tumors initiates the autoimmune response. Although this may be sufficient to trigger PNS in some patients, other tumor- and host-specific factors are likely involved. For example, SCLCs are neuroendocrine tumors that almost always express the Hu antigen, yet only a small number of patients with SCLC develop anti-Hu antibody associated PNS. In some disorders, a prior viral infection can trigger autoimmunity. This has been demonstrated for the development of autoimmune encephalitis in about 20% of patients after herpes simplex viral encephalitis.[16] In these cases, patients develop new neurologic symptoms approximately 4 to 6 weeks after the initial herpes simplex viral encephalitis. Viral studies are negative and serology and CSF are positive for one or more antineuronal antibodies (the most frequent are anti-NMDA receptor antibodies). Patients often respond to immunotherapy with residual deficits related to the prior herpes simplex viral encephalitis. There are increasing reports of patients developing autoimmune neurologic syndromes after the use of immune checkpoint inhibitors for treatment of systemic cancers.[17] Cases of inflammatory encephalitis (in one case with anti-NMDA receptor antibodies), myasthenia gravis, and exacerbation of demyelinating disease have been reported, and inflammatory neuropathies and Guillain-Barré-like syndrome.[18] Discontinuation of the drug and corticosteroids usually result in partial or complete improvement. Considering the efficacy and increasing use of these treatments, the frequency of these autoimmune complications may increase in the future.

TREATMENT OF PARANEOPLASTIC NEUROLOGIC SYNDROMES

The different pathogenic mechanisms involved in PNS explain the variable responses to treatment. In general, for all PNS, prompt tumor treatment is an important contributor to the possible stabilization or improvement of the syndrome.[19] For the classic PNS where the antigens are intracellular and mediated by T cells, there are case reports of responses to a variety of immunosuppressive and immunomodulatory treatments but larger series have failed to demonstrate consistent efficacy. An exception is the limbic/brainstem encephalitis in young men with testicular tumors and anti-Ma2 antibodies; about 35% of these patients show improvement with immunotherapy and tumor treatment (usually a testicular germ cell tumor). The best chance for a response seems to be in those patients whose symptoms are still progressing or who have signs of active central nervous system inflammation (eg, CSF pleocytosis) compared with those whose syndromes have plateaued. In these patients, treatment with any or a combination of intravenous immunoglobulins (IVIG), plasma exchange, corticosteroids, cyclophosphamide, and rituximab, among other agents can be attempted. For patients with cancer, there may be concern that the use of chemotherapy and immunosuppressive therapies can lead to increased toxicity; however, and in large part because of the rarity of these cases, there are no reports supporting this concern.

For antibody-mediated PNS of the peripheral nervous system, such as LEMS or myasthenia gravis, antibody depleting or neutralizing strategies (eg, plasma exchange, IVIG) are effective. However, in patients with antibody-mediated autoimmune encephalitis, these approaches are often less effective because they do not reduce levels of intrathecal antibodies or deplete the intra–central nervous system antibody-producing cells. Current treatment recommendations are based in the experience with patients with anti-NMDAR encephalitis.[20] However, it is not known if these recommendations are equally efficacious when applied to other antibody-mediated encephalitis. In NMDAR encephalitis about 50% of patients demonstrate a response to initial corticosteroids and plasma exchange or IVIG. In this case, continuation with these treatments is reasonable. For the remaining 50% of patients, more aggressive immunosuppression with rituximab or cyclophosphamide should be initiated. Based on their efficacy and data suggesting that treatment with second-line agents improves outcome and reduces the risk of relapses, rituximab is being increasingly used in the initial treatment regimen, especially in those patients with severe symptoms.[20]

SUMMARY

PNS may affect any part of the nervous system. Serologic tests based on the detection of specific antineuronal antibodies facilitate PNS diagnosis and can suggest treatment strategies. Once thought to be poorly responsive to therapies, there is a subgroup of PNS, mostly associated with antibodies against antigens located on the neuronal cell surface, which are highly treatment responsive. It is important that these patients be recognized because early immunotherapy can reduce PNS severity, speed recovery, and for some syndromes decrease the risk of PNS relapse.

REFERENCES

1. Leypoldt F, Armangue T, Dalmau J. Autoimmune encephalopathies. Ann N Y Acad Sci 2015;1338(1):94–114.
2. Graus F, Dalmau J. Paraneoplastic neuropathies. Curr Opin Neurol 2013;26(5): 489–95.
3. Sharp L, Vernino S. Paraneoplastic neuromuscular disorders. Muscle Nerve 2012;46(6):841–50.
4. Rosenfeld MR, Dalmau J. Paraneoplastic disorders of the nervous system. In: Daroff RB, JJ, Mazziotta JC, et al, editors. Bradley's neurology in clinical practice. 7th edition. London: Elsevier; 2016. p. 1196–201.
5. Darnell RB, Posner JB. Paraneoplastic syndromes involving the nervous system. N Engl J Med 2003;349(16):1543–54.
6. Granerod J, Ambrose HE, Davies NW, et al. Causes of encephalitis and differences in their clinical presentations in England: a multicentre, population-based prospective study. Lancet Infect Dis 2010;10(12):835–44.
7. Graus F, Delattre JY, Antoine JC, et al. Recommended diagnostic criteria for paraneoplastic neurological syndromes. J Neurol Neurosurg Psychiatry 2004;75(8): 1135–40.
8. Lawn ND, Westmoreland BF, Kiely MJ, et al. Clinical, magnetic resonance imaging, and electroencephalographic findings in paraneoplastic limbic encephalitis. Mayo Clin Proc 2003;78(11):1363–8.
9. Titulaer MJ, Soffietti R, Dalmau J, et al. Screening for tumours in paraneoplastic syndromes: report of an EFNS task force. Eur J Neurol 2011;18(1):19-e3.
10. Hoftberger R, Dalmau J, Graus F. Clinical neuropathology practice guide 5-2012: updated guideline for the diagnosis of antineuronal antibodies. Clin Neuropathol 2012;31(5):337–41.
11. Blachere NE, Orange DE, Santomasso BD, et al. T cells targeting a neuronal paraneoplastic antigen mediate tumor rejection and trigger CNS autoimmunity with humoral activation. Eur J Immunol 2014;44(11):3240–51.
12. Dalmau J, Geis C, Graus F. Autoantibodies to synaptic receptors and neuronal cell surface proteins in autoimmune diseases of the central nervous system. Physiol Rev 2017;97(2):839–87.

13. Gresa-Arribas N, Titulaer MJ, Torrents A, et al. Antibody titres at diagnosis and during follow-up of anti-NMDA receptor encephalitis: a retrospective study. Lancet Neurol 2014;13(2):167–77.
14. Dalmau J, Gleichman AJ, Hughes EG, et al. Anti-NMDA-receptor encephalitis: case series and analysis of the effects of antibodies. Lancet Neurol 2008;7(12): 1091–8.
15. Graus F, Titulaer MJ, Balu R, et al. A clinical approach to diagnosis of autoimmune encephalitis. Lancet Neurol 2016;15(4):391–404.
16. Armangue T, Leypoldt F, Malaga I, et al. Herpes simplex virus encephalitis is a trigger of brain autoimmunity. Ann Neurol 2014;75(2):317–23.
17. Cuzzubbo S, Javeri F, Tissier M, et al. Neurological adverse events associated with immune checkpoint inhibitors: review of the literature. Eur J Cancer 2017; 73:1–8.
18. Hottinger AF. Neurologic complications of immune checkpoint inhibitors. Curr Opin Neurol 2016;29(6):806–12.
19. Keime-Guibert F, Graus F, Fleury A, et al. Treatment of paraneoplastic neurological syndromes with antineuronal antibodies (Anti-Hu, anti-Yo) with a combination of immunoglobulins, cyclophosphamide, and methylprednisolone. J Neurol Neurosurg Psychiatry 2000;68(4):479–82.
20. Titulaer MJ, McCracken L, Gabilondo I, et al. Treatment and prognostic factors for long-term outcome in patients with anti-NMDA receptor encephalitis: an observational cohort study. Lancet Neurol 2013;12(2):157–65.

Moving?

Make sure your subscription moves with you!

To notify us of your new address, find your **Clinics Account Number** (located on your mailing label above your name), and contact customer service at:

Email: journalscustomerservice-usa@elsevier.com

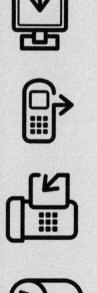

800-654-2452 (subscribers in the U.S. & Canada)
314-447-8871 (subscribers outside of the U.S. & Canada)

Fax number: 314-447-8029

Elsevier Health Sciences Division
Subscription Customer Service
3251 Riverport Lane
Maryland Heights, MO 63043

*To ensure uninterrupted delivery of your subscription, please notify us at least 4 weeks in advance of move.

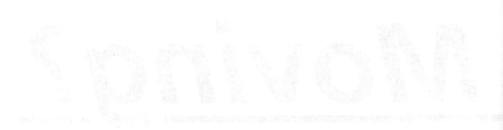